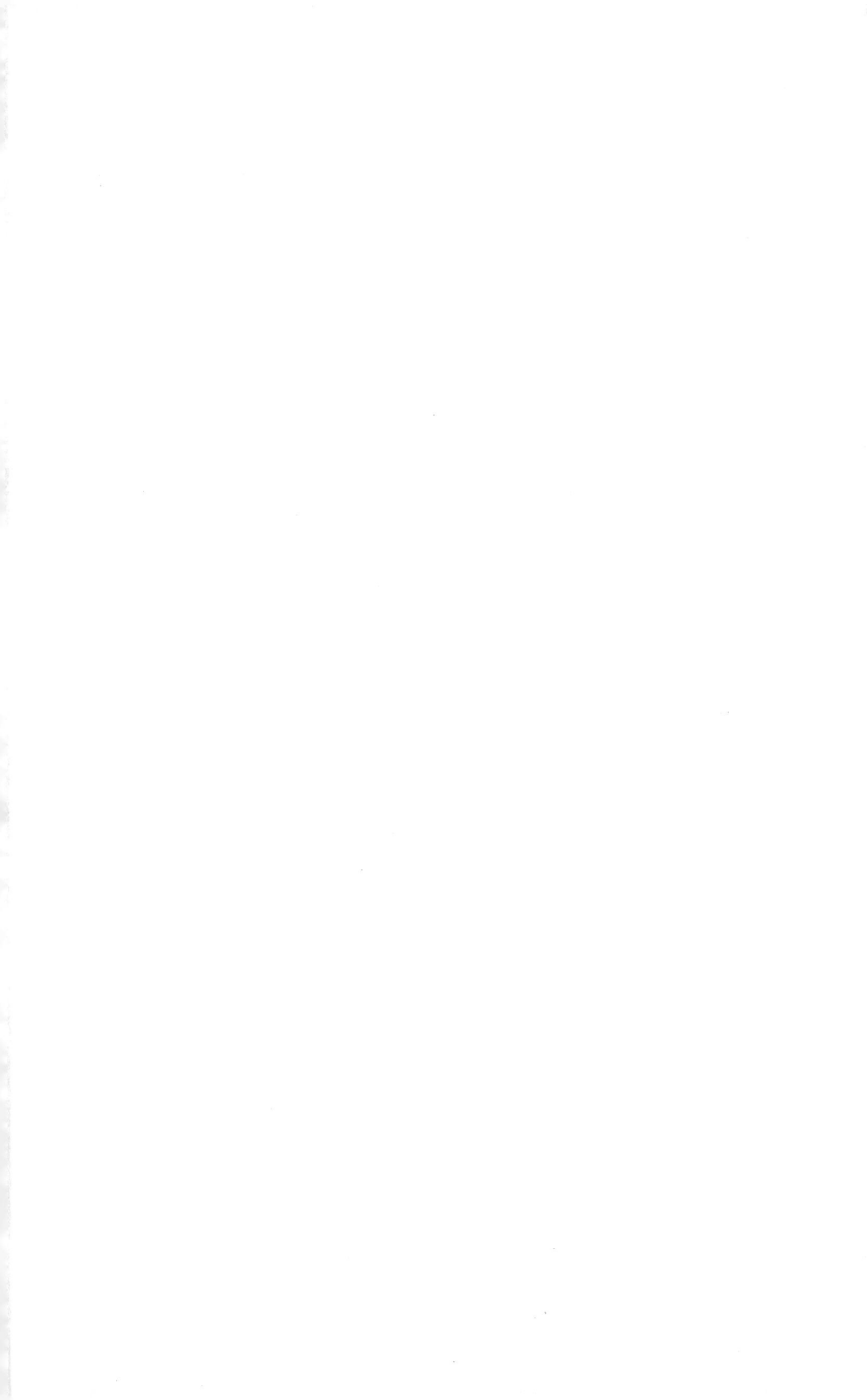

Cancer and Self-Help

Cancer and Self-Help

Bridging the Troubled Waters
of Childhood Illness

Mark A. Chesler

and

Barbara K. Chesney

THE UNIVERSITY OF WISCONSIN PRESS

The University of Wisconsin Press
114 North Murray Street
Madison, Wisconsin 53715

3 Henrietta Street
London WC2E 8LU, England

4   2   5   3   1

Printed in the United States of America

Library of Congress Cataloging-in-Publication Data
Chesler, Mark A.
Cancer and self-help: bridging the troubled waters of childhood illness /
Mark A. Chesler and Barbara K. Chesney.
416 p.   cm.
Includes bibliographical references and index.
ISBN 0-299-14820-3 (cloth: alk. paper).—ISBN 0-299-14824-6 (pbk.: alk. paper)
1. Tumors in children.   2. Self-help groups.   I. Chesney, Barbara K.
II. Title.
RC281.C4C437   1995
362.1'9892994—dc20   95-18996

Contents

Figures

Tables

Cases

Preface

> You know, being in a group with other parents, it's like extending helping
> hands to one another . . . it's kind of like having a bridge to walk over
> rough ground, or troubled waters. Having a child with cancer is tough; it
> hurts you and the kid and lots of other people. It's nice having this bridge
> to support you when you get into this kind of trouble.

This parent's comment about her participation in a self-help group
for parents of children with cancer captures many others' experiences
and reflections. Through connections with peers, many parents reported feeling better able to navigate the troubled waters of their life
experiences as they cared for a child with cancer.

In this volume we report a series of studies of this phenomenon that
we undertook over a fifteen-year period. Throughout that period, we
have been interested in understanding what goes on in self-help groups
for parents of children with cancer, and we have approached this inquiry from the point of view of members of those groups. We hope this
volume reflects and represents their own understanding of the reality of
childhood cancer and of their experiences in these self-help groups.

In the process of conducting this work, we have greatly appreciated the assistance of several organizations and many individuals. The
Candlelighters Childhood Cancer Foundation (CCCF) aided us with
material resources, access to many groups throughout the nation, and
much emotional and intellectual advice and encouragement. This volume would not have been possible without their enthusiastic support
and comradeship. Indeed, without the Foundation's activity, the existence and opportunity for exploration with so many local groups for
families of children with cancer would not have been possible. In addition, we appreciate the gracious hospitality and participation of the
many local groups and group leaders or liaison persons whom we vis-

ited over the years. The Program on Conflict Management Alternatives and the Center for Research on Social Organization, both affiliated with the Sociology Department of the University of Michigan,
provided important financial and logistical assistance. The Department of Sociology, Anthropology, and Social Work of the University of
Toledo did likewise.

Grace Ann Powers Monaco, Minna Nathanson, and Julie Sullivan,
cofounders and long-time leaders of the CCCF, also were especially
helpful throughout these studies, as was the current Executive Director
of the Foundation, James Kitterman, and Group Liaison, Yvonne
Soghomonian. Several colleagues also assisted in the development of
the studies and findings represented here: Oscar Barbarin, of the University of Michigan, contributed many of the ideas presented in Chapter 2; Benjamin Gidron, of the Ben Gurion University of the Negev,
helped conduct and analyze data from Study #3, and his participation is
represented especially in Chapters 1 and 11; Steven Sunderland, of the
University of Cincinnati, also participated in Study #3, and contributed
to the analyses provided in Chapter 11; and Thomasina Borkman, of
George Mason University, read and reacted carefully and helpfully to
several portions of this entire manuscript. We also were aided immea-
surably by research assistants at the University of Michigan, including
especially Toby Ayers, Debra Dermack, Scott Dimetrosky, Sheryl
Lozowski Sullivan, Theresa Norgaard, Jessica Roberts, Timothy
Lawther, Lisa Roth, Nancy Schwartz, Noreen Stillman, and Margaret
Yoak. In addition, research assistants at the University of Toledo included Agnes Caldwell, Debra Groh, and Michael Schuchert. Monica
Johnson's careful and consistent attention to the details of our manuscript and Patricia Preston's last-minute assistance, made it a technical
reality.

Throughout this volume, we have tried to address ourselves to several different audiences: parents of children with cancer who are involved in, or who wish to learn about or organize, self-help groups;
professionals in health care and the social services who wish to understand and work with parent self-help groups; scientists who wish to
learn more about research, theory, and the empirical reality of self-
help for parents of children with cancer, or about self-help groups
more generally; policymakers who want to find ways in which public-
and private-sector resources can assist the development of this grass-

roots phenomenon; and members of the general public—perhaps
friends and neighbors and co-workers of parents of children with
cancer—who want to understand and to be helpful to parents and
children struggling with this illness. We have attempted, therefore, to
write about and present information and findings about these groups
in a language and style that is broadly accessible for a wide range of
readers. With regard to pronoun gender, we have adopted an approach increasingly favored by publishers: the alternation of gender-
specific pronouns in order to avoid phrasing like *he or she, his or her,*
and the like. A series of notes to each chapter contains technical references and commentary that may be more useful to professional and
scientific audiences.

We dedicate this volume to parents of children with cancer throughout the nation. Their struggles with their children's illnesses and recov-
eries, their desires to maintain or advance their own and their families'
quality of life, and their efforts to improve the quality of medical care for
all children and families moved us in this inquiry. The self-help groups
that some of these parents have formed and participate in represent one
way to act on these life crises and encounters, a way that reflects some of
the grand themes of U.S. society: voluntary democratic organization,
neighborly love, and experiential wisdom. That it sometimes takes a
major life crisis to reassert these themes—individually or collectively—
is surely a tragedy; that these themes are rediscovered and reenacted by
these parents is their victory.

Part 1

Introductions and Frameworks for Understanding Self-Help and Childhood Cancer: Laying the Bridges' Foundations

This section provides readers with a series of conceptual frameworks and bases in prior literature for understanding the current inquiry into self-help groups for families of children with cancer. Chapter 1 reviews some of the relevant research on self-help and self-help groups in general, identifying some of the major issues discussed in prior research and articulating the major themes or core dynamics that arise in all or most self-help groups. This helps to set a theoretical context for the current work. We think this material is essential for understanding the particular shape that self-help takes for parents of children with cancer, but we recognize that this chapter may appeal primarily to scientists and professionals working directly with self-help, with more formal social services, or with other types of voluntary organizations.

In Chapter 2 we review some of the relevant research on the psychosocial impact of childhood cancer on the family. This chapter identifies the major stresses faced by parents of children with cancer. Thus, it develops the theoretical basis for exploring these parents' experiences and describes the psychosocial context that self-help groups for these family members try to address. Once again, we think this material is essential background for all readers, but it is most relevant to parents of children with cancer, professionals who are working with them, or scientists trying to understand their psychosocial situation.

Chapter 3 presents the research procedures and the series of specific studies that comprise the empirical basis of this volume. In addition, we discuss the model of participatory action research that guided us in this work. While this chapter may be of primary interest to other researchers and social scientists, we think all readers can benefit from understanding our approach to the methods of studying self-help.

1
Introduction to Self-Help and Self-Help Groups

I went to the meeting and shared my experiences with them. When I see someone else who is going through the same thing I am and they can handle it, then I can conquer it too.

Knowing that other people have gone through it helps. Sometimes I think I felt isolated, like this was only happening to me. It helps to talk to people.

The group meeting lets you know that there are a whole lot of other people in the same boat as you. And I didn't feel uncomfortable if I wanted to cry.

The group with which I am working gives me something positive to do. I feel I am helping someone down the road and changing things in a positive manner.

Other people are going to be experiencing processes that us "advanced parents" have gone through. The whole concept of our group is to help prepare each other to ask questions and learn more about the disease and treatment and understand it better.

It feels wonderful to be able to help! We really opened up some eyes, and I feel we made a difference in hospital policies as well.

These are the voices of parents of children with cancer. They are the voices of parents who are active in their local self-help groups, and they identify some of the themes of self-help group activity. They reflect the availability of specialized experiential knowledge, the importance of meeting and identifying oneself with other parents, the importance of shared experiences and feelings, the opportunity to improve coping, the fulfillment of contributing to the welfare of others, and the advantage of engaging in local efforts for change. These themes and the experience of parents in self-help groups are the core of our inquiry in this volume. We want to understand what goes on in these groups. What activities or programs do they offer? How are they organized? Which parents of children with cancer participate in self-help groups, and why? What benefits do they derive from membership—what are the outcomes of participation? How do the groups produce benefits for parents? How do the groups relate to the larger medical and civic environment within which they operate? Finally, what does inquiry into the nature of self-help groups for parents of children with cancer suggest about self-help in general?

The recruitment and mobilization of peers in an informal, non-hierarchical and voluntary setting, and the sharing of their common experiences, are the basic building blocks for almost all forms of self-help. The unique conditions of a self-help group give members an opportunity to see their personal problems in a new light, to collectivize and legitimize their intellectual and emotional reactions to diagnosis and treatment, and to adopt active and empowered roles in coping with new and stressful life dilemmas. The opportunity not only to receive help from others, but also to provide it to others, is potentially empowering. Self-help underscores the importance and even the indispensability of the human bond among peers as a mechanism of communication around difficult issues, and as a mechanism with healing power. While different groups, and even different forms of self-help, emphasize varied aspects of this process, almost all demonstrate these basic themes.

Although most self-help groups share common elements, there are also major differentiating factors, including the national political or cultural ethos, the focal issue or problem common to a given set of persons, and the local resources available for their organizational effort. Such factors have significant effects on (a) the size and structure of the self-help sector in a nation, the issues around which groups do or do not organize, and their relationships with human-service professionals and formal service organizations; and (b) individual groups' goals, resources, leadership patterns, organizational structures, and activities or programs.

The self-help sector in a nation can be large or small, with groups and organizations structured around many or a few issues, and with varying levels of contact and interaction with formal helping agencies and professionals. In the United States, for instance, Jacobs and Goodman (1989) estimate the size of the self-help sector, in terms of the number of people participating in a self-help or mutual aid group during one year, at 3.2% of the population, and Wuthnow's recent (1994) estimate of U.S. participation is about 5%. Individual groups can focus primarily on individual members' goals of personal change, on social change, or on some combination thereof. Leadership patterns vary among groups that are led externally, mostly by professionals; internally, by one or more members; or by some combination of shared professional and lay leadership (Borkman, 1990; Mellor, Rzetelny, and Hudis, 1984; Yoak and Chesler, 1985). The organizational structures of self-help groups can be formal or informal, with or without elected officers, regular committees, budgetary procedures and rules of operation. Finally, different groups may engage in a variety of programs or activities, including emotional support, member education, public awareness, advocacy, recreation, fund-raising and peer counseling.

The issues and life problems or experiences around which self-help groups organize define their particular membership and programs. For instance, members' physical and mental situation and their relation to formal systems of help and service are the primary basis for group development and maintenance. Several authors have begun to document and examine the varied problems or issues around which people organize to form self-help groups.[1] Indeed, in the United States one can find self-help groups and organizations dealing with practically every social, personal or medical problem. They are most likely to focus on vulnerable situations, where the social system has not responded effectively to people's needs and concerns. They are often concerned with rare or stigmatized events and diseases, where the incidence in the population is small, scattered through a wide geographic area, or relatively invisible. It is under these conditions that the formal medical or social service apparatus, as well as family and friendship networks, are most likely to be inadequate or quite limited. It is common to find several types of groups focusing on the same medical, social, or personal problem, yet targeted toward somewhat different populations (family members of patients versus patients themselves, for instance), or focused on somewhat different ideological and programmatic preferences (a desire for mutual support versus a desire for information, for instance).

In this chapter we first examine some of the general literature on self-help and self-help groups. Thus, we frame our inquiry into self-help groups for parents of children with cancer in the broader context of studies of self-help in general. At the same time, we believe that the particular issue or problem around which self-help is organized plays such a definitive role in the ways groups emerge and organize around these general themes, that we provide in Chapter 2 a review of the psychosocial experience of parenting a child with cancer. This painful and lasting reality provides the second context for understanding how the nature and structure of self-help groups work for parents of children with cancer: it details the nature of the "troubled waters" over which self-help groups provide a "bridge."

What Is Self-Help? What Are Self-Help Groups?

Self-help can be distinguished from several other common forms of help and assistance. Checkoway, Chesler, and Blum (1990) have distinguished it from self-care and community-based care: self-help is more than taking responsibility for oneself and one's own care, and is quite different from community efforts at redevelopment and citizen welfare. Borkman (1990) and Powell (1990) make useful distinctions among self-help, formal professional help, and informal help. *Informal help*, often called natural help, is a generic form of social support, most generally available from kith and kin. It often proceeds on the basis of an exchange theory of human interaction: when you do something for someone, you expect something in return, and when you receive something from someone, you expect (and are expected) to give or do something in return.[2] *Professional help* is aid and assistance from titled and official purveyors of human services, the helping professions. It usually proceeds on the basis of a contractual relationship; the professional is paid or otherwise formally compensated for services delivered. *Self-help* involves voluntary help from peers who are in a common situation. It is more likely to proceed on a communal basis (Clark, 1983). Assistance is provided as an act of commitment to others and to self-growth, and no reciprocation is expected.

As Borkman (1990) emphasizes, the knowledge bases that underlie these three forms of help and support are fundamentally different. For instance, *professional knowledge* is grounded primarily in technical and scientific information; it is general and analytic. In the case of experienced professionals who have worked in a field for many years, this specialized technical information is undoubtedly supplemented by practical nuances and modifications derived from their daily encounters with people and their problems. Informal help and helpers rest on a base of social or *lay knowledge:* general information possessed by ordinary citizens not necessarily well-acquainted with the problem or situation at hand. *Experiential knowledge* is the basis of established self-help groups and group members; it is "grounded in lived experience, concrete, pragmatic and holistic (Borkman, 1990, p. 5)."

Table 1.1, adapted from the work of Powell (1987, p. 127), further distinguishes these three primary forms of help and support, beyond the question of knowledge base. According to Powell's schema, self-help groups constitute one of three types of helping systems, each distinguished by the participants' role. Participants in self-help groups are both providers and recipients of help in mutual, peer-oriented, and self-directed volunteer roles, specifically defined by the groups' functions and individual members' own agendas. The experiential knowledge base identified as common to self-help groups is seen by Powell as leading to referent power, power rooted in the characteristics of the person. In contrast, professional and informal helping systems rely on expert and social power bases, respectively, and the typical roles of participants and help providers differ as well.

A self-help *group* is a somewhat formal entity, composed of and led by people suffering in common from a given condition or problematic situation. In self-help groups people do "for" and "with" one another, generating an alternative to sole reliance on professional expertise and guidance, or on informal family or social support systems. The definition of a self-help group at this general level is relatively standard and

Table 1.1. Properties of three helping systems

Type of system	Role of provider	Basis of power	Knowledge base	Role of participant
Self-help	Volunteer (explicit)	Referent	Experiential	Mutual, self-directed
Professional	Paid (explicit)	Expert	Professional	Nonmutual, other-directed
Informal	Indirectly paid (implicit)	Social	Social	Experiences both mutuality and direction

Source: Adapted from Powell, 1987, p. 127.

consensual, despite some national and cultural variation. However, much of the literature fails to reflect important distinctions consistently. Thus, the terms *support groups, mutual support, groups, small groups, discussion groups, group programs, group therapy, social support,* and *peer support* are often used interchangeably and carelessly.[3]

A core distinction made by Powell (1987) contrasts *hybrid* self-help groups with *autonomous* ones. The hybrid self-help group is sponsored or supervised by professionals, and is really a form of professional help conducted in a mutually supportive manner. In fact, some authors argue that the professionally led self-help group should not even be considered a self-help group at all. The autonomous group is led by the people identified and linked by their common condition; professionals may be involved, but not in positions of primary leadership and responsibility. The dimensions of indigenous power and self-control and of leadership and responsibility are crucial to this distinction. Mellor et al., (1984) elaborate on this distinction, establishing a continuum which ranges from professional-led to member-led self-help groups. Figure 1.1 depicts this continuum, designed to illustrate the "movement of each group toward self-help (p. 98)," but also useful in establishing a typology of individual groups. Although emotional support and member healing may occur at any point on this continuum, the internal dynamics of different types of groups may vary considerably. For instance, participant passivity and dependence, often coupled with low commitment, are likely to characterize groups at the professionally led end of the continuum, while high degrees of mutual support for personal growth as well as social action for change are likely to characterize member-led groups.

Any typology of groups, including the ones developed by Mellor et al. (1984) and Powell (1990; 1987), is a somewhat artificial description of the realities of different groups, and of any single group over time. While any group may be characterized in terms of these frameworks, the lines between the categories, or the points along the continuum, are often blurred in practice, and many groups live between the lines. Moreover, groups may shift categories as their external and internal operations change over time. Despite these cautions, it is quite useful, both as a research activity and as a practical matter, to begin to develop some ways of describing the various orientations and operating foci of different self-help groups.

Figure 1.1 Self-help continuum for groups (from Mellor et al., 1984: 98)

NO SELF-HELP				SELF-HELP
Professionally led groups	Professional leader	Professional leader is resource person and facilitator	No professional present, but reliance on professional contact	Nonprofessional leader or no leader
Dependence on leader	Peer support	No formal leadership	Social action/personal change	Members plan and expedite activities
Lack of sharing	Mutual aid but only within group setting	Mutual aid within and without group setting	Peer support, mutual aid	Social action/personal change
No commitment to group	Leader recruits members	Peer support	Recruits members and accepts referrals	Mutual aid, peer support
Passive	Members defer to leader in decision making	Some social action	Ego reinforcement	Recruits own members
		Recruits own members and accepts referrals		Ego reinforcement

The Crisis That Leads to Self-Help Efforts

In our daily lives most of us are embedded in a series of informal support systems. Indeed, life as we know it would be difficult to imagine without the friendship and support of family members, friends, and neighbors. At certain times in our lives, however, we encounter serious crises—the death of a close family member, serious personal illness, the onset of a chronic illness, recognition of an addiction, sudden unemployment, divorce, or separation. Such crises may escalate the levels of stress and threat in our lives beyond our normal coping capacities, and are often destabilizing, requiring us to respond in new, unaccustomed, and sometimes unknown, ways. Often disempowering, they may render us passive and reactive, rather than proactive, in dealing with difficult situations. They are often disconnecting as well, separating us from the normal routines of our lives, from regular work roles, from accustomed companions, and from established forms of support from friends and family members. To the extent that they are unanticipated and unimagined crises, they may create major conflict between new and old ways of thinking and acting, adding the stresses of adaptation and a search for new coping strategies to the crisis itself.

In these times of crisis our informal support systems sometimes fail to provide the kind or amount of assistance that we need. We may then turn to formal and professional support systems, and seek technical information and assistance or psychological counseling, alone or in a group setting. This channel of support, too, may or may not be appropriate or adequate to our needs. Under the same circumstances, we sometimes elect to meet and talk with other people who are experiencing a similar life crisis. In this case the process of peer self-help has begun.

The Core, Universal Themes or Components of Self-Help Groups

There is a certain "magic" in the operation of self-help processes and self-help groups, as Katz's (1993, p. 17) quotation from a member of The Compassionate Friends (TCF) demonstrates:

The special magic of TCF: that healing comes from sharing yourself with others and all working together for all . . .

Core themes emerge again and again in reports of this phenomenon, across different problem situations, cultural settings, and nations. In Chapters 4 and 5 we examine these themes with specific regard to the activities and operations of self-help groups for parents of children with cancer in the United States in concrete, empirical detail. In the remainder of Chapter 1, we provide a synthesis of some of the outstanding literature on this topic, drawing from other scholars' reports of the types of processes that appear to occur in self-help groups.[4] The following are the most widely reported and verified core processes or themes:

1. The development of different forms of knowledge based upon experiential expertise
2. The recognition of shared life experiences and crises, often associated with new forms of intimacy and an altered social identity
3. The receipt of support and affirmation that eases pain and helps counter social stigma
4. The opportunity to improve coping skills and buffer stress, partly through learning from others and contributing to their welfare
5. The experience of acting collectively in a grass-roots process of creating change in social systems

Experiential Knowledge

In an age of information explosion and increasing specialization of technical information, knowledge is a valuable commodity. In times of personal and social crisis, access to new and relevant knowledge is often critical for effective response. The specialized knowledge base available to professionals permits them to exert substantial and legitimate control over human-service delivery systems by the application of theories or ideologies of cause and effect and through organized systems of professional help and assistance (Chesler, 1990b). Thus, the democratization and sharing of this knowledge base, or the development of an alternative knowledge base, is a critical aspect of any alternative form of empowered action and social support.[5]

In self-help groups, individuals experiencing a common life crisis often search for any and all available and relevant information. Borman (1992) indicates that, as a result, self-help groups become "centers for both scientific and experiential information" (p. xxiv). Groups not only help collect available technical and professionally legitimized knowledge, but also provide an arena for the development and sharing of a new resource—experiential knowledge. As Romeder (1990) explains, self-help groups are places "where members have the chance to learn or practice the art of sharing their life experiences and wisdom they have acquired, commonly referred to as 'experiential knowledge' " (p. 38). As members share their lay wisdom, their own speculations about cause and effect, their own "tricks of the trade" or skills for coping with crisis, they help create a knowledge base that has its roots in experiential encounters rather than technical knowledge. Thus, it is quite naturally a more democratic form of knowledge. It also has its roots in an alternative epistemology, one that has become increasingly popular in the United States. Self-help group members often treat knowledge as something that can be created by individuals who share and analyze their personal experience and life-learning, not solely something that already exists in the minds of professionals (academic or medical/psychological) who then transmit it to lay people.[6]

The articulation, discovery, and elaboration of lay information and knowledge also help to generate a set of specific beliefs about the crisis condition or situation at hand and about relevant coping processes (Borman, 1992). This belief system, or ideology, acts as an alternative guide for individual behavior and group activities, even though it may differ from professional perspectives. The unique knowledge about coping tactics and skills that veteran sufferers generate may differ from the often abstract wisdom of professionals and the well-intentioned ignorance of friends and family members. In the context of newly acquired skills, the "commonsense wisdom" (the experiential knowledge) of ordinary persons is validated as useful and helpful (Klass, 1992; Powell, 1987). Both Borkman (1990) and Marieskind (1984) discuss how this knowledge and its public legitimation confer power on the people who express it. The recognition of such powerful knowledge and the new coping and social skills that may be learned and expressed as a consequence, have also been suggested as ways that self-help group involvement can lead to increased social efficacy (Katz and Bender, 1990b).

Although these forms of expertise are constructed in different ways, they are not necessarily contradictory. Experiential knowledge and technical knowledge may contain the same assumptions and have very similar implications for policy, programs, and services, but they usually have different components and emphases, stemming from the different people and experiences involved in their development. At the very least, their different origins have important implications for the relationships between lay and professional actors, and among lay members of self-help groups.

Shared Life Experiences

Sharing a life crisis with others in the context of a self-help group is an intimate and emotionally bonding experience. In the context of a life crisis, as peoples' lives are altered in fundamental ways, they may need to find new ways of thinking and acting. Belonging to a self-help group puts people in touch with others who share their common problems and life experiences sufficiently to create and share new ways of thinking about themselves. In order to facilitate opportunities for such thinking, most self-help groups encourage openness in the public setting of the group. At the same time, groups develop protective norms to ensure privacy and promote comfortable disclosure. In fact, self-help groups are a unique setting for public disclosure in a private space. Wuthnow (1994) comments on this process:[7]

People must interact with one another long enough to see self-disclosure modeled, learn how the group is going to respond, and know enough about the behavior and expectations of other people to feel assured that nothing terribly shocking is likely to happen. Once that level of understanding is established, people can move across the boundary between the private space and self-disclosure. (p. 203)

Through mutual disclosure and role modeling (Lavoie, 1990), people may begin to see how their individual concerns are not simply troublesome personal issues, but common reactions to a stressful situation. When details of that stressful situation, as well as common reactions to it, are shared with others, a self-help group often becomes an alternative form of community, one created by individuals who have discovered the need for a new or special type of shared human encounter.

Several scholars of self-help have identified how these shared experiences and the resultant sense of community may lead individuals to discover and express a new "social identity."[8] In noting this relatively universal characteristic of self-help groups, Borman (1992) and Mullan (1992) refer to the "instant identity" gained therein. This new identity is borne of the shared experience, or "common problem," that creates immediate interpersonal "resonance" (Romeder, 1990) or "identification resonance" (Klass, 1992). An "identification with fellow travelers" (Klass, 1992) can lead to validation of one's own experience and place in the world through discussion of mutual problems and learning from others' sharing of feelings and modeling of distinctive role behaviors. Borkman (1990) amplifies this phenomenon in her discussion of the process of identity change that often occurs in such an "experiential learning community."[9] Bakker and Karel (1983) also discuss the process of identity change, suggesting that in order for people in crisis to cope positively with their changed life situation, they need to find "a different way of experiencing [their] problems and situations [that] requires different interpretations" of their experience (p. 162).

In self-help groups such as The Compassionate Friends, Klass (1992) suggests, the organizational structure and interaction patterns and the rituals and traditions of the group provide an alternative meaning system that helps people to affirm their feelings about their situations and relate them to their prior experience. These gains are engendered by the deepened sense of support and intimacy often found in a self-help group—a form of relationship akin to that found in other, more established, loving connections. Mack and Berman (1988) apply this orientation to their discussion of the isolation and lack of connectedness experienced by parents of children with rare genetic diseases. They argue that the cohesion and sense of togetherness found in a self-help group can play a curative role in overcoming parents' sense of alienation. Indeed, we are never fully human alone; we only become fully human in the midst of community. A severe life crisis can make us feel alone, and in such an alienating situation, connecting with others who are similarly affected can provide unique benefits. Exposure to and interaction with others navigating the same life crisis can facilitate the discovery of a new sense of self.

This transformation occurs, according to Wuthnow (1994), partly through the storytelling that takes place in self-help groups.

Through storytelling individuals turn their experience into a collective event. They preserve their individuality but at the same time find community in the similarities between their stories and those told by others in the group. Storytelling has become the dominant mode of discourse in small groups. (p. 292).

Thus, the group becomes a particular kind of community, a "narrative community." As people tell their stories, they try out a new "socio-biography," a new social identity, which is in turn affirmed by the group and can lead to new behaviors and attitudes. The notion of a narrative community attempts to capture the way in which the sense of a newly created community helps people try out new identities through the process of storytelling and storylistening. In turn, the process of intimate storytelling or narration helps to create a sense of community among prior strangers. This is a particular kind of community that is integrated by the nature of members' life experiences and their ability to share these experiences through the narrative process. As people live together in a group, over time, they also develop a story about the group's activities, operations, and meaning for them, and this takes the form of a group narrative.

Powell (1987) discusses a closely related process, drawing attention to the ways in which the self-help group may operate as a reference group for people, a setting in which they learn new values and behaviors, and adopt a different cultural frame or meaning system with which to make sense of their collective situation.[10] This process of identity reformation and resocialization into new beliefs and behaviors (Weber, 1982) often leads self-help groups to develop "communities of belief" (Antze, 1976) based on their common perceptions and beliefs about their experiences. Within these varied frameworks for community, self-help groups may be substitutes for the vanishing social structure of small, isolated villages and neighborhoods, and as such may represent "a new form of solidarity in an atomistic society" (Van Harberden, 1990, p. 215).

Support and Affirmation

Kropotkin (1972) argues that mutual aid is a "natural human force" that involves both the social and economic needs of a community and its members. In this view, mutual aid groups or self-help groups are important to individuals because of their potential for providing (1) connection with others who have shared experiences; (2) ongoing interaction with a relatively stable and supportive group of others; and (3) the security of interdependence and mutual concerns (Marris, 1974; Kropotkin, 1972). In times of illness and personal crisis, when traditional helping modes are nonexistent, inaccessible, or marginally useful, these resources may be available in the form of a self-help group. Such resources find expression in interpersonal processes such as emotional bonding and support, affirmation and compassion, empathy and true understanding of another's situation, and identification with a larger social entity.

In the face of continuing strain and tension in our social fabric at the national and local level, self-help and support groups are increasingly popular. They function in ways similar to the family, as surrogate sources of intimacy and affirmation. However, they are not quite like families, but more like expanded social networks or intimate communities.

Analyses of acculturation processes, that is, the introduction of new members into self-help groups, indicate how sensitive most members are to helping each other cope with their particular crisis. Consistently, before suggestions are made for new behavior, elaborate group discussions focus on the crisis or loss at hand, and on individuals' feelings and reactions to these situations. This is the stage when parents of a chronically ill child speak about their dreams and hopes of seeing their child recover and get married, or when a grieving mother speaks about her child in vivid terms, as if she were alive. Others, too, "tell their stories," affirming and identifying with the feelings of new members, and in the process legitimizing these feelings. Several scholars of self-help also discuss the ways in which these processes and activities help establish a new social support system or network upon which people can rely as they attempt to deal with their current crisis and integrate it into their life experience (Borman, 1992; Hedrick et al., 1992; Humm, 1984). Meeting other people who are willing and able to provide help is a central function of self-help groups,[11] and Mullan (1992) makes a particular point of indicating the ways in which "veterans" can support "rookies" by affirming their feelings and reactions and by helping them interpret and respond to their situations.

The benefit of connecting to others with whom one can share perceptions, beliefs, feelings, and experiences is especially important when the life situation or illness people experience is stigmatizing, or when it leads to their being labeled as deviant or as victims. Chronic illness frequently is stigmatized in our society. The type and extent of help or support offered to ill people often depends upon the nature of the illness and the attributions made about it. For instance, Brickman and his colleagues (1983) interpret the dynamics of lay or professional helping processes in terms of two factors: (1) the degree to which the situation is seen as one for which the individual is responsible for having created;

and (2) the degree to which the situation is seen as one in which the individual is responsible for managing a recovery. A situation which a person is not responsible for having created, but from which he or she is responsible for recovering is most amenable to help from others. People in these situations are perceived as most deserving of sympathy, since they have not brought on the situation themselves, and help is presumed to be most effective for them, because they can play a role in their own recovery.[12]

Clearly, perceptions of various problem situations and settings (physical disease of cancer, emotional reactions to cancer, drug and alcohol abuse, accidental injury and murder, self-inflicted damage, mental illness, poverty, immigration) vary on these dimensions, and social beliefs regarding the responsibility for causing and recovering from these situations may vary as well. Perceptions of responsibility for cause and recovery create an especially strong stigma regarding persons with mental illness or families of persons with mental illness. To the extent that public perceptions hold people who are mentally ill responsible for their "weakness," or hold their families responsible for causing these illnesses, compassionate and effective help is hard to come by. Especially in situations of social stigmatization, the company and help of peers who have been through the same illness and the same stigmatizing process is enormously important. For instance, Kaufman, Freund, and Wilson (1989) discuss how support and affirmation helped create a positive social identity for members of self-help groups for mentally ill persons, an identity that was "often distinct from their devalued (or alienated) status in most social groups outside of the self-help community" (p. 7). In a similar vein, Kurtz (1990a) reports how groups organized by the National Depressive and Manic Depressive Association (NDMDA) help counter stigma via the "reconstruction of a positive identity for persons labeled as deviant" (p. 106).

Over time, Powell (1990) reports, self-help groups generally help people expand both the size and density of their social networks. Thus, not only may new friendships be developed through this process, but established friends and contacts may be able to deepen and expand the intimacy and helpfulness of their relationships. For instance, McWhirter, McWhirter, and McWhirter (1988) discuss the ways in which self-help groups organized around a common religious tradition and within a social context of oppression can create increased solidarity among neighbors. Their analysis of Christian Base Communities in Central America provides direct evidence of the different forms that mutual support takes in self-help groups, as well as the broad scope and agendas of such groups.

New Coping Skills to Buffer Stress

Shared intimate experiences, unconditional affirmation, and ongoing support can provide people with the emotional bulwarks and practical skills needed to deal with new and challenging situations. Several scholars have argued that the outcomes of the support provided in self-help groups include a stress-buffering effect on mental and physical health, an improved capacity for solving the practical problems of daily life in new circumstances, and, perhaps, improvements in physical health itself.[13]

Several scholars have focused on the ways in which self-help groups may improve members' coping skills and increase their sense of personal empowerment.[14] One theme has centered on the individually empowering potential involved in proactive coping and "prosumer" orientations to care (Gartner and Riessman, 1977; Powell, 1987). The argument is that groups help increase members' self-reliance, coping ability, personal responsibility for solving problems, personal responsibility for making changes in their lives, and informed consumerism.[15] Self-help group involvement also may lead to reduced dependency on the formal professional system, and thereby may reduce the enormous power differential and disempowering potential that often exists in relationships between service providers and service recipients (Hasenfeld, 1987).

Thus, one of the central dynamics of a self-help group is the provision of an arena in which individuals can strive to meet their needs, pursue their interests, and exert greater self-determination and control over their personal lives (Froland et al., 1983). As people learn more about their own situations and how others in similar situations have coped, they learn new coping skills and tactics. Parents of ill children, in particular, may find themselves more able to move beyond shock and passivity, and to take on active roles in the care of themselves, their children, and other family members. In self-help groups, people often accomplish these coping tasks by adopting and acting on the experiential wisdom of veterans who have weathered a similar crisis.

Several observers emphasize the reciprocal nature of this mutual helping process, indicating that the act of helping others and seeing oneself as a useful and potent helper, can be therapeutic—for the helper as well as for the person being helped.[16] The notion of "helper therapy," or "help as therapy," is one of the most common and powerful dynamics in self-help groups. It emphasizes the ways in which people discover that, despite their crisis situation and despite their prior social status and experience, they may have resources that other people value and cherish. These valued resources may be as simple as everyday information and coping hints and as complex as technical expertise and love. The realization that others may gain from one's own experience often places a crisis experience in a different light, and the realization that one has something to offer others may lessen feelings of hopelessness and lead to more positive social comparisons. It may mean that a person is not as bereft as originally thought and, in fact, must have some spare resources if she or he truly is able to be helpful to others in the midst of a crisis. The *peer-oriented* nature of this helper-therapy process and the experiential knowledge base that lies at its heart reveal the fundamental assumptions of equality and comradeship that undergird self-help.

Considering these potential gains in coping skills and strategies, Rappaport (1993) raises the question of whether we might best view self-help groups as alternative models of service provision or as caring communities. After all, if these groups are providing benefits to individuals, might they not be seen usefully as adjuncts to professional systems of mental health delivery or social service? On the other hand, the apparent "service" is an exchange among peers, an outgrowth of mutual intimacy, commitment, and support, rather than a product of formal role and expertise. Rappaport decides that "the members are not clients getting services and therefore somehow different from the rest of us; rather, they are people, living lives" (1993, p. 246). As we indicate later (see below and Chapter 9), one may also consider local self-help groups—especially those that are focused on improving the environment for their members—as social movement organizations, as communities of special interest acting for change.

Collective Empowerment and Action

The mutually supportive, egalitarian processes described above generate an empowering tradition in self-help that is enhanced by its reliance on indigenous and grass-roots leadership (Borman, 1992). As a complement or an alternative to the professionally dominated medical and social service systems, self-help groups are often consumer-initiated, governed by members, and more or less autonomous from the professional service system. [17] Such voluntaristic, grass-roots and democratic leadership is collectively empowering for members, and has been an essential element in the development and maintenance of our "uniquely American" tradition (de Tocqueville, 1957). This cultural fit may help explain why autonomous self-help groups are so popular in the United States, as contrasted with the less autonomous versions of self-help found in nations with more centralized social service systems.

Not all self-help groups are completely composed of and led by such grass-roots and indigenous leaders. However, even those groups that permit professionals to be members or leaders generally establish a partnership or coalition that guarantees some degree of member and group autonomy and separate spheres of influence and self-control (Yoak and Chesler, 1985). As Borman notes (1992), "The professional may assist members in learning what to do and how to do it, but the members themselves must eventually take the important roles" (p. xxv). As a result, changes in personal efficacy appear to be among the common benefits of self-help group membership and leadership (Chesney and Chesler, 1993).

Democratic participation and democratic empowerment in self-help groups not only have the potential to create individual, internal transformations, but to facilitate collective action and external social transformations as well. [18] The increased knowledge gathered by people active in these mutually supportive and empowering settings and the bonds they establish with peers are resources crucial to the organization and mobilization of any change effort or social movement activity. [19] Obviously, as Smith and Pillemer (1983) note, self-help groups "differ among themselves in having varying degrees of social movement/social change orientation" (p. 215). However, the potential for collective as well as individual empowerment and for collective action exists. For example, scholars have pointed to groups' and members' increased ability to "exert pressure on the environment" and "correct the service system" (Bakker and Karel, 1983, p. 163), by undertaking advocacy vis-à-vis the service system with which they deal or the public in general.

Self-help groups utilize several common tactics to advocate and act upon their members' concerns: reopening clogged communication channels with professional systems or public agencies; engaging in collaborative problem solving that persuades decision makers of the need for change; generating new resources for their own activities or to support service-system changes; creating potent challenges or protests to change policies and practices; and mobilizing press and public opinion in support of their cause. All these tactics require the exercise of some sort of power, either collaborative or adversarial, either newly emergent or tied to preexistent structures. Then structural conflict between groups and the human system often surfaces, and in the face of resistance, some groups may escalate overt conflict in order to gain attention, to engage collaboration, or to force new decisions (Chesler, 1991).

More generally, Reynolds (1982) suggests that self-help can be seen "as a medium of social and economic advancement in a society with limited resources (p. 79)," and Bakker and Karel (1983) argue that, however subtly, all self-help "implicitly criticizes how the welfare state is organized" and operates (p. 160). Particularly in this context, observers have cautioned against the pattern of state support for and potential cooptation of self-help as a strategy to pacify groups with unmet needs or to justify cutting back on public and professional resources available to people in crisis (Withorn, 1980). This is an especially important concern in an age when conservative national governments are attempting to cut back the welfare state and promote the scarcity paradigm of limited expertise, support, love, resources, and power. In such cases, the voluntarism of self-help can be seen and misused as a cheap and privatized substitute for even limited public involvement and response to crisis conditions in the community.

The literature we have reviewed suggests that the above five themes are relatively universal characteristics of self-help groups. As Biegel and Yamatani (1987) also argue, "Self-help groups share a common helping focus regardless of the problem area" (p. 1197).[20] Dynamics such as empathy, exchanging experiential wisdom, mutual affirmation, encouragement of sharing, skill development, and normalization seem to be common across all these groups. Similarly, other authors agree that it is the opportunity to tell one's stories and "to meet with others with similar problems that is the most beneficial aspect of group participation."[21]

Particularistic Aspects of Self-Help Groups

Despite the existence of these common core themes or processes in the vast majority of self-help groups, there are differences among groups as well. Different national, cultural, and social background factors may create different beliefs and traditions about the responsibility of the person, family, community, and nation in dealing with stressful life situations, different traditions about local and grass-roots mobilization of kith and kin, and differential access to state-supported services. In addition, the common life situation, issue, or problem that brings people together in a particular group creates differentiation within the larger phenomenon of self-help, even within a given nation or culture. For example, whether or not a situation is a medical problem, as contrasted with a lifestyle issue or a social advocacy agenda, makes a major difference in the orientation of group members and their relationships with the non-member public. Especially within the medical context, the nature of the illness situation (age of onset, chronicity, treatment character, stigma, seriousness, probability of personal or social causation/blame) affects, by definition, the potential membership and posture of the group. These factors determine the age and social strata from which members are drawn, the depth and length of their crisis, their need for or attraction to self-help, their skill and energy in local initiative and leadership, their experience with and openness to professional leadership, their energy, their personal and group goals, and their readiness to invest in collective action. These factors also find expression in the organizational characteristics of self-help groups, for instance, in the types of group activities, resources, ideology, leadership patterns, and duration and type of involvement. Thus, the specific problem or situation will account for much of the variation of self-help groups within a given nation and culture, and even within a given subculture or demographic subpopulation.

Emerick (1990) extends this argument, noting that

Some structural factors may be generic to all self-help groups, but conditions that facilitate or impede the establishment of partnerships between self-help groups and health care professionals vary with the type of group—that is, with the nature of the problem the group addresses. (p. 401)

Emerick argues that groups for people with particular physical health problems, such as heart conditions, will differ from groups for people with other health problems, such as AIDS: the differential assignment of moral responsibility, as well as treatment regimens, are critical. Moreover, groups for people dealing with either of these well-defined physical ailments will differ from groups for people dealing with mental health problems, such as schizophrenia or manic-depressive disease. They will also differ from groups for people dealing with normative life-cycle transitions, such as divorce or death of a spouse. These differences occur precisely because people with these problems or illnesses are dealing both with issues that are seen differently by the public and with treatment systems and professionals that have different philosophies and resources for care.

Several scholars have attempted to categorize self-help groups in terms of the problem situations or life conditions to which they respond.[22] These categorizations can be helpful in creating a typology of self-help groups that integrates properties of the situation or problem around which the group organizes, and the likely impact of that situation on its organizational characteristics. Madara and Meese (1990) provide, as shown in Figure 1.2, a list of self-help groups that is representative of the scope and mission of groups organized around the problem-specific commonalities of their members. This list is part of their work in establishing and maintaining an east-coast self-help clearinghouse that provides individuals with information about the availability of groups and lends technical support to the growing self-help movement. It can be, and has been, duplicated or expanded and fine-tuned to local realities by other clearinghouses in other parts of the nation.

A five-part schematic for classifying self-help groups by their primary situational focus, provided by Katz and Bender (1990c), is reproduced in Figure 1.3. According to this typology, disease or illness-specific groups and groups organized around life situations are labeled *therapeutic* groups, with social support and stress reduction being their major goals and programmatic agendas. Collective action and social change are the priority agendas of the second category, social advocacy/action groups, which are composed of people who share a given problem or social background and identity. These groups focus much of their energy on advocacy for change in the surrounding social context—its allocation of social resources and its policies. Katz and Bender delineate a third type of group with a narrower focus of providing support for

Figure 1.2. Self-help group listing (from Madara and Meese, 1990, pp. 5–7)

Adoption
Aging/Older
Adults
AIDS
Alcoholism
ALS
Alzheimer's Disease
Amputation
Anemia/Blood Disease
Anorexia/Bulimia
Arthritis
Autism
Battering
Blind/Visually Impaired
Breast Cancer/
  Mastectomy
Burn Survivors
Cancer
Caregivers
Cerebral Palsy
Child Abuse
Childbirth/Cesarean Birth
Co-Dependency
Crime Victims/Offenders
Deaf/Hearing Impaired/
  Tinnitus
Death of a Child/
  Miscarriage
Death of a Loved One–
  General
Death of a Loved One–
  Spouse
Death of a Loved One–
  Suicide
Debt

Diabetes
Disability—Physical
Divorce/Separation
Drug Abuse
Employment
Epilepsy
Foster Parents/Children
Gambling
Head Injury/Brain Tumor/
  Coma
Heart Disease
Herpes
Infertility
Inflammatory Bowel
  Disease
Kidney Disease/
  Hemodialysis
Laryngectomy
Learning Disabilities
Life-Threatening Illness
Liver disease
Lupus
Marriage/Family
Men
Mental Health—General
Mental Health—
  Consumers
Mental Health—
  Depression
Mentally Ill—Families of
Mental Retardation/
  Developmental
  Disability
Multiple Sclerosis
Obsessive-Compulsive

Ostomy
Overweight
Pain, Chronic
Parenting, General
Parenting—Single
  Parents
Parenting—Stepparents
Parents of Disabled/Ill
  Children
Parents of Premature/
  High Risk
Parents of Twins and
  Triplets
Parents Troubled by
  Teen Behavior
Parkinson's Disease
Phobia
Respiratory Disease/
  Emphysema
Sex/Love Addiction
Sexual Abuse/Incest/
  Rape
Sexuality/Gay and
  Lesbian
Short/Tall Stature
Skin Disease
Smoking
Speech/Stuttering
Spina Bifida
Stroke
Veterans
Women
Women's Health
Youth/Students

Figure 1.3. Classification scheme of self-help groups by primary focus
(from Katz and Bender, 1990c, p. 27)

Type I Therapeutic

A. Mental Health organizations: overcoming specific psychological-physical problems. Recovery, Inc., National Alliance for the Mentally Ill, G.R.O.W., Neurotics Anonymous, Emotions Anonymous.
B. Addiction organizations: e.g., Alcoholics Anonymous, Alanon, Alateen, Narcotics Anonymous, Overeaters Anonymous
C. Physical Health Groups:
    (i)   Disease-Specific: e.g., Make Today Count, Mended Hearts, The Lost Chord Club, Renal Dialysis
    (ii) Parents of Children with Learning Disabilities, Candle Lighters, S.I.D.S., Friends and Family of Schizophrenics
    (iii) Multi-Diagnostic: e.g., Centers for Independent Living
D. Life Transition Groups; e.g., Widow-Widower groups, Alone Again, Alone Together, Retiree Groups, Divorce Groups
E. Stress Reduction; e.g., Santa Monica Senior Peer-Counseling Center

Type II Social advocacy/action

A. Groups created to overcome a single problem: e.g., Mothers Against Drunk Driving, Welfare rights organizations, Coalition for the Rights of the Disabled
B. Groups created on a basis of age: e.g., Gray Panthers
C. Groups created to further ethnic/minorities: e.g., Alianza Hispano-Americana, Black Single Mothers Association

Type III Groups created to support alternative lifestyles

A. Gay Liberation groups
B. Urban and Rural Residential Communes

Type IV Groups to provide outcast/havens through a 24-hour live-in situation

    Daytop Village, Delancy Street, Battered Women's Shelters

Type V Mixed types (more than one primary focus)

A. Ex-prisoner associations: e.g., the Fortune Society, the 7th Step Foundation
B. Social-Therapeutic (family-oriented): Parents without Partners, Families Anonymous
C. Economic:
    (i)   Food banks
    (ii) Self-help housing organizations
    (iii) Consumer/producer cooperatives: e.g., Amish, the Doukhobours, Hutterites
    (iv) Other economic: The +40 Club, Debtors Anonymous, Checks Anonymous

people with alternative lifestyles, and, on occasion, helping them create change in the external environment as well. This category reflects the themes of social support, affirmation, and shared life experiences, as well as the reduction of stigma and the facilitation of collective action that are identified throughout this chapter. Their final two classifications are extremely specific groups: outcast havens for the support and protection of particularly vulnerable populations, and mixed types with more than one primary focus.

Powell (1987) offers an alternative scheme that presents five examples of self-help group missions and parallels Katz and Bender's typology as well as our discussion of the five major themes that characterize self-help groups. As he notes,

The typology is organized by the five basic missions of self-help organizations. They are to change a highly specified behavior; to modify a broad range of difficulties and coping patterns; to reform society and/or validate a lifestyle; to relieve the burden of family caregivers; and to sustain the physically disabled.[23] (p. 149)

These schemes for group categorization point to both variation and commonality in the goals and foci of a wide range of self-help groups.

Self-Help Groups at the Center or the Periphery?

Several of the dominant themes of the self-help movement and of local self-help groups are distinguishable from some of the core values and central organizational processes of contemporary Western society. For instance, our U.S. society operates largely from a cultural ethos of highly specialized technical knowledge. Expert knowledge is gained through specialized training processes and credentialed by official state and professional sources. Whether in the medical field or in other technical areas, such knowledge is part of the system of status and privilege that denotes power—power of position, power to make decisions that affect others, and power to establish and implement preferred moral norms. The *experiential knowledge* base that is so critical in the framework of self-help groups implicitly challenges the technical base (and sometimes the content) of the prevailing professional knowledge and its related cultural ethos. In suggesting that traditionally nonexpert, yet viable, knowledge can be produced and utilized by lay people, such groups raise questions about the epistemologic base as well as the uniqueness of traditional knowledge and its claims to privileged status and power.

In a society that emphasizes the privacy of deeply emotional experiences and that also values rationality in life planning, the kinds of public *sharing of intimate feelings* that often accompany self-help group activity stands in marked contrast to traditional emotional postures and styles. In addition, the possibility of people developing *new social identities* related to their experience in coping with problems challenges the notion that demography and socialization firmly establish individual identities that do not and should not change over time. As people identify firmly with their new status and bond to the common identity forged in the self-help group, the interpersonal, familial, community, and occupational relationships that have been constructed over time are challenged, reorganized, and at times even replaced.

Bellah and his colleagues (1985) summarize many observers who argue that individual autonomy, self-reliance, and personal accountability for one's successes and problems are among the root values of U.S. society.[24] Yet it is harder and harder, amidst the advances of the welfare state and bureaucratic capitalism, to live up to these traditional values. Moreover, the great geographic mobility of contemporary families combined with the depersonalized and alienating structures of modern economic life have greatly weakened traditional ties to kith and kin. The new forms of *support and affirmation* discovered and created in the context of self-help activity offer an alternative family or community environment to people facing crises. Moreover, patterns of societal discrimination against poor or less powerful citizens and people who need help (i.e., are non-self-reliant), including chronically ill children and their families, are challenged by the *stigma-countering* activity of self-help groups. Efforts to counter stigma, by definition, are efforts that counter societal norms and seek to build new ones.

Many people in this society feel that they are not able to cope effectively with some parts of their lives—that their lives are out of their control. In the context of self-help groups, people attempt to *learn new ways of coping with and buffering stress.* If this can be accomplished by people undergoing considerable stress and distress, why can it not happen for people everywhere in this society? The notion that our personal lives can be brought under better control and that the stresses of modern life can be buffered through peer support and the exchange of experiential knowledge challenges reliance on the official organs of the welfare state and its control of people's daily lives and options; it also counters the assumed alienation and anomie of a mass society.

Feelings of powerlessness are rampant in a society characterized by large and distant governments, massive and impersonal economic institutions, and vast, depersonalized neighborhoods and communities. Less and less frequently do we encounter real popular trust in democracy as a form of government, or in local or voluntary initiative as a way to solve community or public problems. Local efforts at *collective empowerment* and community-building through a process of grass-roots mobilization renew our democratic heritage. The *action for change* undertaken by previously powerless and distressed groups of people presents an alternative vision of the balance between crisis and opportunity. It also challenges our prevailing notions of dependence upon large institutions that organize and implement social action and social service from the top down.[25]

Thus, self-help groups present and highlight contradictions in values and processes that are central to our culture and society. Wuthnow (1994) provides a cautionary note, however, arguing that since small groups are well suited to deal with the problems created by our increasingly complex social environment, they may not be counter-normative. Instead, they may support evolving norms and social structures that will help individuals adapt to the social fragmentation reflected in the above trends. In such circumstances, self-help group values and processes are reminders of some of the historic values of our society—values and life priorities that have been pushed to the periphery of our common life—and help recapture some of these traditions. In the face of these contradictions, it is no surprise that self-help groups now are growing rapidly; they represent the best visions of our past operationalized in present forms of association and organization.

Moreover, it is not surprising that there is so much ambivalence and criticism about self-help. The very organizational elements and group dynamics that attract members may be the very factors that fail to appeal to other individuals in the same crisis situations. These elements at least implicitly challenge the belief systems and operating styles of many traditional centers of service and power in our society. It is no wonder that so many professional systems (individuals and institutions) seek to control the self-help movement and interpret it as simply another form of human-service delivery or "treatment," and that so many governmental agencies and large corporations seek to co-opt the self-help movement, treating it as simply another form of voluntary activism that can be brought under the control of dominant organizations and organizational processes. Those who represent the center—those who occupy and champion the natural superiority of expert and specialized knowledge, and of rational and linear forms of expression and problem-solving, traditionally alienating economic and political formats, and nondemocratic power bases that reify the status quo—seek to control the resolution of these contradictions. In so doing, they attempt to control the definition and operation of the self-help movement. From their point of view, and in the interest of preserving their power and privilege, self-help—and the values and processes it represents—must be kept at the periphery of our common life. To place the core notions of self-help at the center of our common life would require major transformations of our current values, as well as organizational and community practices.[26]

As we explore self-help within the particular context of childhood cancer, we focus both on members' direct experiences with self-help groups and with various public images of these groups. We argue that the basic ethos of self-help demands an alternative paradigm both for studying and understanding the operations of self-help groups for families of children with cancer, and for working with such groups in practice. Self-help groups, with agendas aimed at knowledge development, mutual support, emotional sharing, consciousness-raising, and empowerment, use their collective knowledge and resources to respond to the individual and institutional problems they encounter. Given this mission and these operating styles, self-help groups can be viewed as departing not only from many of our society's current central beliefs and practices, but from the mainstream medical system's view of psychosocial responses and resource usage.

Since we are concerned primarily with the ways in which the particular situation or life crisis may influence the shape and character of self-help, we ground the inquiry in this volume firmly in the particular realities of childhood cancer. In the next chapter we explore the stresses associated with being a parent or family member of a child with cancer and lay the groundwork for the analysis of self-help groups formed by or for these family members.

2

The Challenge of Childhood Cancer

Stress, Coping, Social Support, and Empowerment

A serious and chronic illness, childhood cancer is the major nonaccidental cause of mortality in children under fourteen years of age (U.S. Department of Health and Human Services, 1992; Sutow, 1984). Approximately one-third of the children diagnosed with childhood cancer will not survive five years (American Cancer Society, 1990; Green, 1989). Despite considerable medical progress, every child diagnosed with cancer faces the possibility of relapse and death, and all parents face the reality of seeing their children suffer. Treatment varies by the specific nature of the illness and by its stage, but often lasts for several years and is frequently painful. Although an increasing number of procedures can now be performed on an outpatient basis, lengthy hospital stays are not uncommon. Temporary side effects, such as hair loss and fatigue, are very common. Permanent side effects, such as loss of a limb, neurologic dysfunction, or a compromised immune system, can have debilitating and serious impacts on the lives of long-term survivors as well as on children undergoing therapy. These medical and physical realities are accompanied by psychosocial and logistic dilemmas for young people and their families, including stress, financial loss, and social isolation. These are the "troubled waters," the deep and dark depths of shock and stress, of fear and despair, that face parents of children with cancer.

There is good news as well. Over the past thirty years, significant medical advances have enabled many more children with cancer to become long-term survivors, perhaps to be "cured." In the 1950s, only 5–25% of children diagnosed with cancer could reasonably expect to have a normal lifespan. Survival proportions had changed to 20–80% by the late 1970s, and by the 1990s estimates for long-term survival for different types of childhood cancer reached 40–90% (American Cancer Society, 1990). Rates differ according to the specific nature of the cancer involved; for instance, for Wilms' tumor (a disease primarily of early childhood), the survival rate approaches 90%; for acute lymphoblastic leukemia, the rate is approximately 70%; for other forms of childhood leukemia, the survival rates drop to 50% or lower; and they are still lower for brain tumors. There is still much to know about how best to treat the medical problems of children with cancer. In addition, we have even more to learn about the psychosocial care of these children and their families. The growing long-term survival rates are accompanied by new psychosocial dilemmas, including concerns about long-term social/emotional adjustment and potential insurance and employment discrimination.

In this chapter we explore the major psychosocial stressors associated with childhood cancer, identifying the stresses and struggles which self-help groups for these families try to address. We set the stage for examining the responses to crisis and stress that develop from new knowledge and coping skills gained through shared life experiences, and the unique social support and individual as well as collective empowerment that may reduce or buffer these stresses. At the conclusion of this chapter we mirror the discussion of the themes of self-help outlined in Chapter 1, linking the kinds of stress that families experience to the coping, support, and empowerment resources potentially available in self-help groups. This chapter provides the disease-specific background and theoretical framework for our empirical exploration of self-help for families of children with cancer.

Major Stresses of Childhood Cancer

The immediate stresses and challenges of a serious and chronic illness, including the threat of death, face all families who experience the diagnosis of childhood cancer. These issues are not necessarily unique to childhood cancer, and are probably reflected, in different degree and character, in the experience of people encountering other serious and chronic childhood illnesses. However, because we anticipate that each particular problem situation has some unique characteristics, and that these may significantly affect the kinds of self-help groups that are formed in response, here we provide some background on the particularities of the childhood cancer experience.

A "family disease" that disrupts both the balance of a family and its rules for interpersonal behavior (Cassileth and Hamilton, 1979), childhood cancer invades not only the patient's life, but the lives of all of his or her loved ones and friends. Parents and other family members often join in the battle to fight the cancer, helping and supporting the ill child and each other. Thus, family members often "must be viewed as second-order patients in their own right" (Rait and Lederberg, 1989), as they struggle with childhood cancer, the needs it creates, and the unique responses it demands.

The first encounter with the diagnosis of childhood cancer is generally shocking and overwhelming to parents (Chesler and Barbarin, 1987). Several parents in our studies reported their initial reactions upon hearing the diagnosis as follows.

When I was told of the seriousness of the diagnosis I was devastated. I remember shrinking in back of the room. I felt like a truck ran over me. My husband didn't think I would get through the day.

I didn't know where to start, who to talk with, what to ask. I didn't understand what the doctors said. I was confused, nothing made sense.

I was petrified at first. I knew nothing about the disease. You hear *leukemia* or *cancer* and immediately think of death. He was only nineteen months old when he was diagnosed. It seemed so unfair. At the beginning I took it very hard.

While the stresses of childhood cancer begin at, or sometimes prior to, the initial diagnosis, they continue through various stages of the child's illness: full diagnosis, hospitalization, initial treatment, side effects, ongoing checkups, ongoing medication, the potential for relapse, and the possibilities of death or long-term survival. Reports from parents indicate that their greatest periods of stress occur at diagnosis, and at relapse if one occurs (Chesler and Barbarin, 1987). Moreover, the stresses they encounter are not rooted solely in the biological or physical aspects of the illness and treatment itself. Just as patients with nonchronic illnesses can feel dehumanized and stripped of their identity as they deal with the medical system (Coe, 1978), families of children with cancer can feel that the very cores of their familial and social roles are being compromised. Parents attempt to continue their roles as caregivers to their children, adding to that role the new demands of being the parents of an ill child. When those demands are compounded by the complexities of new forms of interaction with friends, family members, neighborhood agencies, and the medical staff, parental stress can be overwhelming.

Patients and families confronting childhood cancer face unique stresses that challenge them at various levels.[1] Especially at the early stages of diagnosis and treatment, *intellectual* and *informational* issues can be stressful, as illustrated below by parents' own words.[2]

I needed more information to increase my feeling of control. I wanted to know as much as I could so I could be part of the process.

I wanted to read and educate myself in order to eliminate much fear.

It has been difficult to find out about problems the hard way—by experience— because the doctors failed to inform us, or there was no material available for us to read.

Confronted with their ignorance about childhood cancer, with much new and terrifying information, and often with an unfamiliar vocabulary, parents need to reestablish some sense of equilibrium and control—of themselves and their situation. As front-line caregivers, parents must become familiar with medical terminology about their child's illness, and with the names and dosages of the numerous drugs and treatment protocols established for care. In addition, a lack of information about where things are in the hospital, where needed resources can be obtained, and who key staff are, can be both frightening and confusing. Parents of newly diagnosed children also may find it hard to learn enough information quickly enough to clearly and accurately explain their child's diagnosis and prognosis to family and friends.

Instrumental and *practical* stresses also challenge families' abilities to maintain normal and stable lives. For those without adequate medical insurance, the financial burdens of treatment and ancillary expenditures for travel, lodging away from home, and childcare may pose extraordinary problems. In addition, logistic demands at home can be overwhelming, as family tasks may have to be reallocated and reassigned. Daily needs such as meals, housecleaning, and care of siblings may be delayed or accomplished only with help from extended family members, friends, neighbors, or community agencies. Arranging transportation to and from the child's treatment center alone can become quite stressful for some families. Finally, it may be necessary to communicate and engage in problem-solving with employers, schools, and community agencies for resources and support—yet another time-consuming part of the parents' new role. Some of these stresses have been reported by parents as follows:

The logistics of meals, driving to the hospital, and the day-to-day nitty gritty issues.

I got intimidated by small details and new procedures I had to learn in caring for my child—for instance, using syringes, IV procedures, schedules for administering medications, side-effects, or returning symptoms to watch for.

We had to leave our home area for five months to get my child's treatment out of state. She just had a $150,000 transplant, and we're waiting for the bills.

I was working full-time because I had been divorced, and I had a real hard time all the way through. I wanted to get back to work because I had all these bills, but I also needed to stay close to my baby. I wanted to make everything normal, but I was also running to the city every day exhausted.

For parents of children who are dying or who do die from cancer, additional practical stresses arise in the form of having to make hospice or terminal-care decisions and arrangements, and dealing with funeral and burial issues.

While practical and logistic issues are crucial, stresses also come in the form of emotionally laden *interpersonal* issues. The new social role of a person with cancer, or a family member of a cancer patient (or the parent of a child who has died from cancer), involves dealing with potential stigma, isolation from others, and new social expectations. Co-workers, friends, and family members may mean well and be concerned but be unable to face and deal with the diagnosis and illness; thus they may become additional sources of worry rather than helpers—stresses rather than resources. The needs of family members other than the child with cancer (especially siblings) may be compromised, and consequently they may feel ignored and alienated, precisely at a time when their worries and needs for attention are escalating. The immediate need to develop good working relationships with the medical and treatment staff can be difficult for parents who already feel overloaded, or who may not be experienced in dealing with medical professionals. Some parents reported such stresses:

We have marital problems. There is a lack of communication on my husband's part, and he wouldn't help much with the other kids.

My relationship with my husband's parents is not good. They made a lot of negative remarks about us and make me feel responsible for my son's illness and the long-term outcome. I suppose I have guilt over their remarks, but I feel their attitude accentuates all the negative possibilities, and I am uncomfortable around them.

I felt like everyone was disowning me. My best friend never called—she is no longer a friend. People seem to have a thing about cancer. Like a lot of people, they think that cancer means death.

Parents of normal kids, kids without cancer, were detrimental. I got frustrated with the stigma from uneducated individuals.

It was hard to deal with some of the doctors' noncaring attitudes. I had to rehash the whole story to each of many residents, who were strangers.

These excerpts make it obvious that sometimes family members and friends not only failed to be helpful, but at times they added to parents' stress. The entire interpersonal situation surrounding childhood cancer is one in which both public and private roles and relationships with others are in great flux.

Certainly all of these stresses associated with childhood cancer include an *emotional* component. The sheer shock of diagnosis and the realities of treatment and prognosis challenge parents' ability to control their feelings. Parents and families can experience feelings of hope, fear, anger, sadness, and powerlessness all at once, and throughout the various stages of the illness, treatment and possible recovery or death. Some examples of this intense and continuing emotional trauma are provided by parents:

It has been like a nightmare, and I still haven't woken up. All I could do was cry for a long time. The diagnosis and treatment have made everything else in the world seem so unimportant.

Initially it seemed overwhelming to watch my daughter suffering physically as well as emotionally. To this day I resent that she has given up most of her teen years and socialization to this illness. You can never give this back to her. So I have had to deal with my anger and frustration.

It has been hard to stay optimistic and have positive thoughts.

My own coping style was a problem. I tend to feel that I should be able to handle almost everything, when, in fact, at times I can feel completely overwhelmed and losing control.

And in the case of a child who died, one parent reported:

I have long-term anger and sadness at my son's death. I accept it and have built a new life after the fact, but I remain sad and angry—probably for the rest of my life.

The results of such long-term and intense emotional stress, and the roller-coaster effect of good and bad news, of joys and fears, can lead to psychosomatic and physical illness. Especially when added to the search for useful information, the attempt to reestablish a network of social relations and provide direct care may result in decreased health and well-being.

Finally, the stresses of childhood cancer affect many parents on an *existential* level. It is common for parents to wonder why their particular child has cancer, or what they have done to deserve this fate. The threat of a child's death and the suffering of "innocent children" challenge many people's commonsense conception of the proper order of things and the place of God and religious commitment. Childhood cancer can provoke a wide range of spiritual and existential struggles. For example, some parents' traditional forms of spirituality are highlighted, as exemplified by informants' reports of "feeling closer to God" and the following excerpt from a parent of a child with cancer:

I felt at first that God had abandoned me. Later I trusted in God. He was in control.

For others, these stresses are not necessarily linked to traditional spirituality as such, but to being "more honest and open with yourself," and having "a better ability to forgive others" (Wuthnow, 1994, p. 227). The report of a parent of a child with cancer highlights this aspect of an existential and potentially spiritual struggle:

When my son was on treatment, I knew something was being done. When he went off treatment, I wondered what would happen next. The unpredictability of his response, and the uncertainty about the future, and how we should live our life, is still difficult.

Plans for the future and stable notions about faith, fate, or a just world may give way to great uncertainty and significant changes in life plans, careers, and images of one's personal and familial future.

The stresses associated with the childhood cancer experience also lead to a unique set of specific concerns about the future for patients and families, creating long-term, often intense anxiety (Davis et al., 1990). For example, the literature and these excerpts from our interviews and conversations with parents indicate that parents worry about their child's immediate response to treatment, about a relapse of the illness, about future painful or disfiguring treatments that might become necessary, about the possibility of death, and about long-term psychosocial adjustment and health should he or she survive. Other worries involve family concerns; relations with grandparents, siblings of the ill child, and one's spouse are all affected by the illness situation and its intense practical and emotional demands.

Since interactions with the medical staff are such a major component of any family's response to childhood cancer, parents naturally worry about getting along with the staff, how much and how often to ask questions, whether concerns they voice will upset the staff, and whether their child is receiving the best possible treatment. Other likely causes for worry are family financial needs, such as budgetary crises that the illness has brought about, maintenance of an adequate work schedule, and life and health insurance for a child during and after treatment. Parents also worry about their own personal health, as they continue to focus on and monitor the health and well-being of their ill child and other family members. They worry about seemingly simple occurrences that can threaten their role as caregivers, such as getting headaches, being tired, getting a cold, or getting enough rest. They also worry about complex issues such as their own and other family members' mental health.

The five major categories of stress experienced by parents of children with cancer, and some of the specific worries associated with each stress category, are summarized in the left-hand column of Table 2.1

Table 2.1. Stress and related social support

Categories of stress	Forms of social support	Sources of social support

Intellectual
Confusion
Ignorance of medical system
Ignorance about who the
  physicians are
Ignorance about where things
  are in the hospital
Lack of clarity about how to
  explain the illness to others
	Information
	Ideas
	Books, newsletters
		Medical Staff
		Social service staff
		Scientists and
		  researchers
		Other parents of ill
		  children

Instrumental
Disorder and chaos at home
Financial pressures
Lack of time and
  transportation
Need to monitor treatments
	Problem-solving
	  activities
	Practical assistance
	  at home or work
	Financial aid
	Transportation to
	  the hospitals
		Social service staff
		Family members
		Friends
		Neighbors and
		  co-workers
		Community agencies
		  (e.g., school)

Interpersonal
Needs of other family
  members
Friends' needs and reactions
Relations with the medical
  staff
Behaving in public as the
  parents of an ill child . . .
  and stigma
New social expectations
	Affection
	Listening
	Caring
	Being there
		Family members
		Close friends
		Medical and social
		  service staff
		Other parents of ill
		  children
		Religious congregations

Emotional
Shock
Lack of sleep and nutrition
Feelings of defeat, anger,
  fear, powerlessness
Physical or psychosomatic
  reactions
	Affirmation
	Counseling
	Clarifying
		Close friends
		Spouse
		Social service staff
		Other parents of ill
		  children

Existential
Confusion about why this
  happened to me
Uncertainty about future
Uncertainty about God, fate
  and a "just world"
	Reflection on God and
	  fate
	Creating a community
		Clergy
		Religious congregations

(adapted from Chesler and Barbarin, 1987, p. 51). Parents do cope with these stresses and, as later discussion will show, generally cope quite well. As they cope, they often build bridges of self-help and mutual support. We turn now to a discussion of parental coping strategies, and to their use of various forms of social support, for these are the foundations of self-help.

Coping with the Stresses of Childhood Cancer

Coping refers to the reactions of individuals to a potentially negative or stressful situation, and implies that individuals respond in ways that can influence their own feelings or behaviors, as well as the outcomes of events (Silver and Wortman, 1980). It includes ways of thinking as well as ways of acting, and has been broadly defined by Lazarus and Folkman (1984) as "constantly changing cognitive and behavioral efforts to manage specific external and/or internal demands that are appraised as taxing or exceeding the normal resources of the person." As parents experience the stresses described above, they seek to respond—to cope—in various ways.

Coping responses may be physiological, psychological, or social in nature. Their major aim is to maintain a positive sense of self, manage distress, and reduce the conflict between oneself and the environment (Menaghan, 1983). In addition, positive and effective coping responses can help a person alter, influence, and control a given stressor or crisis (Pearlin and Schooler, 1978). The specific manner in which individuals cope with stress differs as widely as does the nature of those stresses. According to the theory of learned helplessness, for instance, some persons may react in an increasingly passive manner, one that actually decreases their potential for dealing with and having a positive effect on the outcome of their situation (Silver & Wortman, 1980). Others may focus only on the potentially harmful effects of a crisis, constantly imagining the worst possible situations and outcomes. Still others may identify those aspects of the crisis that represent a challenge, one that can energize them and provide a potential for mastery and gain (Lazarus, 1981). Given the need in a medical crisis to both manage their emotions and direct their efforts toward solutions to their problems, some people may cope with both tasks simultaneously, while others will view these two coping options—emotion management and practical problem-solving—as mutually exclusive.[3]

Coping is best seen not as a static process, but as an ongoing one, so that any particular coping strategy may have a different utility at any given time during a crisis or during the development of a person's response capacity (Lazarus, 1981).[4] Aside from questions about any individual's choice of coping strategies, and the timing of these choices, it is clear that what constitutes good coping for one person may be dysfunctional for another. For example, venting anger may be stress-relieving for one person in one kind of situation, and stress-escalating for another person, or for the same person in another situation.[5]

As they attempt to cope with the stresses associated with their child's illness, parents of children with cancer face grave threats to their social and psychological functioning. As reported earlier in this chapter, great pain often accompanies the stresses and disruptions facing the family. It is important, however, to avoid the assumption that families cannot cope successfully and that they will fall apart in the face of these threats. Parents' own appraisals of their coping adequacy and strategies provide important and poignant assessments and insights into their situations (Stewart, 1990). Even though parents are often temporarily overwhelmed by such stress, they just as often report having coped with it successfully.[6] The childhood cancer experience obviously poses a challenge to prior living patterns, but it is a challenge that can also bring about positive life change. No one would deliberately seek such a challenge, but "making the best of a bad situation" has promoted personal growth for parents in many families.

The extent to which parents and other family members can maintain or improve their social and psychological functioning depends on the effectiveness of their particular coping styles and strategies. Some people may prefer to cope privately (e.g., by going off by themselves, by reading alone, by praying alone); others may cope more publicly (e.g., by seeking out friends to talk with, by joining groups or organizations, by organizing a family support network). Some may adopt active strategies, while others may opt for passive roles. Passive coping is characterized as rare by much of the general literature (Wethington and Kessler, 1991), but it is frequently employed by parents of children with cancer, who are witnessing a life-and-death struggle in the context of a very complex and technological medical-care bureaucracy. In fact, some have argued that the medical bureaucracy operates in ways that systematically disempower people and require them to behave in relatively passive ways (Taylor, 1979). Despite these personal and bureaucratic pressures, other parents adopt active forms of coping, attempting to learn about the illness, dealing vigorously with the medical staff, and playing an active role in restructuring their crisis environment.[7] Still others may use a combination of active and passive modes as they respond to the stresses of their child's illness with the coping strategies that work best for them.

Social Support for Families of Children with Cancer

Both the research and social service literatures are rich with ongoing debates regarding the conceptualization, measurement, and effects of social support. While a number of valuable definitions of social support exist,[8] some are especially relevant to an exploration of support systems for families of children with cancer. A two-dimensional construct for social support with objective-subjective and tangible-psychological dimensions is offered by Caplan (1979). The actual provision of aid is defined as *objective* support; in contrast, *subjective* support involves the perception that aid has been received. These two forms of support may occur simultaneously, as a person accurately perceives help being provided and herself actually receiving it. On the other hand, a person may feel she is receiving help when it is not actually forthcoming; and still others may fail to perceive assistance that is actually being delivered. Caplan (1979) makes a further distinction between physical or material resources as forms of *tangible* support, and *psychological* support in the form of feelings, values, and emotions.

Throughout this discussion of social support, we employ the concept of social support primarily in its subjective and psychological forms. However, at certain points, we also provide evidence of more tangible forms of support. We choose such a priority in the light of prevailing literature that points to the correlations between individuals' subjective assessments of their own social networks and their own reported well-being.[9] This view argues that help only matters if it is experienced as helpful. In addition, this definition is preferable because it potentially embodies the experiential expertise and informant subjectivity that is vital to the mutual support processes found in self-help groups. We can only explore the potential contribution of self-help to parents' efforts to deal with the crisis and stresses of childhood cancer through their own reports and voices. Their perspective enables us to identify the sources and types of support that are most successful and empowering to them as individuals.

Sources of social support are as integral to any discussion of helping and support as are types of social support. As discussed in Chapter 1, *formal* sources of support are usually expert and specialized; in the case of families of children with cancer, they are likely to include doctors, nurses, social workers, psychologists, and other health care, social service, and community professionals. *Informal*, or *lay*, sources of support usually exist as a function of an individual's everyday social network or life, and usually include family members, friends, neighbors, co-workers, and school companions. *Experiential* sources of support, a special form of lay support, include the fellow parents and self-help groups of families of children with cancer which are the focus of this volume. These sources and types of social support involve different bases of expertise, different kinds of role relationships between givers and receivers of help, and different organizational forms (Powell, 1987; 1990).

Taking advantage of the benefits of social support is, however, no simple matter. Our society reacts in conflicting ways toward help-seeking behavior, and socializes us into having competing notions about giving help, so that the notion of social support involves problems as well as promises. In an atmosphere of identifiable societal negativism and stigma toward help-seeking and dependency, any individual's pursuit of aid may endanger his sense of self-reliance, independence, or self-esteem and social status.[10] Even in a time of acute stress, people in dire need of assistance may ignore, avoid, and stifle those needs. Moreover, giving aid can be as difficult as seeking it, again because of socially constructed notions about how to respond to one's own and others' needs. Often victims of tragedy or illness are blamed for their fate, because of the belief in a "just world" in which people get what they deserve and deserve what they get.[11] Practical considerations such as time, energy, and resources can also limit helping behavior (Nadler, 1983). In addition, expectations about reciprocity and worries about how giving help may compromise others' feelings of competence and independence shape our posture toward giving support.[12]

In particular, Chesler and Barbarin (1984a) have explored some of the dynamics of informal helping systems for families of children with cancer. Parents who sought assistance from their close friends reported a series of dilemmas in the help-seeking and help-receiving process; their friends, in turn, reported a similar series of dilemmas. Among the major issues parents and their close friends both reported dealing with was managing the emotional impact of the illness, an issue which was very powerful for friends as well as parents. For instance, Chesler and Barbarin quote the following parents and their close friends on this dilemma of helping:

I didn't want to talk about it because it was something I wanted to shut in the back of my mind and have go away. It doesn't go away, but I want it to. I didn't want to talk about it because that brought up my unconscious fears (parent).

It was difficult talking about it with them because our real close friends were really shocked. They were shocked and cried and didn't want to believe it. It was just like us at first (parent).

I felt absolutely like someone had hit me. I was just very shocked (friend).

This wasn't just a one-month crisis. We're talking about a couple of years as an intense period of crisis in which the thing was really impacting on their family and anyone they were relating to, including us (friend). (pp. 123–24)

Chesler and Barbarin also report that some parents of children with cancer, as well as their friends, expressed concerns about intruding on a family's privacy and on the prior boundaries of a close relationship. In addition, parents and their friends worried about avoiding the creation of a new or additional stigma for parents, and creating an increased aura of weakness and non-normality. Friends' often voiced concern about finding ways to help that truly were effective, and about getting the kinds of feedback, or "cues," that indicated effectiveness. For example, two friends of parents reported the following:

Sometimes the family said, "People are afraid to ask us because they don't want to bring up the negative topics, so they rely on us to do it." So they gave us clues to know what they did want people to notice and talk about.

It was clear that we were useful and helpful. They've been very direct and open about their appreciation of our support. (p. 126)

Families dealing with childhood cancer may require intense and enduring social support, support that has long-term as well as short-term potential for improving well-being and emotional adjustment. Indeed, social support has been found to be related positively to effective coping and psychosocial adjustment for parents of chronically ill children, and specifically for parents of children with cancer.[13] However, this potential for long-term assistance, and its benefits, is challenged by the problems involved in seeking ongoing assistance from any part of a person's social network, and by the danger of "burning out" valuable sources of support. Moreover, certain sources and types of support may be most helpful in specific instances of need. Doctors and nurses may be most helpful with needs for information, the clergy may be most helpful in dealing with existential stress, psychologists or social workers may be most relevant for assistance with emotional stress, and friends and neighbors may be most useful for relieving interpersonal stress.

Whether in addition to formal counseling or in place of professional assistance, veteran families of children with cancer can also provide social support. Their support may be as timely and informed, and even more uniquely sensitive, than the support that formally trained but experientially distant professionals are likely to provide.[14] An ideal social support model for families of children with cancer includes the potential benefits of all of the above sources and styles of help: both formal and informal, as well as uniquely experiential. Ongoing debate in the practice literature on social support recognizes that formal and professional helpers, such as psychologists, social workers, and other clinicians, may differ in their supportive potential from informal or experiential networks that include family, friends, and—the focus of this volume— mutual support groups. All these sources are useful and necessary, and our focus on the unique nature of self-help groups should not be taken as depreciation of other forms.

The two right-hand columns of Table 2.1 list the variety of forms and sources of social support that might be available to and used by families of children with cancer. The table links these forms and sources to the major psychosocial stresses of childhood cancer identified earlier in this chapter.

Disempowerment and Empowerment of Families of Children with Cancer

Several scholars have argued recently that concepts of active coping and self-generated healing can empower patients and their families

(Cousins, 1979; Rappaport, 1985; Siegel, 1986). Rappaport (1985, p. 17) notes that a definition of empowerment may be difficult and elusive, but he observes that "empowerment is a little bit like obscenity; you know it when you see it!" Minimally, a working concept of empowerment implies an ongoing process of mastery over both internal and external problems; it implies both a sense of psychological control or internal healing and a capacity for social influence.[15] Useful working definitions of empowerment exist at both the individual and organizational levels of analysis (Schulz et al., 1993). Feelings of personal efficacy and control, efforts to exert control over one's life, and participatory behavior all may represent *individual* empowerment. A more *organizational* notion of empowerment implies shared attempts at group control or leadership, skill development and expansion, and community-level impact. Whichever notion we adopt as a focus, it is clear that empowerment does not happen alone. People need to be engaged with others in order to feel and act empowered. Both forms of empowerment are involved as parents cope with childhood cancer, especially if and when they participate in the collective activities of self-help groups.

The scope of the potentially *dis*empowering aspects of childhood cancer is, unfortunately, quite broad. We identified, earlier in this chapter, a variety of stresses normally associated with childhood cancer, and many parents have expressed their concerns about feeling "a loss of control" with regard to these stresses. Direct challenges to the very core of the role of parent or family member come from the emotional and logistic demands of the illness. The realities of the illness itself, its treatment, and the rules and regulations treatment entails, often create a sense of powerlessness for parents and their children.[16] For parents, who are accustomed to caring for their children, isolation from a direct role in the healing and caregiving process—at least in the initial stages of treatment—may be disempowering. Disempowering actions on the part of medical system personnel, community agencies, and other social institutions, even if they are not intentional, may further erode parents' and families' emotional stability and sense of control over their own lives and those of their children. The actions of family, friends, and significant others, usually well-intended but often rooted in misunderstanding and fear about the illness, its origin, and the prognosis, can also be disempowering.

Within the traditional medical model, parents are socialized into relatively passive and compliant roles as medical consumers, and this often results in limited views of their behavioral options for gaining new knowledge and negotiating authority. From the Lewinian (1939) standpoint of a minority group, people facing crises find themselves—or the loved ones for whom they are advocates—deviant and disabled in a socially constructed sense (Fine and Asch, 1988). In reality, they neither have to view their "disability" as a negative problem, as society does, nor to see their situation as helpless. They can overcome the reflected appraisals of others and the associated stigma. Not as victims but as advocates, people experiencing crises may empower themselves, taking a new view of themselves as agents of personal and social change, and helping others like themselves to develop changed self-images.[17]

Empowering roles and relationships can successfully create or reinforce the notion that a person can and must take action to achieve or protect personal and familial goals. When these goals are realized through activities in which a group of like-experienced people engage, they can be the roots of an "identity politics" approach to individual coping and to social activism (Anspach, 1979; Melucci, 1985; Touraine, 1988). In this context, individuals who discover that they have a shared social identity may work together to identify common stresses that shape their lives and common targets or objectives for change. Through collective activities, people may adopt a structural perspective that points to necessary changes in the social order that may facilitate individual adaptation and growth.[18] Such a perspective is crucial for the study of the empowerment of medically or socially stigmatized and disadvantaged groups.

Self-Help and Stresses of Childhood Cancer

Just as childhood cancer can present uniquely stressful challenges for families, self-help groups for families of children with cancer can offer uniquely empowering antidotes for those stresses. In terms of the typologies of self-help groups identified in Chapter 1 (see Figures 1.2 and 1.3), groups for families of children with cancer generally represent therapeutic groups (Katz and Bender, 1990c), but it is a special type of therapy designed for parents (significant others or caregivers) of people experiencing trauma and illness (Powell, 1987). A brief overview of how these groups operate and how they may benefit parents of children with

Table 2.2. Relationships between categories of stress and self-help themes

Self-help group themes	Categories of stress				
	Intellectual	Instrumental	Interpersonal	Emotional	Existential
Experiential knowledge	**	**	*	*	
Shared life experiences (and identity formation)		*	**	**	**
Support and affirmation (v. stigma)			**	**	*
Coping skills (giving and getting)	*	**	**	*	
Collective empowerment and action		*	*	*	*

** = Major focus
* = Minor focus

cancer is provided below; empirical elaboration of this perspective is the focus of the rest of this volume.

Parents of children with cancer may use self-help groups to reduce stress and cope more effectively with the crises of their child's illness by developing feelings of control over their lives and related environmental pressures.[19] For instance, many studies of voluntary organizations indicate that they can benefit members through the development of shared consciousness, shared experience, and shared ideology about a common problem (Scotch, 1988). A self-help group of persons in a similar situation may provide a "cognitive antidote" to feelings of decreased control and powerlessness. Parents of children with cancer can develop and maintain new sources of information, a new social network, a new identity as members of the larger social category of parents of children with cancer, additional coping resources, and the capacity for taking organized action with others to change or improve the service delivery system in their community or medical treatment center.[20]

Table 2.2 illustrates some of the potential links between the five categories of stress associated with childhood cancer and the five themes of self-help discussed in Chapter 1. With regard to *intellectual* stress, self-help group participation can provide access to the uniquely valuable experiential knowledge and expertise of others with similar experience. Such expertise can promote both individual parents' understanding of their child's illness and treatment and the group's collective knowledge. In addition, group activities can provide information about coping options and about some of the "tricks" parents use to deal with their own and others' practical problems, feelings, and concerns. As they search for new and essential forms of knowledge, self-help group members also can gain access to professional expertise about these matters.

Involvement in self-help groups can produce *instrumental* and *practical* resources to help parents respond to the stresses they encounter. Through the sharing of life experiences that occurs in these groups, parents can learn about how others dealt with daily dilemmas, develop new coping skills for solving personal and family problems, and learn how to deal more effectively with staff members and the organizational structure of the medical system. The dynamics of self-help and mutual support groups are especially useful in helping parents of children with cancer develop new, effective coping strategies, or redevelop preexisting coping skills that respond to the new demands of their child's illness.

Through the unique process of sharing their experiential knowledge with others in the self-help group, parents can increase their own knowledge and self-awareness, and identify the limitations of their own current coping skills and of their existing family communication and coping systems (Mantell, 1983). For example, through sharing narratives of family experiences and coping strategies, parents may learn that special care and attention should be given to the siblings of these children, or to grandparents. Parents may also get direct help in making accurate attributions about the events they are experiencing (Wortman and Dunkel-Schetter, 1979), thus enabling them to develop new coping strategies more successfully, and to feel less isolated as they do so (Lynam, 1987). Moreover, by participating with other parents, self-help group members can act collectively to empower themselves to make changes in the medical care system, especially changes that increase access to practical resources, psychosocial services and effective treatment. These actions represent an expression of voluntary and grass-roots efforts, in this case by a particularly vulnerable population.

In response to the *interpersonal* stresses they face, families who get involved in self-help groups can obtain various types of assistance. Parents of children with cancer often feel unfairly burdened by their child's illness relative to others, and the self-help group provides an arena for comparing oneself with others in a similar situation—a comparison that is likely to better reflect new realities. It also helps counter the social stigma so often associated with cancer, with families experiencing any chronic childhood illness, and with people needing assistance in general. Through sharing experiences and pooling resources in self-help groups, parents can gain support and affirmation for their own feelings and responses. Contributing to the welfare of others, even in the midst of one's own stress, can protect against feelings of individual and interpersonal isolation and powerlessness.

Sharing one's life experiences, experiential knowledge, and support with a group of others who are navigating the same crisis can help parents develop a new sense of identity, one grounded in their newly emerging role and expertise as parents of children with cancer. They can (and often must) become advocates for their own children and for other children as well.[21] This new social identity and accompanying role behaviors can help to reduce the sense of loneliness and confusion that parents so often experience, and can increase their positive sense of self.[22]

As parents extend their social network through group contacts and conversations, and as they become actively involved in a group, they may participate in local efforts at self-help group leadership (Yoak and Chesler, 1985; Yoak, Chesney and Schwartz, 1985). For some parents this requires learning and practicing new skills in organizational management and public representation. Moreover, some parents extend their new sense of social identity as parents of a child with cancer, and as members of an organized collectivity of such parents, to join in the group's effort to take collective action for organizational change in the medical system or community. Parental entrepreneurs (Darling, 1988), or simply parent advocates, in search of information, control over their situation, desire for communion with others, concern about the quality of medical and psychosocial services, and tools for challenging authority, may often choose social action as a strategy. Successful or not, such social action and efforts for change can validate parents' new identity and role and the renewal of voluntary democratic processes. It can also move parents into more active roles in a variety of other community activities and enterprises, broadening the base of active, democratic citizenship.

Self-help groups are unique in comparison to other types of support groups in that they bring together people encountering the same problem or enduring a similar crisis in a setting where they can help themselves and one another (Smith and Pillemer, 1983). Being together, talking together, and acting together in ways that begin to feel normal, given their unique situation, challenges the social stigma of abnormality, strangeness, and weakness that these families so often face.

The sharing dimension of self-help membership also provides a response to *emotional* stresses, as parent members exchange emotional experiences and connect to one another on an intimate basis. The group setting generally encourages disclosure and self-revelation, and the support gained thereby often promotes self-reliance and personal as well as interpersonal competence. For many, the self-help group provides the first safe, encouraging opportunity to test one's new identity as the parent of a child with cancer. Once this opportunity occurs in a semipublic context of mutual support and affirmation, parents can test that social identity further in public interactions with outsiders—friends, neighbors, and health professionals—and can receive further support from group members for the results of those tests.

As an alternative form of social support, parent groups may provide emotional resources and benefits that are not available elsewhere. Those benefits can come in the form of direct sharing and emotional venting, supported by the opportunity to develop such openness in a trusted atmosphere of common need.[23] Emotional benefits may be realized in the group through increased consensual openness and mutual acceptance, and through validation of feelings.[24] Such positive results occur despite the skepticism of some practitioners and researchers that such sharing may lead to inappropriate and increased emotional burdens (Wortman and Dunkel-Schetter, 1979). In fact, emotional benefits from group participation have been linked to greater utilization of psychosocial services (Kartha and Ertel, 1976), suggesting that perceived benefits of group involvement can lead to positive changes in health behaviors. They can help counter the self-imposed or internalized stigma or guilt too often associated with being the parent of a child with cancer, a guilt that is exacerbated by ignorance about the true causes of childhood cancer and by isolation from others struggling with similar issues.

The capacity of self-help group involvement to help parents respond to the *existential* stressors of childhood cancer is realized as they share new perceptions and common understandings of the uncertainties and the underlying meaning of their situation. As self-help group participants, many parents feel part of a larger group with an agenda of helping and sharing, which can be as comforting as it can be functional. Moreover, it is fulfilling to realize the ability to contribute to the welfare and growth of other parents. Part of parents' test of their new social identity may involve reexamination of both old and new sacred or secular beliefs and practices that are challenged by the crisis of their child's illness and treatment. Although social and emotional support may be the key ingredients in all self-help groups, this support can take many forms and respond to many stresses. Wuthnow's (1994) study of Bible-study groups demonstrates how support helps members respond to their spiritual or existential struggle and their experience of "trying to figure out what is really important in life" (p. 119). Many parents of children with cancer also report that their child's illness has required them to rethink their life priorities. Through interactions with others in similar situations, parents can develop new role definitions, new views of their own and their child's options, and new life opportunities. This is one more way in which such groups provide a unique forum for mutual aid and growth.[25]

3

Action Research
with Self-Help Groups
Methods Used in This Volume

Five different research efforts and sets of data, carried out over a fifteen-year period, constitute the empirical bases of this volume. First, in the late 1970s we conducted a lengthy participant-observation investigation of a single local self-help group for families of children with cancer, and a comparison of the experiences and attitudes of those group members with those of other parents who had not elected to join this group (Chesler, Barbarin and Lebo-Stein, 1984). That inquiry was part of a larger study of the psychosocial impact of childhood cancer and of the core stresses and struggles of childhood cancer which gathered questionnaire and personal-interview data from 95 parents and 30 children in 55 families. [1]

A second study, conducted during the early 1980s, entailed an organizational-level investigation of fifty self-help groups for families of children with cancer located throughout the United States. Data were gathered for this comparative organizational study by means of field visits to each site, personal and group interviews with participants and medical staff members working with these groups, questionnaires to members of local groups, and the collection of organizational records and materials. In the course of these visits, interviews of varying depth were conducted with over 275 parents of children with cancer and with 85 medical professionals; questionnaires were gathered from 146 parents and 50 professionals. These efforts provided data on group structures (size, operating procedures, leadership patterns, degree of bureaucratization), programs, and activities.[2] The results of this study are reported primarily in Chapters 4, 5, 8, and 9.

In the late 1980s a third study combined both organizational-level and individual-level approaches in field visits to eight self-help groups for families of children with cancer. In addition to collecting organizational data similar to that gathered in the second study, we conducted individual interviews with group members and with nonmembers, and group interviews were conducted with group members. We also gathered individual questionnaires from a total of 116 parents of children with cancer, some of whom were group members, and some of whom had not participated in the local group. These questionnaire responses provided additional data on the personal characteristics of both members and nonmembers, detailed the benefits members felt they derived from participation in these groups, and permitted comparisons of members' and nonmembers' perspectives and experiences on a number of dimensions. Individual and group interviews were also conducted with professionals, and questionnaire responses were obtained from professionals at each group site.[3] The results of this study are reported primarily in Chapters 4, 5, 6 and 7.

A fourth study, conducted in 1992–93, involved follow-up inquiries with current group leaders and liaisons in the fifty self-help groups from the second study. This longitudinal effort to assess the changes over time in these organizations utilized telephone interviews that replicated as closely as possible the questions asked in field visits conducted ten years earlier.[4] The results of this follow-up inquiry are presented primarily in Chapter 10.

A fifth source of data is the result of our long-time personal associations with many local self-help groups of families of children with cancer, mainly through the auspices of the Candlelighters Childhood Cancer Foundation (CCCF). Founded in 1970, CCCF is a Washington-based networking and clearinghouse organization linking over 400 local self-help groups of families of children with cancer throughout the United States and other nations. It has extensive files of newsletters, reports, and information from these local groups, and provides a variety of services to them. These materials, and our visits to local groups, meetings with numerous parents, conversations or presentations with and to health care professionals and professional

Figure 3.1. Timeline and flow of studies used in preparing this volume

Study #1 1978–80	Study #2 1981–84	Study #3 1986–88	Study #4 1992–93	Study #5 1978–93
Participant observation in one group	Field visits to 50 groups	Field visits to 8 groups	Telephone restudy of 50 groups visited in 1981–84, via interviews with parent or professional leaders	Continual examination of group newsletters and other materials
	Group interviews with parent members	Questionnaires to parent members, and non-members		
	Interviews with professionals	Group interviews with parent members		
		Interviews with parent members, nonmembers and professionals		

1978 ———————————————————————— 1993

associations, and consultations with varied medical centers have created an excellent firsthand database of anecdotal information on local
groups. The materials and insights gathered through this process are
reported throughout this volume.

Figure 3.1 indicates the methods, content, and sequence of these
five data-collection efforts.

Research with Self-Help Groups

The research studies reported here used several different techniques of data collection and analysis. In all of this work we were
driven by a set of epistemological and methodological guidelines reflected in a research paradigm most closely identified as participatory
action research (P-A-R). This approach requires that informants (and/
or representatives of the informant population) participate actively in
the research process, that key decisions be made with and in the interests of the informant population, and that action for change be part of
the endeavor.

Participatory action research (P-A-R) is quite consonant with the
highly participatory and experiential culture and goals of self-help.
Moreover, it employs technologies of data collection and analysis that
are congruent with the reliance on local wisdom and lay leadership that
characterizes the self-help movement. Grounding data collection efforts and theory in the experiences of the informant population and
inductively deriving findings from field reports turns investigators' attention to the field, rather than to prior academic theory and literature
(Glaser and Strauss, 1967). Finally, the ways in which participatory action research utilizes research findings are more consistent with the
organizational structures, action needs, and empowerment potential of
self-help groups. What does P-A-R entail, and how did we implement it
in these studies?[5]

The Conventional Social Scientific Model

There are many versions of the scientific method, and different versions are more or less applicable for different researchers in different
situations studying different phenomena. The social scientific academy,
however, is dominated by one version of the scientific method. Drawing
heavily on the physical sciences' positivist and deductive approach, it
stresses the search for general laws, formal and a priori hypotheses,

neutrality with regard to moral issues, standardized assessment devices, reduction of observed reality into constituent parts, and establishment of "distance" and nonintervention between the investigator and the field of study.[6] Various advocates and critics of the positivist and deductive approach at the heart of this conventional method differ as to particulars, but almost all would agree about the emphasis on these central canons (Lincoln and Guba, 1985; Rowan, 1981).

Alternatives to this conventional model of academic research include "applied research," "action research," "feminist methodology," and a variety of inductive or phenomenological and qualitative approaches. Some of these latter approaches utilize methods that are more appropriate for generating both academic and practically useful knowledge for researchers and for self-helpers.

An Alternative Paradigm

In *action research,* a commitment by the researcher to personal action and to improving the human social condition directly is an integral and necessary component of the knowledge-generation process. The central features of action research involve a repetitive and cyclical process of diagnosis, analysis, action, and evaluation; a high degree of cooperation and involvement between researcher and practitioner, with constant feedback loops; and a commitment to use findings to solve social problems.[7]

Participatory action researchers emphasize conducting action research on a more fully participatory basis with subjects—often called co-researchers.[8] As Gaventa (1988) suggests, "Research is seen not only as a process of creating knowledge, but simultaneously as education and development of consciousness and of mobilization" (p. 19). Such action objectives are built into the research design from the beginning, with the initiative and participation of the co-researchers.

This style of scientific work stresses respect for and reliance upon the needs and expertise of practitioners and citizens involved in the issues, sites, or problems under study, and involves them in the direction of the entire endeavor from start to finish. Indeed, it often emphasizes the need for "member validation," "getting feedback from informants" (Miles and Huberman, 1984) or "member checks" (Lincoln and Guba, 1985), and argues that people who are the direct informants in and beneficiaries of research can help inform and direct the work, monitor it, improve its validity, and make the best use of it in efforts for change. Through participation, local informants, citizens, and activists can increase the researcher's knowledge base directly and consciously. Through participation, informants can also learn new skills in gathering and analyzing information, thus laying bare the workings of the social systems of which they are a part and enabling them to play a role in improving those systems' strategic decision-making capacities.[9] Such participation in knowledge creation is often consciousness-raising and empowering.[10] According to Brown and Tandon (1983), the focus on participation and empowerment and on dealing with issues of institutional control, conflict, and change are major characteristics that distinguish P-A-R from other forms of action research. In contrast, the conventional researcher is most likely to exclude "subjects" from significant knowledge of or participation in the research project (except as required for human-subject consent processes). He is also likely to maintain distance from the field of inquiry, and to avoid direct efforts to alter the field. These approaches are justified in order to maintain "objectivity" (called "objectivism" by Keller, 1985) through tactics of detachment and control—control of oneself and one's research subjects or field of inquiry. Conversely, we constantly remained close to, in fact often a part of, the objects of our inquiry.

Since the participatory character of P-A-R involves subjects in becoming co-researchers, it also requires researchers to enter the world of those being studied, and to trust informants' willingness and ability to tell them about this world. One way to do this is to use the techniques of narrative analysis. For instance, in this volume we often present quotations, vignettes, and case studies in which parents of children with cancer tell their own stories—stories of their experience with their child's cancer and stories of their self-help group involvement and activity.[11] In these stories parents attempt to understand and articulate their sense of what happened to them throughout the crisis, and what life-meaning they make of it. In addition, they talk with one another about how their groups function, often creating together a narrative of their collective experience—or perhaps several different narratives, depending on who is telling the story. Since storytelling is a core activity in self-help groups, this technique seems appropriate for conducting research with such groups as well. The subsequent thematic ordering and analysis of parents' stories about their self-help group experiences helps us place their unique narratives in a more general context and understand their experience from theoretical as well as descriptive standpoints. Taken together, parents' stories also highlight the way these groups operate as normative narrative communities.

The conventional deductive research paradigm generally places less trust in informants' abilities to fully participate in research and to tell their own and their groups' stories, and thus usually poses a specific and detailed inquiry agenda prior to entering the field. In the case of self-help groups, social service agencies and governmental funding sources, and social scientists sponsored by them, primarily want to know whether groups work—whether members have better mental or physical outcomes as a result of participation—or whether they work "better" than professional service systems (Jacobs and Goodman, 1989). They are also usually interested in testing a priori theories that can explain the characteristics of group participants and group operations. The central foci of P-A-R studies are more likely to evolve inductively from interactions with members and groups in the field. Primary concerns of group leaders seldom focus on the generic assessment of effectiveness—they already know how effective they are! They are more interested in solving particular problems of group functioning: leadership, recruitment, maintenance, fund-raising, programming to meet members' needs, and working with (or changing) medical and social service agencies.[12] Moreover, centering inquiry on these informant concerns means that subsequent conceptual principles and theory are more likely to be grounded in and derived from field realities, and that findings can be generated that better inform and explain member choices and group dynamics, as well as direct future actions.

Research conducted within the conventional paradigm may or may not lead to action for change; such research often concludes with articles in appropriate scientific journals or a technical report filed with agency or governmental offices. The very concern for detachment and disengagement generally precludes action-taking, especially action that might challenge established agencies' policies and procedures. Participatory action researchers may have undertaken action or worked for change prior to or concurrent with the research endeavor. Acting with or on behalf of the groups with which they are conducting research, they are usually personally engaged in helping to utilize the findings from research studies and to organize and participate in efforts for change.

While participatory action research has these many advantages for certain types of inquiry, it also has some potential drawbacks: the very commitment to empathy, collaboration, and action with informant groups may draw the researcher too deeply into this world to be able to see it clearly. A meaningful form of objectivity depends on the researcher's ability to both enter the subjective field of inquiry and stand apart from it sufficiently to be able to "test" inside information against external realities. This stance helps ensure that the commitment to informants does not result in only narrow images of their world—images that conform to their (and the researcher's) preferred ways of being seen.

Participatory Action Research with Self-Help Groups

This brief discussion of alternative paradigms for social scientific research and public action is particularly relevant to research concerning self-help groups. Such groups are distinctive social phenomena; they are more like voluntary grass-roots organizations or nascent social movements than rationalized bureaucracies (Katz, 1981; Killilea, 1976). Moreover, as Borkman (1984) suggests, "Each self-help group constructs its own experiential paradigm—of the problem and the means to resolve it" (p. 208). The tremendous variety in organizational form and function, even in local units of a single national umbrella organization, means that pre-established and standardized research questions, measures, topics, and approaches may fail to adequately tap or be relevant to real-life heterogeneity (Levy, 1984). For instance, in his discussion of "collaborative" forms of self-help group research, Kaufman (1993) emphasizes why researchers must rely on participants' experience in guiding the research process:

Reliance on experience has direct implications for the field of self-help group research. If the researcher enters the field with pre-established definitions of self-help, he or she could miss important instances of peer support activities. (pp. 264–65)

The processes that occur in self-help groups are more like private interactions in a family or intimate relationships than public social relationships. Thus, researchers' access may require clear identity or identification with the condition at hand, and intimate knowledge of the language and styles that code in-group/out-group perceptions. Jacobs and Dopkeen (1990) argue that a researcher may improve her access and learn more by becoming a member of the groups being studied, and then "studying . . . herself" (p. 171). In our work with groups formed by/for families of children with cancer, it has been very helpful for the senior investigator to be a parent of a child with cancer, an organizer and former leader of a local self-help group, and a national officer of the Candlelighters Childhood Cancer Foundation. It also has been important that other staff members had lengthy personal experience with self-help groups and with the medical and psychosocial realities of childhood cancer. These personal histories provided us with special knowledge of individual and group situations and with the collective identification and legitimacy to ask and to be told about intimate personal and organizational details. They also provided credibility that allowed us to vouch for or sponsor other staff members who did not have this personal background.

Since issues of personal and collective empowerment are crucial in self-help groups, inquiry methods and actions for change that explicitly seek to empower participants become extremely relevant and important. For instance, P-A-R often self-consciously attempts to counter researchers' monopoly over the knowledge-generation process, and thus over the cultural forms, language, and policies that are derived from research. In fact, several researchers discuss the many ways in which control of the means of knowledge production by scientists and the elite may help disempower people who have few resources, are under great stress, or are in dependent relationships with powerful agencies.[13] This orientation is certainly compatible with self-help groups' concern about dealing with the orientation and power of professionals' expert knowledge, and their investment in the development, use and legitimation of parents' experiential knowledge (see the discussion of this issue in Chapter 1).

Both the structure and process of self-help organizations suggest that their reality cannot be known or predicted ahead of time or from "the outside." Standardized or highly controlled research designs are not often feasible; or, in order to be feasible, they overlook or inappropriately categorize group realities into oversimplified models.[14] Small grass-roots organizations responding to people in pain may create a buzzing confusion of interactions and events (late-night phone calls, crying and hand-holding sessions, time spent shopping or painting houses together, etc.). These events, while suited to people's unique needs and circumstances, may be invisible or incomprehensible to the outside observer or the short-term visitor.

The principles underlying P-A-R fit quite well with the desired goals of self-help group involvement: member/informant participation in the design and operation of activities, local and grass-roots orientation, freedom from professional control, opportunities to learn new skills, participation in new social processes, and attaining outcomes of consciousness-raising and empowerment. For instance, P-A-R emphasizes the existence of a "sharp bifurcation between expertise, based on the study of a problem, and experience, the subjective living of that problem" (Gaventa, 1993, p. 29). The fundamental culture and ideology of the self-help movement has been described in similar terms (Borkman, 1990). Respect for the personal struggle, experiential wisdom, and emergent social dynamics embodied in the self-help process requires researchers to cast a skeptical eye on professional expertise and power—including our own. Thus, both participatory action research and narrative analysis represent inquiry approaches that are (more) consistent with the nature of self-help phenomena. They both privilege the reality of the informant population rather than the researcher population. As Rappaport (1993) notes:

By its very nature, narrative analysis is an antidote to professional hegemony. It forces us to ask questions, such as "Who has the right to speak for this person?" It requires us to learn about both the structure and content of the stories that people tell about their own lives and of the lessons they learn from their communities of membership. It highlights (albeit imperfectly) their views of themselves rather than emphasizing our views of them. (p. 244)

The practical value of these approaches in studies with self-help groups has been borne out in the work of a small but growing group of researchers.[15] These principles, and our use of them in this volume, do not suggest that participatory action research is the only research method suitable for studying self-help groups, nor that it is an easy method to apply rigorously; but it does appear to have unique advantages, especially when investigators work with phenomena that are outside the mainstream of formal organizations and want to adopt action roles as well as inquiry roles.

At the same time, its disadvantages, or potential limits, must be observed and accounted for. As scholars and activists working inside and outside these groups, we tried constantly to protect ourselves against uncritical acceptance of the information that group members and professionals provided. We tried also to avoid biasing what people told us by the over emphatic sharing of our hunches, ideologies, hopes, or a too great sense of collaboration with them and their self-help ventures. We did so in several ways: researchers with varying levels of involvement with childhood cancer and self-help participated in gathering and analyzing the data; different methods of inquiry were used, including more traditional modes of "objective" paper-and-pencil questionnaires; results were shared with, and feedback obtained from, other scholars in the field; and, informants with different personal and group experiences were constantly involved in hearing and reacting to the information and findings.

In these explorations we were not driven primarily by a dominant theoretical perspective or by "theories of self-help groups." Rather, we were guided by a desire to answer relatively practical questions of group operations:

- What do groups do?
- How do they do it?
- Who participates in groups?
- What differences can groups make for people?
- How do groups relate to professionals?

Along the way to answering these questions, we do generate theories about how and why groups did the things they did.

Access to Groups and Individual Informants

The research literature on local voluntary organizations, and especially on self-help groups, often addresses the difficulty of investigator access to these organizations. Members of these groups generally express little interest in serving as scientific subjects, and have little motivation to spend their time and open their lives to an outsider from the distant social scientific community. Disease-specific medical self-help groups may be expected to pose a special problem in this regard, since they occupy a sensitive emotional sector of members' lives. Meaningful access to the private lives of people suffering from an illness, or from some socially stigmatized condition, is a matter of carefully negotiated privilege. Access to these private contexts is not easy to obtain, is delicate to maintain, and generally implies some reciprocal moral or ethical exchange. The Federation for Children with Special Needs, a coalition of self-help groups of parents of children who are ill or who have disabilities, explicitly warns against participating in research under pressure, or when the research purposes are unclear, or when it is not clear how the results will be used (Anderson, 1988; see also *Report of Consensus Conference on Principles of Family Research*, 1989).

We suggested in Chapter 1 that the core phenomena and ideologies of self-help groups often are counter-normative to some mainstream assumptions about self-care and social service. Moreover, since many self-help groups develop explicitly to fill gaps or create change in the service delivery system, they are not likely to trust establishment-based researchers, even action researchers, and especially not researchers embedded in the professional bureaucracy responsible for delivering services that people feel are inadequate.[16] Groups and individuals struggling for legitimacy and influence, or simply wishing to preserve their privacy, may insist upon some degree of control over researchers' freedom to investigate, to interpret and publish their results, and some evidence of researchers' commitment to their partisan cause.

Our approach to the access issue was to immerse ourselves deeply in groups' lives, and to enlist group members as active participants in examining an area about which they, also, wanted to know more: how and why their groups work. Chesler's experiential credentials helped establish a special relationship of trust with group members, a relationship which other staff have been able to maintain, given their own commitment to the research paradigm and goals. He is the parent of two adult daughters; one is a survivor of childhood cancer, and the other has experienced the dilemmas of a sibling of a child with cancer. His eldest daughter was diagnosed with acute lymphoblastic leukemia in late 1976. In 1978 he and his wife, together with three other families of children with cancer and aided by a member of the medical staff, formed a local self-help group (leading to Study #1 in Figure 3.1). In 1981, Chesler became active in the Candlelighters Childhood Cancer Foundation (CCCF), and has served as an elected member of the Foundation's Board and Executive Committee (as President of the Board, Chair of the Board, Research Consultant to the Board) from 1983 to the present. In these roles, as a parent in a family experiencing childhood cancer as well as a university-based social psychologist, he has had immediate and open (even welcoming) access to discussions with parents, professionals, and local groups. His 1987 book, *Childhood Cancer and the Family* (with Oscar Barbarin) and his many articles on the psychosocial impact of childhood cancer have made him a sought-after speaker at meetings of local groups, clinic grand rounds, and parent and professional conferences.

Chesney is the daughter of a man who died from cancer. She worked with the national CCCF to create a guide for parents who wished to be peer-counselors to other parents of children with cancer (Bogue and Chesney, 1987), and through this process became acquainted with, and trusted by, members of the national staff. They also facilitated her entry into local groups in the eight-group comparative study (#3), and these visits led to a doctoral dissertation examining the impact of group membership on parents (Chesney, 1989). Over a period of eleven years she has presented research findings at various group conferences and professional scientific meetings.

With specific regard to the field visits, various strategies were devised to ensure that different members of the research team would be able to enter groups and carry on conversations with a high level of trust and openness. In our studies, successful access was attained by the combination of careful introductions to certain groups (including sponsorship by the national officers and staff of the CCCF), joint visits by several staff members to some groups, personal contacts, and all staff members' special training and background in the literature on childhood cancer and in group and organizational work. In addition, over the years several staff members were family members of people with cancer themselves or long-term survivors of childhood cancer; the latter were especially attractive and welcome investigators in the eyes of parents of children with cancer. Open and trusting relationships with local groups were indicated in various ways: in conversations about intimate details of childrens' illness and family coping; in open discussions of sensitive areas in parents' and groups' relationships with the medical system; and in several instances of informants' willingness to reveal sensitive information after requesting that the tape recorder be turned off during part of the interview. Successful access is also reflected in the low refusal rate: only one group out of all the groups contacted in *all* of the studies declined to participate in the study (a professional leading a group refused access to members of the parent group).[17]

Data-Collection Procedures

Our primary research aim in the field study of 50 groups (#2) was to identify commonalities and variations in group activities and structures, organizational relationships, and professional roles within self-help groups of parents of children with cancer. We chose the sample of 50 self-help or mutual support groups from a national pool of more than 300 such groups made available by the CCCF, by children's medical centers, and by other state and national organizations and programs. Groups were selected to achieve variation with respect to geography, characteristics of the treatment center or community base, and the structure of relationships among each group and the professionals in its local health care system. Although no systematic way exists to verify retrospectively whether the sample was representative of the numerical distribution of such groups across a variety of dimensions, our prior and subsequent experience, as well as the empirical evidence presented in this volume, has convinced us that it does represent the range of parent groups organized to deal with the experience of childhood cancer. In the later study of 8 local groups (#3), we targeted some groups we had visited earlier (in #2) and some groups that had been identified as conducting especially interesting programs. Thus, the latter study is not representative of the population of self-help groups for parents of children with cancer in general; however, data gathered in this effort do highlight the differences between members and nonmembers of local groups.

The first contact with groups in all our studies was a letter explaining the study and requesting that the group contact (a parent leader or sometimes a nurse or social worker) return a form indicating their own and their group's willingness to participate. In the case of groups affiliated with the national CCCF, the director of that network also provided a personal letter of introduction. Access to groups not formally affiliated with CCCF was facilitated through personnel at local treatment centers and other personal contacts. Upon receipt of responses, interview sessions (usually taking a total of two to three days per group) were scheduled according to geographic location and interviewers' travel plans.

Informants for questionnaires and interviews were selected and scheduled by local contacts, usually a member/officer of the group or an associated professional. These contacts were given the following guidelines in setting up an interview schedule: to allow at least two hours per interview; to solicit some current and former leaders of the group; to include some parents of children with cancer who were not members of the local group; and to arrange for appointments with those people in the medical system who worked most closely with or were most important to the group (nurses, doctors, social workers). A call back shortly before each trip confirmed the details of interview scheduling.

Since the key foci of the studies were on group as well as individual phenomena, some interviews were held with more than one person at a time. This was most often true of interviews with parents, where from three to ten parents might be present and responding in one group interview. Professionals were interviewed separately from parent members, and those conversations were most often with individuals. Individual and group interviews averaged between one and one-half and two hours, with some as long as three hours, and the shortest one about fifteen minutes. Group interviews were tape recorded using a semi-structured form, so that the interviewer could make notes about responses. After the interview, the interviewer used the tape recording to complete a full set of written notes entered onto this form. Those notes did not constitute a transcription, but an accurate reconstruction of the interviewees' responses. In addition, field notes were prepared which documented interviewers' impressions and reflections apart from the interview content itself.

Questionnaires were distributed to group members (Studies #1, #2, and #3) and nonmembers (Study #3) by the local contact person. They were returned, sealed, to that contact person, and then shipped in a block to our offices at the University of Michigan.

Multiple Methods for Gathering Group-Level Data

For the group-level data, several different information-collection strategies were used in order to complete a multi-method data base and reference file on each group studied. An in-depth group interview with parents served as the basic information source. Individual interviews with parents and with professionals, self-report questionnaires, group materials and records, and (in the case of Study #2) a follow-up "group information" instrument provided supplementary data.

An unstructured interview schedule (Denzin, 1970) guided us in our individual and group conversations with informants in Studies #2 and #3. Deviations from this schedule were common as we sought to follow informants' leads in discovering and narrating their own realities and in trying to develop a sense of group reality based on several interviews. The same interview schedule was used for both parent members and professionals, with slight variations in emphasis and probes. Notes were taken on the interview schedule during the conversation; each interview also also taped, in order to capture greater detail and to allow the researcher to concentrate on the flow of the interview. Taping was also discovered to be essential in a team research undertaking, as the field staff and the office staff were able to share in the experience of each group by sharing the tapes.

The general pattern was for the researcher or research team to enter a group intensively and to spend several days conducting interviews with group members and professionals. Once the interviews and all associated material had been organized and reviewed, an informal case study was prepared on each group. Each case study was considered complete when the investigator(s) felt they understood the group's activities, operating structure, and narrative "storyline"—its social puzzle. In some cases, this required several callbacks to resolve contradictions, inconsistencies, or gaps in the data collected. For example, in order to complete and verify information in Study #2, a group-level form was developed and mailed back to a group liaison after initial analysis was begun on each group. This form summarized the factual data we had gathered on a group and asked the contact person to respond to gaps or ambiguities in concrete (non-opinion) information that were discovered. Some of these issues had not been addressed clearly or completely in the verbal interviews, due to the detailed and varied nature of the responses sought.

Measures and variables used for group-level analyses were taken from various information sources available in the study; from composite responses to the interview questions, from the follow-up information form, and from materials provided by the groups (by-laws, budgets, annuals reports, brochures), as well as from standard records and secondary sources (American Hospital Association, 1980; U.S. Dept. of Commerce, 1980). When there were discrepancies in information, the researchers went back to primary sources to determine their nature and causes.

In Study #4, the information gathered in Study #2 was used as baseline data for telephone interviews seeking updated information on the same sets of variables inquired into earlier. In addition, specific questions focused on changes that had occurred over time in groups' activities, organizational structures, membership patterns, and relationships with the treatment staff.

Methods for Gathering Individual-Level Data

In Studies #2 and #3, all parent informants completed questionnaires asking about their experiences and attitudes, about the activities the group did or did not perform, about how the group operated, about how the group related to the local environment—including the medical system—and about their perceived levels of satisfaction with various aspects of the group and the medical/social service system. Personal interviews with four or five of the most active members/leaders of each group covered aspects of their experience with the crisis of parenting a child with cancer, with the aim of rooting the study within the stressful life situations and coping responses that can give rise to self-help participation. In addition, interviews explored in depth the reasons these members became and remained active in the group. In Study #3, additional questionnaires were mailed to a larger number of active members and nonmembers in each group. These questionnaires inquired into their experiences with relevant family crises via a series of structured questions relating to specific stresses, coping patterns, and social support mechanisms. Questions also were asked about their participation in the self-help group, as well as their perception of group activities and group benefits to individuals. It is from 116 of these individual self-help group members' and nonmembers' questionnaires that the data reported in Chapters 6, 7, and 11 were derived.

The potential loss of personal meaning and information occasioned by the use of an impersonal and prestructured questionnaire was compensated for by intensive and open-ended interviews with a small subsample of group leaders. In turn, potential selection bias, given the small number of interviews, was compensated for by the larger sample and wider range of people responding to questionnaires. In addition, in several groups it was possible to identify, from clinic or group lists, names of parents of children with cancer in the local area who were not active in the group. These parents were also sampled and asked to complete the questionnaire. While there was a lower response rate from this nonmember population, data that were collected provide unique and important comparisons.

Because of our prior knowledge of the variety and distribution of the local groups from Study #2 (Yoak and Chesler, 1985), we are confident that the participant population in Study #3 is sufficiently similar to the national population of participants in such self-help groups. No similar claim is suggested with regard to the population of nonparticipants. Problems of defining the population of nonparticipants, gaining access to them, and their refusals to participate in Study #3 mandate caution in this regard. Such problems are not unknown in studies on self-help, where difficulties in creating control groups are well documented (Powell, 1987).

Other data reported in Chapter 11 are based on 100 questionnaires from members of self-help groups for parents of murdered children in the United States, and interviews with parents in five self-help groups for parents of children with mental illness in Israel. These data also were gathered as part of the comparative investigation referred to as Study #3 in Figure 3.1 and in endnote 3 to this chapter.

Feedback and Use of the Research Findings

Consistent with the P-A-R approach, we have been directly involved over the past decade in the application and use of these findings to improve the workings of self-help groups. Engagement in this process of change began early in the research process, and research and action proceeded in a recursive and reciprocal manner throughout. Rather than treating action for change as a potential contaminant to the research process, we saw it as a series of opportunities to share, test, and enrich our knowledge development; rather than dealing with application solely at the end of the research chain, we saw it as coterminous with and integrated into the research itself; and rather than seeing application as a skill and commitment distinct from knowledge development, we saw these roles as synthesizable, although not unitary. Thus, these action efforts also were data- and theory-generative, and added to the data base via a reflexive P-A-R approach.

Networking   Early in the research process, as our staff visited various local self-help groups to gather data, we often shared information discovered about one group with other groups. For instance, when a group in New England wanted information on how to run a certain type of fund-raising event, we shared information gathered from a New York group's efforts to run just such an event. Similarly, when we visited two groups in Southern California, we discovered that one of them was run by a parent member in a semitherapeutic manner; she and the group members felt that dealing with deeply held (or withheld) emotions was critical to coping and healing, and that other activities were denials and distractions. On the other hand, another local group was almost completely focused on fund-raising for parents and their local hospital; they felt that dealing with feelings was a waste of time when there was so much work to do to help others. Our staff suggested that these two groups connect and network with one another—that they had much to learn from one another. In addition to "seeding" the linking and networking process, these efforts often generated important data, as groups reacted not only to their own realities, but to others' experiences and responses.

Consulting   Some local groups were struggling with issues of personal member trauma, leadership development, meeting process, group dynamics, or intraorganizational conflict at the time of our field visits. To the extent that we had expertise in group and organizational development, we offered our services to help solve these problems.

Leadership Training   A network of California and West Coast self-help groups, aided by the Candlelighters Childhood Cancer Foundation and the Northern California Division of the American Cancer Society, involved us in leading a weekend workshop for current and potential leaders of local self-help groups for families of children with cancer. This workshop utilized the data from Study #2, as well as a variety of experiential training sessions, to focus on ways of recruiting parents, running meetings, working with medical facilities, counseling bereaved parents, and dealing with educational systems. (Ayers and Chesler, 1987).

Organizing Groups   On several occasions our staff met with local parents of children with cancer who wanted to start a group but did not know how, and helped them initiate and organize groups.

Educating or Challenging Medical Staffs   Some medical staffs resisted (overtly or covertly) the formation of local self-help groups of parents of children with cancer, or were reluctant to work with local groups that had formed. Our staff sometimes made presentations to medical staffs that informed them of the potential value of self-help groups. In addition, we sometimes helped local groups plan how to overcome such resistance (getting lists of parents of newly diagnosed children, getting access to hospital meeting rooms, presenting their needs/demands to hospital staff, being seen as a legitimate part of the coping process). Some groups asked our staff to help lead their challenges, or to join them in informing, influencing, or otherwise pressing for change in local staff policy and practice (see Figure 9.1). Sometimes this activity relied upon the action-research strategy of presenting data and findings; at other times it involved mediation or assistance in generating political or economic pressure rather than information.

Mediating Parent-Group/Staff or Institution Conflict   In some cases where local parent groups and local medical staffs or community organizations (or at times local affiliates of the American Cancer Society) were engaged in disputes that were difficult to resolve, our staff was asked to intervene to help establish dialogue and facilitate local problem-solving efforts. Problem-solving efforts involving parties of dramatically unequal power and resources are difficult, but are essential to staffs' abilities to adequately serve children and their families, and to families' (or groups') abilities to work effectively with medical institutions.

Disseminating Findings   The findings of these studies, as well as lessons from other relevant literature, have been disseminated to parents of children with cancer in both written and oral form. Articles describing these findings have appeared in CCCF publications and in other media. In addition, staff members have presented findings to various parent group meetings and conferences. Findings also have been published in journals and magazines normally read by those professional practitioners who are likely to work most closely with parents of children with cancer and with their self-help groups. In addition, staff members have been speakers and presenters at practitioners' meetings, have served on working committees of these associations that examined their policies and practices with regard to self-help groups, and have presented grand rounds at several local medical centers. Articles reporting findings from these studies also have appeared in a variety of scholarly journals and have been presented at meetings of scientific communities.

Influencing CCCF Policy   CCCF has made use of these findings in their own programs of providing support to local groups. Excerpts from this work have appeared in the Foundation's newsletters and in Foundation handbooks and guides (e.g., Nathanson, 1987) for local group leaders. We are pleased to publish this volume in order to continue that process.

Part 2

The Activities and Operations of Self-Help Groups: What the Bridges Look Like

In this section we present empirical findings related to an organizational-level analysis of self-help groups for parents of children with cancer.

In Chapter 4 we examine the activities and programs of the fifty groups in our comparative group sample. In addition to describing these activities, we discuss their relevance to the core themes of self-help discussed in Chapter 1 and the major stresses facing parents of children with cancer discussed in Chapter 2. Further, we analyze the occurrence of these activities in terms of certain of the groups' central features.

In Chapter 5 we examine the operating structures of the fifty groups. In addition to describing their organizational operations, we use features of their governance patterns and degrees of formalization to explore how operational styles and structures may be associated with particular activities and programs.

4

What Self-Help Groups Do

In this chapter we examine the activities and programs of self-help groups organized by and for families of children with cancer. Since self-help groups are formed and sustained in response to particular needs faced by members, we continue to ground this exploration of group activities in the needs and stresses of parents of children with cancer identified in Chapter 2. People facing different life crises, or people dealing with a common life crisis in fundamentally different ways, will be drawn to groups emphasizing different programs and activities, even within the general childhood cancer framework. From interviews, examinations of materials and records, and participant observations with over fifty groups across the nation, we illustrate in detail the major self-help group activities and programs. These are the activities that contribute to the magic of self-help groups for families of children with cancer.

Self-Help Groups as Responses to Stress and Need

Table 4.1 suggests the relationships between the five categories of stress typically faced by families of children with cancer (see Chapter 2) and the major categories of activities that occur in parent self-help groups. The *intellectual and informational stresses* that parents faced, combined with the need to comprehend the culture and jargon of the medical system, often led to group activities designed to provide information and education. The *practical or instrumental stresses* of childhood cancer forced parents to deal with the demands of treatment and hospital rules and regulations, often exacerbated by issues of transportation, childcare, household maintenance, and other logistic demands of everyday life. Self-help groups often responded by providing programs that delivered practical assistance and much-needed monetary or other

Table 4.1. Stress and self-help activities for parents of children with cancer

Category of stress	Self-Help group activities
Intellectual	*Information*
Confusion	Staff presentations
Ignorance of medical system	Handbooks
Ignorance about who the physicians are	Library of articles
	Newsletters
Ignorance about where things are in the hospital	Information-sharing among parents
	Education of the general public
Lack of clarity about how to explain the illness to others	Share experiential knowledge
Instrumental	*Practical*
Disorder and chaos at home	Collect and distribute funds for wigs, prostheses, parking
Financial pressures	Provide transportation
Lack of time and transportation	Arrange parent lodging
Need to monitor treatments	Improve local medical care
	Raise funds for research or added services
	Discuss coping skills
	Take collective action
Interpersonal	*Emotional and Social*
Needs of other family members	Identify with others in the same situation
Friends' needs and reactions	Meet new people
Relations with the medical staff	Find someone to talk with
Behaving in public as the parents of an ill child . . . stigma	Social events, parties
New social expectations	Share life experiences
Emotional	*Emotional*
Shock	Find professional counseling
Lack of sleep and nutrition	Share intimate feelings with people in the same situation
Feelings of defeat, anger, fear, powerlessness	Mutual support
Physical or psychosomatic reactions	
Existential	*Existential and Spiritual*
Confusion about why this happened to me	Talk about religious beliefs
Uncertainty about the future	Share the struggle
Uncertainty about God, fate, and a "just world"	

Source: Adapted from Chesler and Barbarin (1987, p. 214).

tangible resources. A third major set of stresses that parents faced centered on their *interpersonal relationships*—their social lives and connections to others in their families, neighborhoods, and workplaces. Self-help groups not only provided an arena for conversation about such relationships, but also offered parents opportunities to meet new people and to broaden their circle of friends and helpers. A fourth major source of stress, the *emotional trauma* of childhood cancer, often generated in parents a need for emotional and social support, and the need to cope with newly aroused, strong emotions. Most self-help groups provided structured as well as informal opportunities for parents to share their feelings, validate their emotional responses, and connect meaningfully with others "in the same boat." Finally, parents often faced the *existential stress* of making sense out of the childhood cancer experience, and of reconciling the diagnosis and treatment with their preexisting world view, orientation to the future, and life plans. Sometimes that reconciliation involved significant alterations of their world views and personal agendas. For some parents, only the experience of a child's terminal situation sparked such conversation, while for others the general stress of diagnosis and treatment led to such questioning and exploration. Although seldom the major focus of any self-help group, such emotional and often spiritual—sacred or secular—concerns commonly arose in the context of discussions of "Why did this happen to me?", "Where is a benevolent God when it comes to children's pain?", or "How do I wish to spend my time in the future?" Whether such exploration occurred between individuals or as part of focused group activity, it involved members seeking greater spiritual development or bonding.

What Did Groups Actually Do?

Table 4.2 lists the five major categories of activities undertaken by self-help groups of families of children with cancer, and the percentages of the fifty groups studied that reported conducting each activity. In addition, it indicates the priority that each of the fifty groups studied placed on each of these activities, as well as the frequency of their occurrence at group meetings. Table 4.2 indicates that the activity with the highest priority and greatest frequency across meetings of all groups was the provision of emotional support. The next most highly prioritized and frequent activity was information and education. Social and

Table 4.2. Major categories of activities in self-help group meetings (N = 50)

Activity category	Percentage of groups with this activity	Percentage of groups with 1st or 2nd priority for this activity	Percentage of groups frequently engaging in this activity (a lot or some)
Information and education programs	82	62	76
Emotional support programs*	72	94	90
Social and recreational events	84	22	68
Fund-raising programs	66	24	36
Making changes in the medical system	38	10	34

*Although only 72% of the groups reported emotional support programs, 94% reported such support as a high priority, and 90% reported it as occurring frequently. Thus, even in groups where emotional support was not a formally designed activity or program, it took place on at least an informal basis or as part of other programs, and was seen as the most important priority across all groups.

recreational events were third in terms of priority and frequency, while fund-raising and making changes in the medical care system were much less common. Of course, individual groups differed on these priorities and frequencies, but the overall priorities of emotional and informational agendas are quite clear. However, even these five major categories of activities did not exhaust the programs and events that occupied group members and meetings. Many groups also established one-on-one network and phone contacts among members outside of meetings (84%), visited hospitalized children and families (40%), and conducted organizational maintenance activities (58%).

Emotional Support/Help Programs

The provision of emotional support and help for parents in crisis lies at the heart of the self-help movement, and reports of this as the most important activity in groups of parents of children with cancer echo previous research.[1] Such activities were designed to help parents respond to the emotional stresses of childhood cancer, although they often addressed interpersonal and existential stresses as well. However, the kinds of emotional support provided, and the means of its provision, varied considerably throughout the groups we studied. For example, support sometimes involved a few parents talking with one another before, during, and after a group meeting. It also occurred during a relatively formal "rap" session, where parents took turns discussing their anxieties and responding caringly to one another. As several parents noted,

Just talking, this is the real purpose of the group, sharing and supporting.

The meeting is where parents can cry and discuss things that bother them.

At most meetings, in most groups, a common introductory activity included a "check-in" process. People often went around the room, stating their names and bringing others up to date on their child's status and progress, major events in their lives, and their major concerns or worries. This process signaled everyone as to who had what current needs, and who needed special support during the current session. At times, of course, the process stopped for a while, and someone who needed support and help got it right then and there—in the form of a conversation, a question, a sharing of a common experience or even a solution, a hug, or simply a knowing shake of the head and a smile.

If a professionally trained social worker or psychologist was leading the group, either on a temporary or permanent basis, the emotional support process often appeared quite similar to group counseling or therapy.[2] In some instances, self-help groups led by social workers and nurses, especially those that met in and were closely tied to particular medical centers, struggled with problems related to lay versus professional control. These struggles centered on the distinctions presented in Table 1.1 (Chapter 1), and included alternative definitions of parents' needs, bases of leadership power and knowledge, kinds of programs and services provided, and autonomy from the medical system.[3] Self-help groups with parent leaders usually were oriented less to therapy or counseling, and more to informal sharing and the expression of mutual concern and support. This may, of course, have been "therapeutic" for participants, but did not constitute professional "therapy." The overwhelming majority of parents of children with cancer, as verified in most of the literature on this topic (Adams, 1979; Chesler and Barbarin, 1987), are not psychologically disturbed or suffering from pathology, and do not need psychological "treatment" or "therapy." They are relatively normal parents and families experiencing tremendous emotional stress and trauma; as such, they do require caring and loving social support.

An example of a parent group that focused almost all of its energy on informal emotional support was located in a small city in the northeastern United States. Here, four mothers of children with cancer met once every two weeks for several hours for coffee, cake, and conversation. They met in a restaurant, in order to get some time away from their households and children. They often cried and held each other while they talked. They met at four o'clock in the afternoon, in the back of the restaurant, partly to avoid the noise and stares of the noon lunch crowd, which had made them uncomfortable about crying and touching. They talked about their children, about the treatments their children were undergoing, about their husbands, about their own time and energy, about their fears, and about their hopes. This group, which met regularly for over a year, had no formal charter or by-laws, no money, no office, and no formal agenda. What they did have on a regular basis— and it was all they needed—was their mutual caring and commitment to one another. The members also had access to a medical social worker, if and when anyone needed her.

Some groups created subgroups at meetings, in order to deal with especially potent or sensitive emotional issues. A common example involved occasional separations of men and women, mothers and fathers, in order to discuss their unique concerns apart from their spouses. For instance, in one large midwestern group, a special meeting was held to focus on "spousal issues." After a common introduction, the men/fathers were asked to meet in one room and the women/mothers in another. Parent leaders in each room asked those gathered to think about and share their problems and experiences in relating to their spouses. The men talked about their physical and emotional pain and their difficulty in expressing their feelings to their wives. They also directed significant attention to issues of sexuality and sexual interaction with their wives: "How often should we?" "We don't anymore; both of us are drained." "How can I think of pleasure when our child is so sick?" "She never wants to anymore." The women talked about their desire for more feeling-based conversations with their husbands and worried that their husbands kept so much of their pain inside. They also had almost exactly the same conversation and questions about their sexuality and sexual interactions with their spouses as did the men. When the two subgroups reassembled, they shared substantial portions of their discussions, but only referred obliquely to the fact that, in both groups, a great deal of attention and energy had been focused on sexual matters. No one wished to raise these issues in a cross-gender public session, where they could be identified with particular spouses. On the other hand, much personal material had been shared and made accessible to everyone attending, perhaps to be dealt with in later, more private conversations within couples.

Emotional support for parents and families did not take place only in specially designed sharing sessions; it often occurred within the context of other group activities. For example, fund-raising often served more than one purpose; in addition to raising money for group activities, or for expanded hospital or social services, self-help group fund-raising efforts involved parents working closely with one another on a common agenda. While parent members were planning fund-raising projects and campaigns together, they were also sharing feelings and concerns about other matters. A similar dynamic usually occurred in social or recreational events, such as parties, dances, or "evenings out." Whatever else was occurring, and whatever the manifest or announced agenda of such events, parents constantly sought each other out and engaged in supportive and meaningful conversations about themselves and their children.

In addition to the personal contacts and interaction at group meetings, group newsletters provided another means for parents to support one another and their children. For instance, Figure 4.1 presents a page from the newsletter of the Candlelighters of Columbia, Missouri. By defining support, the Columbia group advertised their own activities and suggested some coping strategies that readers—whether or not they were members and attended meetings—could find helpful.

Information and Education Programs

Most groups shared information with their members and provided some formal educational programs, another programmatic priority echoed in the existing literature on self-help groups for parents of children with cancer.[4] Typically, families of children newly diagnosed with cancer sought information as a way of relieving the intellectual stresses discussed earlier. Seldom were their needs met fully by the formal medical system, and disagreements about the amount and timing of medical

Figure 4.1. Excerpt on support from a self-help group newsletter (Reprinted from Candlelighters of Columbia, Missouri)

SUPPORT

We can help.

What is a support group?

SUPPORT, v. 1. keep from falling; hold up 2. give strength or courage to; help: hope supports us in trouble 3. assist or protect in combat 4. put up with; bear, endure 5. assist, aid, help 6. person or thing that supports; prop.

The above definition comes from the dictionary, but fits what the support group has become to its members. Members said the group has helped them in these ways.
1. Provides a setting to discuss scary or sad issues.
2. Facilitates positive coping mechanisms.
   A. Male/female relationship (It's okay to leave the kids and go out together).
   B. Okay to feel (be) angry. Ways to handle anger and resentment.
3. Provides a safe outlet to ventilate fears, and anxieties with others who "really" understand.
4. Provides a feeling of an extended family. Members call each other between meetings and have fun and social activities together. Some exchange babysitting.
5. Provides friendships which are maintained through clinic and makes this time emotionally easier to bear.
6. Enhances insight into self, patterns of communication and relating to others.
7. Provides a support network when a child dies.

---

information that should be shared with parents have often been points of conflict between the medical staff and many individual parents or self-help groups. Group members often argued that more adequate information helps lower parents' level of anxiety, helps them care for their children at home, and helps them be better prepared to make difficult treatment choices. Additionally, information that can be shared with friends and family members may make it more possible for the extended family to be involved rather than isolated from the coping process, and to understand and monitor medical practice, and thus provide added support to overloaded parents. Some staff members agreed that parents should be provided with a lot of information, while others disagreed.

Of course, not all parents of ill children wished for a great deal of information, and finding the appropriate level of detail to be shared was not an easy task for members of the medical staff or for group leaders. Given variations among parents on this issue, as well as occasional disagreements between parents and the medical system, it often fell to self-help groups to fill the gaps in the information some parents felt they wanted and needed. One format for providing information to parents involved inviting a medical or social service professional to speak to the group; following are some common topics that staff members were asked to address in various groups:

- Recent advances in treatment
- The effects of chemotherapy and radiation
- Late effects of therapy on survivors
- Nutrition for the child with decreased appetite
- Bone marrow transplants
- Reintegrating the child with cancer into the school
- Coping with childhood cancer
- Keeping the family together
- Dealing with stress
- Problems with siblings
- Insurance
- Coping with death

Several parent group leaders also indicated that outside speakers, especially local medical and psychosocial experts, were good drawing cards for their group, and that attendance was usually greater for such meetings. Some used such events to help recruit new members and to interest staff members in working with the group. In a number of situations, videotapes, movies, slides, or other media accompanied such lectures. In addition, many groups had their own libraries of books and materials for parents seeking information, or had access to special libraries for parents in the hospital or clinic.

In addition to invited medical experts and library materials, some groups used their own members as experts to educate others. Figure 4.2, from the newsletter of the Cincinnati self-help group, describes such a panel presentation of "experiential experts" (Borkman, 1990)—in this case, children with cancer themselves. Obviously, this sort of panel discussion, followed by a general and open discussion, combined both informational and emotional support.

Group newsletters were also a good way to provide information to parents. Most group newsletters featured articles providing general in-

Figure 4.2. Excerpt on programs from a self-help group newsletter

---

THE COPE TORCH

BULLETIN OF THE CINCINNATI ONCOLOGY PARENT ENDEAVOR

July, 1982. Vol. 6, No. 7

REGULAR COPE JULY MEETING***
DATE: July 21, 1982
LOCATION: Children's Convalescent Hospital
                 Pavilion Building, Room 115
PROGRAM: A PANEL OF YOUNG PEOPLE *** A PANEL OF PATIENTS

The July COPE meeting is very honored to present a program that has never been offered before. The program for the evening will feature a panel discussion composed of children, ages from pre-teen to late-teen all of whom have cancer or leukemia. The panel will discuss different aspects of the disease, treatment and their feelings. At the conclusion of the panel you will have the chance to ask questions.

Have you ever had questions that you wanted to ask your own child about his illness or about the way he feels about life? Have you ever wondered what a child with cancer fears the most? This will be your chance to think of those questions and listen to the panel members answer them.

The young people who are going to participate on this panel are very special. They have agreed to face our group and tell us how they feel about topics such as these. If you are hesitant to really speak to your child and question, this is your chance to hear the truth. Perhaps this can be the most important COPE meeting that you could ever attend. I just wonder if the children will have any questions for the parents.

Plan on attending this meeting. Remember July 21st at 7:30 p.m.

---

formation on the above topics relevant to childhood cancer, sometimes written by medical professionals and sometimes by parents themselves. "Dear Dr." columns, parent hotlines, and original stories and poems were all common. The Candlelighters Foundation's *Quarterly Newsletter* typically reprinted articles from local newsletters, and gave permission to local groups to reprint its articles, thus multiplying access to informational resources for groups throughout the nation. Several large, well-established, and well-funded groups created "parent handbooks."[5]

These looseleaf collections were created in conjunction with local medical staffs and were intended to orient parents of newly diagnosed children to their situation and its possibilities. Handbooks typically included information about the diseases of childhood cancer and their treatment, a map and directions to the hospital and to local eating and lodging establishments for the out-of-towner, a list of names and addresses of important people in the medical system and the parent community, coping tips, and information about the self-help group itself.

Social and Recreational Programs

Groups often sponsored social and recreational events that provided families with opportunities to meet, talk with, and support one another in informal settings. Families gathered for these parties, potlucks, or celebrations in a relaxed atmosphere, somewhat removed from the stress and gravity of their everyday lives, yet surrounded by others who were experiencing similar medical and social stresses and altered realities. One of the underlying purposes of these social events was to provide parents of children with cancer with a new circle of friends, and to help overcome their feelings of loneliness, isolation from friends, and social strangeness or awkwardness. These activities clearly were designed to address the interpersonal stresses identified in Table 4.1. They are less intense activities than intimate emotional support sessions, but it was clear that emotional support did occur in such social settings as well.

Some groups organized relatively formal social events, such as Christmas or holiday parties, Easter egg hunts, summer picnics, and family outings, potlucks, and barbeques. For instance, a parent support group in a midwestern city organized a regular night for fathers of children with cancer to attend a major league baseball game together. In another city, the group organized a "mom's nite out": sixteen mothers traveled to a downtown restaurant for a spaghetti dinner—and much talk. These events sometimes drew a large attendance, and some parents who came to these relaxed and "fun" outings never showed up at other types of activities. On the other hand, they also were excellent recruiting arenas for new members and opportunities for the group to share information about its activities with a wide audience. Parties and picnics, especially, were occasions for promoting informal interaction between parents and the hospital or clinic staff, since these practitioners usually were invited and often brought their own families.

In addition to formally organized events, many groups encouraged parents to gather with one another informally. This took the form of one-on-one parent visits, multifamily potluck dinners, birthday parties, trips to zoos or amusement parks, and camping trips. Indeed, some parents of children with cancer reported that the only people with whom they could really relax were other parents of children with cancer. As two parents said:

When we laugh a lot our friends who do not have children with cancer wonder what we have to laugh about. They look at us as if we are strange. But with other parents of children with cancer we can laugh and cry all we want. We all know we have to in order to survive.

I love a party! There's nothing more satisfying than seeing someone forget their troubles for a moment, and as a result draw some strength from that moment with which to face another day.

In the context of meeting parents whose children had a similar diagnosis, in the midst of attending clinic sessions and sitting in waiting rooms together, sharing deeply felt concerns, many parents became close friends with others in the group. Sometimes these new friendships became lifelong ventures, outlasting the treatment process, the cancer, or even the child. In one midwestern town, for example, four couples continued to get together once a year for dinner for ten years, despite the fact that all their children were diagnosed with cancer over fifteen years ago. In their joint attempt to create and sustain a local self-help group and to support each other through difficult times, these four couples became "emotionally bonded" to one another; they cared deeply about one another and about their children's progress. Even though the children with cancer of three of these four families died several years ago, they all still gather to share stories about their living children, their own lives, and their memories of their children with cancer.

Fund-raising Programs

While almost all groups did some type of programming for emotional support, information and education, and social activities, fund-raising was less common. Only six groups reported fund-raising as a first or second priority, but these groups did raise a substantial amount of funds—for their own operations, to support their own or the treatment center's services for families of children with cancer, or to support research into the medical treatment for childhood cancer. Most groups, however, raised only small amounts of money, just enough to support mailings and other minimal demands on their own organizations. Some groups eschewed fund-raising completely.

Groups that did engage in major fund-raising usually did so as a means of responding to some of the practical burdens associated with childhood cancer. Several studies have documented the substantial "incidental" and nonreimbursable costs of dealing with childhood cancer (Lansky et al., 1979). By providing families with even small amounts of funds, these group programs were able to make a difference. For instance, the Las Vegas and Houston parent groups provided parents in need with funds for local transportation services, for special transportation to major treatment centers, for medicine for uninsured families, for wigs and prostheses for children, for in-hospital televisions, and for emergency household needs. Even families whose income levels made such added resources practically unnecessary appreciated the "community giving process" behind them.

A few groups were also very active in raising substantial amounts of money to support local hospitals' research efforts in childhood cancer. For instance, a group in Detroit regularly provided funds to support research conducted by staff members at Detroit Children's Hospital. This was not a singular occurrence; groups played a similar role in Buffalo and Indianapolis. Other groups that raised considerable funds used them for other purposes. For example, a parent support group in the northeast was faced with what they felt was a lack of adequate social work services for their children, and the unwillingness of their local hospital to allocate resources for that purpose. They raised sufficient money to support half the salary of a social worker for two years, and offered those funds to the hospital on the condition that the hospital would support the other half of the position, and would continue to fund it full-time thereafter. The group was successful in this negotiation. Through similar efforts, other groups were able to support expansion of the social work, child life, and outreach staffs serving their children.

The variety of uses to which funds were put was expressed in the words of several parents active in different groups' fund-raising activities:

We helped families out on a personal level: bought tires for a poor family, bought a sofa bed for a family that lost a child and then the mother developed cancer, distributed Christmas baskets.

Funds just for organizational needs. Money goes for reading materials, fees for speakers, parties, newsletters and group activities.

Our main purpose is funding for research and equipment.

We raise money to pay a nurse practitioner's salary.

The sources of funds raised by local self-help groups were numerous. A few local groups created relationships with major corporate sponsors and foundations, or recruited star athletes or entertainers to spearhead public fund-raising efforts. Others participated in United Way or similar municipal campaigns, or received funds from the American Cancer Society's local affiliates. Still others sold cookbooks, T-shirts and candy, and conducted bowl-a-thons, pizza parties, charity fairs, craft sales, dances, raffles, and garage sales. Some groups assessed membership dues and solicited memorial donations in the names of children who had died or who had successfully completed treatment. As one parent noted,

We do a lot of fund-raising. We do a Skate for Life, a New Year's Eve dance, a nut sale, an annual dinner dance, a craft bazaar, T-shirt and sweat-shirt sales, Tupperware parties and a Race for Life.

However, not all groups that tried to raise funds were successful at it, according to another parent:

We tried fund-raising, but the group was so spread out it was unsuccessful. Members did not have enough time. We raise money to keep going from member dues.

Indeed, in some cases, decisions about whether or not to engage in fund-raising, or at what level and for what purposes, spurred major internal debates within parent self-help groups. Reflecting upon one such debate in a group located in a small midwestern city, a parent who was heavily commited to the group's original focus on emotional support sessions said,

Some people are real worried about raising money. But I don't feel that that's the real thing of the group. Money is the root of all evil. That is the only time when we have problems in our group, when it comes to money. Parents have enough on their minds . . . they don't need to be selling tickets.

It was not uncommon for groups that focused heavily on fund-raising to experience substantial conflict in the process. In some cases, this was due to internal conflict over how funds should be spent. In other cases, however, the conflict was caused by the groups' relationships with powerful external agencies—hospitals, the American Cancer Society, and local sponsors of Ronald McDonald Houses. Sometimes these agencies felt groups' fund-raising efforts would compete with their own. As a result, group members sometimes felt used and manipulated by these agencies, even when they supported their local goals and helped raise funds for their causes. Strained relationships occurred within parent groups when certain group members were selected and publicized by these agencies as "spokespersons." In fact, more than one local group reported that it actually or nearly fell apart from the internal conflict associated with "successful" fund-raising programs.

Whether the fund-raising efforts of groups were large or small, the result of a group consensus or a cause of internal conflict, fund-raising seldom had a singular focus and impact. To the extent that it was planned and conducted in common, it was at least temporarily a bonding and support activity, over and above the generation of funds. Thus, fund-raising was one more way in which parents hoped to contribute to the improvement of their children's chances of survival, and to the quality of their children's and their own lives. It also was a way of contributing to the lives of others who were less fortunate. Above all, it was one more example of an active role that parents played in their own struggle with the stresses of this disease.

Making Changes in the Medical System

Although most parents of children with cancer have expressed general satisfaction with the medical care their children received (Barbarin and Chesler, 1985; Chesler and Barbarin, 1984b), many wanted to see changes and improvements in the form and nature of care. Such apparently contradictory views were not necessarily contradictory; they reflected the simultaneous existence of satisfaction and of a desire for improvement. Similarly, many self-help groups reported that they had established good working relations with the medical care system, even when they actively sought to make changes in this system.

Individual involvement in change-related activities may have been an expression of parents' desires to exercise control over this important part of their lives—a part that they often felt was spinning out of control. As one parent said,

It's important to feel needed and productive outside of the life and death of our own child's care and support. *If one can't change science*—and is therefore feeling useless in terms of the outcome of the disease—one must be able to feel important and effective in some other concrete manner.

Such activities also spoke clearly to parents' instrumental or practical need to get what they considered to be more appropriate treatment. But many parents lacked the energy to maintain active engagement; others feared retaliation by the staff for criticism or intrusion onto their "turf." In such endeavors, the collective structure and sometimes autonomous nature of the group served to both encourage and protect individual parents. As one parent noted,

We do not discuss hospital changes we would like to see in front of the social worker in the group.

Although some groups obviously felt the need to talk about changes privately, the professional staff sometimes acted as public and trusted intermediaries between the group and other hospital staff members.[6]

One target of self-help groups' social action or efforts for change was the nature of medical practice itself. As one parent noted,

Our group's job is to educate the hospital staff as to the needs of parents.

Sometimes more than education was required, and significant influence or pressure had to be brought to bear. In many settings, parent groups called special meetings to inform the staff of parent complaints, including a session at a midwestern treatment center where the parent group took the lead in pressing the hospital to move all the pediatric oncology patients into a separate wing. The Portland, Oregon, group pursued such issues by drawing wide community attention to them. In a city with several treatment centers, the local parent self-help group published a monthly newsletter; each month they *named* an outstandingly good practitioner and *described* an outstandingly bad practice or medical occurrence. They did not name the perpetrator of the unfortunate event, nor the institution at which it occurred, but simply described what happened. Their purpose, of course, was to alert staffs more fully to parents' needs and to the staff's responsibility to be aware of and to police peer practices. Figure 4.3 presents their guidelines for these awards.

Figure 4.3. Excerpt from a self-help group newsletter (from the Portland Candlelighters Group)

Guidelines for the Portland Candlelighters Compassionate Care Award

1. The award is to be made to an individual involved with the care of children who have cancer.
2. The individual who receives the award works in a medical setting or has a medically related job.
3. The majority of parents at Candlelighter regular meeting(s) vote to award this individual the Candlelighter *Compassionate Care Award* for exceptional qualities of skill, compassion, and empathy.
4. The local Candlelighter parents can provide three reasons specifically why this individual is deserving of the award and submit them to the Newsletter editor by deadline.
5. Local groups will take turns presenting this award in their area so that only one group is presenting the award in any one month.

Guidelines for Portland Candlelighters Bogie Situation Award

1. The *Candlelighters Bogie Situation Award* will be made in reference to a situation and not a specific individual.
2. Every attempt should be made to eliminate any identifying information with regards to a specific individual or faculty.
3. Agreement by Parent-Members on the appropriateness of this selection should be evidenced by a vote taken at a regular meeting.
4. Suggestion(s) for improving the situation should be included. If possible, consult appropriate professionals for their advice.
5. The Bogie Award, with its suggested remedy, should be written up and submitted to the President or other individual appointed by the Board or President for that purpose. This should be done in plenty of time—for example two weeks before the Newsletter deadline of the month that it is to appear.

Groups' efforts to alter the nature of medical social services included, as noted earlier, efforts to increase the quantity and quality of social work, child life, health education, and recreational services. In a few institutions, moreover, leaders of parent groups, or parent advocates, have been accepted as more or less full members of the medical staff, where they are better able to present parental needs directly (Pitel et al., 1985). In some cases, the existence of a self-help group, in and of itself, requires some changes in social service practice. For instance, an active and successful group must gain continuing access to the lists of names of parents of newly diagnosed children. For many centers, making such lists available, or gaining the permission of a parent to pass on his or her name to the group leader, necessitated a shift in professional practice. Other hospitals, to this day, have refused to share such information. In the name of protecting the rights of individual parents, these institutions have made it more difficult for parents to gain the potential benefits and options for growth available in a self-help group. In attempts to circumvent overt conflict and yet gain access to parents of newly diagnosed children, some parent groups have posted members in clinic sessions, or on wards, and engaged the parents they met there in supportive conversations and recruitment efforts.

A third focus of group efforts for change centered on the practical resources available from the caregiving system. For example, some groups sought to improve hospital food for children, sleeping-in or living-in arrangements for the parents of very young children, and free parking for parents of children hospitalized for long periods of time.

In addition to trying to make changes in the medical care system, some self-help groups actively attempted to influence the health and life insurance industry and their state and federal governmental agencies. Gaining low-cost, reliable insurance for children living with—and beyond—childhood cancer has become a serious societal problem, especially since the number of survivors of childhood cancer has increased so substantially. Information sessions, lobbying efforts, and other means of advocacy have been used by various groups and their representatives. Advice on lobbying from the national office of the Candlelighters Childhood Cancer Foundation is presented in Figure 4.4.

Figure 4.4. Self-help groups working for change (from Nathanson, 1976, pp. 37–38)

CHANGING THE SYSTEM

Potential problems

Activism can be a source of danger for the group. If the group is sponsored, even in part, by a treatment center, support agency, or larger organization, the goal may not be shared or as highly valued by the sponsor.

Before a program of pressure and activism is developed, a group should examine if it will jeopardize a sponsorship or affect funding or referrals. Weigh the risks/benefits carefully. It may be that the group will decide to pursue its goals, and that's fine. But the decision should be made with an awareness of what the costs may be. If sponsorship may be lost, the group must be prepared to make up its losses.

Lobbying

Lobbying government to produce change requires particular techniques. General handbooks on lobbying are available from organizations such as the League of Women Voters and Common Cause. A useful, effective, and essential resource for parent groups is:

How to Organize an Effective Parent Group and Move Bureaucracies:
For Parents of Handicapped Children and their Helpers
Co-ordinating Council for Handicapped Children
220 S. State Street, Room 412, Chicago, IL 60604

Its chapter on "Making Your Group an Action Group" has sections on planning action and on strategies for organizing registration drives, marches, rallies, boycotts, teach-ins, camp-ins, public hearings, and picketing. The chapter, "Moving Bureaucracies," discusses negotiation tactics, ways of staying informed on legislative action, lobbying campaigns, strategies to get a bill passed or defeated, and support publicity in every form of media.

Be sure to know how lobbying may affect the group's tax-exempt status. . . . A separate lobbying group may be needed to protect the group's tax-exempt status. Check with a tax lawyer. Try to find a volunteer attorney through the group's membership, the treatment center, community legal aid, or pro bono programs run by local law firms or bar associations. A national organization or agency may be able to advise the group on this. Also get advice before the group supports the election of any official. Such support may also be prohibited if the group has tax-exempt status.

Personal contact is the most powerful way to use influence. Try to have members visit legislators. Another way to use influence is by mounting letter-writing campaigns. Because a letter requires some personal effort, it conveys a greater sense of sincerity than a telephone call or telegram. (Telegrams, particularly the low cost "Public Opinion" telegrams, may be effective when time is too short for a letter-writing campaign.)

(figure continued on following page)

93

Figure 4.4. Self-help groups working for change (from Nathanson, 1976, pp. 37–38) (*continued*)

Legislators do not read each letter themselves, but they do pay attention to the most thoughtful, legislation-oriented ones from friends, important local citizens, major associations, and voters in their district. And, they do count the numbers of pros and cons they receive. Letters are most effective when they:

Are addressed to the legislator's office, not home;

Include the writer's full name, address, and phone number;

Include the name and number of any pending legislation about which the group is concerned;

State the issue clearly and briefly in only one page;

Use the writer's own words;

Give specific personal examples of how the legislation affects the writer, the group, and the community;

Use facts from local researchers, physicians, and educators;

All facts are verified and accurate;

The writer keeps a copy for future reference;

The writer thanks any legislators who vote to support the group's position.

The group should know its legislators. Find out which of them have had personal experience within the group's children's condition or a related experience. This personally shared experience could be of value in identifying an ally.

Practical Assistance

Faced with the often overwhelming time and energy demands of childhood cancer, many self-help groups tried to provide families with practical or instrumental assistance. Some of this assistance came in the form of financial aid, as discussed previously. In addition to financial support, however, other forms of practical assistance were available through groups' efforts to provide personal services such as "respite care," visitation programs for hospitalized children, a day at Disney World for the terminally ill child and family, special housing arrangements for families traveling long distances for treatment, blood donor drives or bone marrow donor searches for children in need, and wig banks and prosthesis exchange systems. Several parents reported their pleasure in taking part in such practically helpful programs:

I usually helped with food. Being a mother of a large family, I get a lot of practice. I'm helping to support others the way we were helped. Some nice friends come from it.

I feel that system getting better for other families; a sense of accomplishment—*housing* a family. That's *everybody's right*—a place to live no matter *what's* happened!

Several groups located in large cities, or near major children's cancer treatment centers, successfully led drives to fund and build "homes away from home" for families. When a family had to travel long distances for repeated or extended hospitalizations, the provision of local housing at minimal cost was a great advantage. In some cities, local McDonald franchises joined hands to help groups build Ronald McDonald Houses: 10, 20, or 30 rooms or apartments in a single building have been made available at minimal cost to families of seriously and chronically ill children. With washer and dryer facilities and kitchens, these houses provided important practical assistance to families. Given opportunities to meet and talk with other families of seriously ill children, parents in these houses shared information with one another and also generated emotional and social support.

Another form of practical assistance to children and their families was a summer camp or a one- or two-week recreational experience with other children with cancer or their families. In these settings, children with cancer—and sometimes their siblings, parents, or entire family—got away and experienced the joys of camping generally available to physically healthy children and their families. With adequate medical supervision, youngsters with cancer experimented with swimming, horseback riding, "rough play," and other forms of physical recreation that they might otherwise have missed out on. They wore their wigs or took them off, showed their amputated limbs or wore prostheses, carried around their IV lines and took their pills, safe in the company of many other children with similar disabilities or temporary disfigurements. Typically, local treatment centers provided on-the-spot medical and nursing care, and social workers and older survivors of cancer often were available as counselors and discussion leaders at these camps.

Outreach to the Community

A few self-help groups were concerned with raising public consciousness with regard to childhood cancer. Part of their agenda was to make more people aware of the reality of this illness and of the societal and public resources necessary to prevent and treat it. Another concern was to inform the public of the essential normality of children with cancer, of their increasing likelihood of survival and, thus, of their ability to live normally in the community and society. Groups working on this agenda usually established and published the existence of a "speakers' bureau" of members available to make public presentations. Other outreach activities took the form of public educational campaigns, including radio and TV spots.

Some parent self-help groups took the lead to educate educators about the needs and realities of children with cancer, and to ease the reentry of these children into their schools (Barbarin and Chesler, 1983). Figure 4.5 provides an example of a workshop a self-help group sponsored for educators and parents.[7] Although a few hospitals employed trained health educators or other staff members to link families to the local school system, and to help prepare local educators to work with children with cancer, many did not. Moreover, individual parents often found it difficult to accomplish this linking and educational task by

Figure 4.5. Excerpt on a teachers' workshop from a self-help group newsletter (Reprinted from *Chicagoland Candlelighters Newsletter,* 1981 [April])

REPORT ON TEACHERS' WORKSHOP, MARCH 14

In the schools we must look upon students with cancer as children who are LIVING with a chronic disease, not dying of a terminal illness. This was the positive approach stressed during the March 14 workshop "The School Age Child With Cancer," sponsored by the Illinois Cancer Council.

Joan Davis represented the CHICAGOLAND CANDLELIGHTERS at the well-attended workshop. In her dual role as parent and former high school teacher, Joan was able to offer comments from both perspectives.

After an encouraging presentation by Dr. Elaine Morgan on recent advances in childhood cancer treatment, participants heard social worker Cathy Erickson speak on school re-entry and possible problems a student, teacher, classmates or family might experience.

After lunch Joan gave a short presentation on CHICAGOLAND CANDLELIGHTERS, followed by Social Worker Mary Kay Foley's presentation on school adjustment. Many thoughtful questions were raised, evidencing the concern and helpfulness of the teachers present. Flexibility was stressed for dealing with a student with cancer. Perhaps most important, close communication among school, family and medical personnel was emphasized—something we parents can certainly assist in.

---

themselves; some felt uncomfortable and vulnerable asking for "special privileges." In the context of organized self-help group activity, however, these issues could be pursued and seen in a collective rather than individual context, and often led to new school policies and programs. Thus, educational events organized by local groups not only informed parents, teachers, and principals of their options for responding to children with cancer, they also dealt with some of the practical problems of children's transitions from hospital or home to school that occupied many parents' energies.

Personal Visitation Programs and Networks

Most self-help groups tried to ensure that members stayed in contact with one another outside of group meetings. In addition, many sought to make and sustain contact with parents who, for whatever reason (preference, distance, energy, life situation), did not attend group meetings on a regular basis. Visitation programs often took the form of especially committed parents taking the time to call or visit other parents, either at their homes or in the hospital. A few groups, in fact, developed specialized training programs to prepare parents to fill these roles with skill and insight (Bogue and Chesney, 1987). In some treatment centers, social workers helped train parents for these roles, and further legitimized their efforts within the medical system and the community. One parent reported on her group's visitation training program:

Our parent training program enables us to provide support for others. A professionally run six-week session certifies parents as helpers to aid others to open up their feelings.

A California-based group established a "duty roster," and made sure that parents continually were in the hospital to "walk the wards" and stop in at outpatient clinic sessions to meet other parents, especially parents of newly diagnosed children, and to offer them conversation, support, and assistance. In one treatment center, such support was complemented by coffee, juice, and doughnuts—one more way parents tried to ease the burden of long waiting periods and loneliness in clinic waiting rooms. Such activity also aided the group's recruitment efforts.

Other groups developed parent outreach programs that involved personal visits to the homes of families of children with cancer. This was an especially effective technique when children were being treated on an outpatient basis but were too ill to attend school, or when, for a variety of reasons (e.g., other small children at home), parents were homebound. In one group, veteran parents were able to spend several days and nights in the home of a family whose child was terminally ill and had elected to die at home. This "death watch" provided both practical and emotional support for the family, as visiting parents were able to help care for the child, do cooking and shopping chores, help find nursing care, and provide constant love and companionship to the dying child and his parents.

Telephone networks were another way in which some groups helped parents make and maintain contact with one another on a regular basis. This was an especially important program in areas of the nation where parents were separated from each other and from local treatment centers by long distances. For example, a self-help group in rural Texas used an active phone network to substitute for regular group meetings. Once a month designated members called one another to ask about their own and their child's health. A formal "telephone tree" insured that everyone concerned received a call, but that no single member was burdened with calling many members. Several times a year many of these parents also met each other personally at hospital events, and renewed the face-to-face contacts made so difficult by distance.

Business Meetings—Operating the Self-Help Group

An activity seldom reported or discussed as a regular group program, but which was essential and common nevertheless, involved ensuring the smooth operation of the local self-help group itself. The necessity of planning for the group's operations included solving leadership problems, deciding whether to organize more or less formally (e.g., establish by-laws and committees), and managing the group's relationship with the hospital and other agencies. Formal discussions of these issues, as well as committee reports, sometimes coexisted with other activities, such as emotional support and sharing sessions, and information and education programs, but they sometimes competed for time and space. Parents who attended meetings primarily to share their feelings or gain information often became disenchanted with a group that spent considerable time on committee reports and other business and vice versa.[8]

How Are Core Processes of Self-Help Groups Realized in These Activities?

It is not accidental that the above activities were common in self-help groups for families of children with cancer. Indeed, we suggested earlier (Table 4.1) that the parental stresses of childhood cancer required groups to conduct activities and programs that were responsive to these specific stresses and consequent needs. In addition to these connections, examination of some of the core elements of self-help groups suggested other factors and processes at work. While we explore these issues in more detail in later chapters, as "outcomes" or "benefits" of self-help group participation, we can identify here how some of the core social processes in self-help groups (identified in Chapter 1) might have been present in these activities. Table 4.3 describes some potential connections between the five sets of stresses of childhood cancer,

Table 4.3. Stresses, self-help group themes, and activities

Stresses/Needs	Core self-help themes: "The magic"	Self-help group activities
Intellectual	Experiential knowledge Coping skills	Information and education Public outreach Emotional sharing sessions

Instrumental	Experiential knowledge
	Shared life experiences
	Coping skills to buffer stress
	Help others
	Collective action
		Fund-raising and financial
		  assistance
		Making changes
		Educational program for the
		  public

Interpersonal	Shared life experiences Support and affirmation Collective action	Social and recreational events Personal visitations
Emotional	Shared life experiences Identity and community Support and affirmation Coping skills	Emotional sharing sessions Personal visitations
Existential	Shared life experiences Support and affirmation	Making changes Emotional sharing sessions

the core elements of most self-help groups, and some of the self-help activities described in this chapter.

In attempting to cope with the experience of childhood cancer, many parents discovered that they had to find, create, or adopt a new social identity that included their role as a person coping with emotional trauma and potential tragedy or potential recovery. The reality of their child's illness and of their new obligations and life paths was often so great that it could not be ignored even in casual social settings. It came up whenever they were asked about their children or family. In self-help groups, parents met and shared their life experiences with others who had struggled with this problem of identity formation and public presentation. In group rap sessions and networking activities they often found role models and examples of behavioral options they could pursue. Moreover, as active group members, some parents took on this new identity as a parent of a child with cancer quite vigorously and acted upon it in public educational sessions and visitation activities.[9]

In elaborating on group rap sessions and discussions, we have already referred to the ways in which sharing life experiences and crises may create new social networks and emotional bonding among parents. As parents who were strangers found themselves in a new and threatening—but common—reality, they communicated with one another on an intimate level; they also found new friends—friends who understood immediately and fully many of the new dimensions of their lives. As groups attempted to deal with the chronic nature of childhood cancer, such intimacy needed to be sustained over time. Some parents became quite close to their new friends, joining them in celebrations of recovery, in bedside watches at times of serious illness, in discussions of treatment options and risks, and in sharing childrearing or respite care opportunities.

Moreover, as parents shared their feelings and ideas and engaged in peer counseling with one another, they exchanged information about the illness and about coping responses—strategies for handling the practical and emotional aspects of the illness. In so doing, they gave and received help simultaneously.[10] It was often potentially therapeutic, even healing, for parents to learn that despite scarce resources, drained energies, and worries, they had been able to help others who were enduring a similar crisis. The ability to help oneself or others was based, in part, upon acquisition of a great deal of new information—about medical terms and treatments, about bodily functions and reactions, about psychosocial stresses and coping strategies, about the particular hospital and its staff and procedures. Some of this knowledge was available from the medical and psychosocial staff; some of it came only (or primarily) from parents whose wisdom was derived from their own experience. Parents were often their child's single most constant caregiver, since doctors and nurses necessarily rotated. The experiential knowledge parents gained was a crucial resource for meeting the challenges of caring for their ill child and for managing their own and their families' lives.

The decision to become involved in a self-help group represented in part a parental decision to become active in their own child's care. Far beyond the role of being a "good treatment recipient," active involvement in the reestablishment of some degree of control over one's own and one's family life was active and potentially empowering behavior. It also promoted involvement in other people's lives and in the organized medical system. For parents who took leadership roles in these groups, a particular form of voluntary association, additional opportunities arose to learn new skills in social and political organizing. This was especially true when the group attempted to act on parents' behalf in interactions with the medical system or public community agencies.

Which Groups Did What?

Not all groups engaged in all of the activities categorized in Tables 4.1 and 4.2 and discussed in this chapter. For instance, 40% of self-help groups in the fifty-group study offered only from one to four of the following sets of activities; 60% of the groups offered five or more of these activities:

- Information and education programs
- Emotional support sessions
- Business meetings
- Substantial fund-raising
- Social and recreational events
- Making changes in the medical system
- Visiting in the hospital
- Parent networking activities

Moreover, groups that offered some of these activities were more or less likely to offer certain others as well. For example, groups that spent more time conducting organizational business were significantly more likely to do fund-raising, perhaps since fund-raising necessitated time spent discussing how to manage the process of raising funds as well as what to do with them. Similarly, groups that more often focused their meetings on making changes in the medical system were more likely to raise funds and to conduct organizational business at meetings. These activities often occurred together in groups because they called for similar skills and commitments. Groups that planned to challenge the medical system obviously had to plan these activities carefully, so that they would be effective and yet not dangerous to the group's reputation and existing links with the staff and hospital. Well-run and relatively formally organized business meetings aided this process of decision-making and planning. Similarly, formal and fiscally accountable business meetings were required for fund-raising campaigns, which also had to be planned and organized carefully. Both these priorities required good "organizational sense," the same kind of expertise evident in the business meetings and planning sessions of any organization. On the other hand, groups that often held emotional support sessions were significantly less likely to do fund-raising or to conduct organizational business at the same meetings. And some groups held separate meetings for conducting business (once or twice a year) and for doing emotional sharing (once a month). It was hard to conduct business and provide intimate emotional support at the same time or at the same meeting; these two activities called for very different interpersonal commitments and skills, and quite different group atmospheres.

Certain aspects of the history and nature of these self-help groups were also associated with the kinds of activities they offered members. Table 4.4 indicates that the age of self-help groups was associated with their focus on conducting business at group meetings and whether or not they were engaged in substantial fund-raising activities. Both group business and fund-raising activity patterns were closely related, since a group that did substantial fund-raising also had to deal with these issues in meetings. Groups that conducted more business at meetings and raised substantial funds were likely to have been in existence for between three and five years; older groups and younger groups were less likely to spend meeting time on business activities. Perhaps the younger groups were primarily concerned at this stage of their development with getting organized, finding members, and connecting them to one

Table 4.4. Relationships between group demographic characteristics and activity patterns (*N* = 50)

Group activity offered	Group age (%)			Chi-square
	0–3 Years (*n* = 31)	3–5 Years (*n* = 14)	Over 5 Years (*n* = 5)	
Information and education	81	93	60	NS
Support sessions	77	71	40	NS
Business meetings	45	93	40	*
Substantial fund-raising	55	100	40	*
Social and recreational	77	93	100	NS
Making changes	36	50	20	NS
Hospital visits	39	43	40	NS
Networking	87	79	80	NS

*Chi-square statistically significant at *p* < .05

another. Older groups may have worked out a set of procedures that made it unnecessary to spend much time on group business, or had lost the energy to raise funds and challenge the medical system. Other group activities were not associated significantly with this aspect of group history.

Parental Criteria for Effectiveness of Specific Group Activities

In order to explore the effectiveness of these self-help groups' activities, we asked members to respond to a series of open-ended questions identifying what specific activities they felt made their group most effective. The largest proportion of parent informants in the fifty-group study (34% of all responses) mentioned aspects of emotional support and sharing. An additional 16% of the responses identified educational activities, 10% noted the practical benefits of fund-raising programs, and 8% each mentioned change-related activities and social or recreational events.

Reports of several types of emotional support and sharing emerged from these informants' responses. For instance, an important distinction was apparent between informants' views of informal support based on sharing and friendship-building versus support provided with a more organized emphasis on intense emotional discussion.[11] Most comments emphasized the value of friendship, informal support, and talking with others in a similar situation. Social events such as parties and picnics provided a supportive atmosphere in which friendships could develop; later, when people were more comfortable with one another, and sometimes outside the formal setting of group meetings, open discussion of more intimate and emotional issues often occurred.

Parents are much easier with themselves now . . . not strained. There is caring, physical contact, nice things said, we touch and hug . . . not as fearful about our interaction.

We hoped an informal network would result (from educational and support workshops), and it has . . . we have begun to share and support each other.

I felt mothers particularly needed to talk to—to share feelings with. We didn't have this when I started. I hope it has helped someone—if only one person—then it is worth it.

Men get together for card games and talk about kids and feelings.

In response to a similar open-ended question about what group activities were not effective, informants made it clear that not all efforts at providing support were viewed as positive or successful. Difficulty in deciding how to deal with feelings and how to provide emotional support were cited as reasons that some activities were ineffective. Some participants believed there was insufficient emphasis on emotional support in their groups, and too much emphasis on other matters such as business or fund-raising. Others wanted to avoid excessive discussion of the threatening and painful emotions surrounding the experience of childhood cancer.

Meetings with discussion of marital stress had the least attendance; though it's very common, you just can't talk about it in front of others.

Some say the group is too social and doesn't talk about painful issues. Yet, others say the group brings up too much sorrow and pain. They don't want an emotional meeting.

Thus, it was often difficult to achieve a good fit between the emotional styles and personal needs of individual members and the general approach taken by the group toward providing emotional support for a large and diverse constituency.

As an alternative to overtly announced and intense, emotionally focused programs, social activities brought larger numbers of people to meetings, and provided casual settings for meaningful emotional support and sharing.

Picnics and parties give support and friendship; they are fun and supportive. They were not morbid, but good for modeling.

Right now the group is functioning as a social element. People meet . . . and find out about each other. If they want to do serious talking, they might do it someplace else—call each other later, or work on a committee and spend much of the time talking.

With regard to informational and educational programs, parents identified staff members' or parents' presentations regarding illness, treatments and their effects, nutrition, siblings, child rearing, and schooling as effective means of teaching members and reaching out to nonmembers. Some groups also provided information to parents through newsletters, brochures, libraries, and specially created handbooks. Educational programs and materials often drew additional people into the self-help group community, resulting in the eventual establishment of extended friendship and support networks. As one parent noted, "Information and education programs open the door for offering help."

Activities which served to provide practical help, increase resources, and foster positive changes in the medical system were less often reported as effective. Although successful advocacy efforts to urge the staff to alter or improve operations of the medical system were noted as important by only a relatively small number of members (8%), they were very important to some parents; for them, informal and formal change strategies resulted in their becoming "aware of their rights" and able to work for changes in the norms and rules of hospital care.

We educated the hospital to the need for psychological support for families . . . that it is especially important the entire family be dealt with, not just medical treatment of the patient.

Parents are now aware of their rights . . . work through problems with medical care staff.

Parents use an informal change strategy. For example, we find out they have a real oncology nurse; informally find out they can assign this nurse to a child, or put oncology kids in rooms next to each other. The parents just spoke up.

Perhaps, as the above quotations demonstrate, these activities were highly valuable yet not highly visible, with a more subtle impact on feelings about group effectiveness. Advocacy efforts designed to help the staff meet parents' needs sometimes created problems in the relationships between group members and local professionals, and many parents wished to avoid doing anything that might offend the staff. Indeed, poor relationships with the medical staff and a lack of support from these professionals were noted explicitly as two of the major reasons for the ineffectiveness of efforts for change.

Parents' existential stress, feelings of loss of control over their lives, loss of a sense of "normalcy" and community, and general confusion about the personal meaning of their fate and faith, appeared closely linked to each of the other four stress categories; each may increase feelings of confusion and lack of control. Informants' comments about their groups' effectiveness implied that some self-help group activities also serve to offset existential stress by providing an arena in which to explore questions of religious faith and fate. Outside the normal realm of religious observance, both sacred and secular notions of the "meaning of life" and of the role of hope were discussed. As one parent noted, "The group is a place of hope."

Some parents indicated that their experience in a self-help group had empowered them to express their needs, reassert active control over their lives, and play active roles in the care of their children. Several comments also focused on the effectiveness of helping others and verified the importance of the "helper-therapy" concept, as both benefiting those helped and empowering the helper.

Helping helps us. Doing for others combats powerlessness.

Others spoke of the autonomy of the self-help group and the new knowledge and skills they had gained from participating in the group, from exerting group leadership, and from representing the group to the hospital and wider community.

The evidence reviewed here indicates that local self-help groups engaged in a wide variety of programs, all attempting to provide information, support, and assistance to families with varying personal needs and styles, and diverse medical circumstances. In the next chapter, we consider the structure and organization of these self-help groups, specifically focusing on *how* groups conducted the activities and programs discussed in this chapter.

5

How Groups Are Organized
and Operated

In order to plan, carry out, and sustain the kinds of activities described in the previous chapter, self-help groups must organize themselves. In this chapter we examine the various ways in which self-help groups for families of children with cancer solve typical organizational problems. We first examine the processes of group origin and formation, and how groups find or recruit members. Then we examine where, when, and how often groups meet. Issues of leadership and leadership development are central for all voluntary organizations, and they often raise problems of internal competition and transition. Different self-help groups solve these problems in different ways, and we examine here their leadership structures and choices. The fifty self-help groups studied differ from one another in their degree of formal organization and in their procedures for accomplishing tasks such as creating various committees, election procedures, and rules. An important aspect of any group is its relationship with the external environment, and we begin here an examination of the relationship between the group and the local medical and social service system in this context. Looking beyond the local medical system, we also examine aspects of these groups' relations with other community agencies and resources. Finally, we report members' perceptions of their local group's level of overall effectiveness. The distribution of the fifty groups for parents of children with cancer on a number of these organizational variables is shown in Tables 5.1 and 5.4. We refer to these tables throughout this chapter. We also include several composite case studies.[1]

Forming a Group and Recruiting Members

Table 5.1 indicates that 42% ($n = 21$) of the self-help groups in the sample of fifty groups were initiated by parents themselves; almost exclusively, this was a bottom-up effort with little organizing assistance from the national Candlelighters Childhood Cancer Foundation (CCCF). Another 46% ($n = 23$) of these groups were started by professionals, usually members of the local medical or social service staff. Specifically, six of the twenty-three groups started by the medical staff were initiated by physicians, six by social workers, two by nurses, and nine by members of local agencies or community organizations (e.g., American Cancer Society, Self-Help Clearinghouses). Finally, 12% ($n = 6$) were started by a mixed cadre of parents and professionals. The

Table 5.1. Diversity in self-help group internal structures ($N = 50$)

Internal structure		Percentage of groups
Initiation	Parents	42
	Professionals	46
	Mixed	12
Size	Large (large attendance and mailing list)	18
	Active core (small attendance, large mailing list)	32
	Small (small attendance and mailing list)	50
Age	Stage 1 (3 years or less)	62
	Stage 2 (3–5 years)	28
	Stage 3 (over 5 years)	10
Formalized structure	High (incorporated, differentiated)	32
	Intermediate (semiformal)	24
	Low (informal gatherings)	44
Budget size	Small < 1,000	62
	Medium 1–10,000	22
	Large > 10,000	16
Retain parents as members after child dies	Yes	70
	No	30

variety of parents, professionals, and parents and professionals starting these groups is consistent with the literature on this topic: Borman (1982), in particular, has drawn attention to the large number of medically oriented self-help groups that have been started by professionals, and Nash and Kramer (1993) report that 86.7% of the sickle-cell groups they studied had professionals involved in their formation.

Parents who initiated these groups did so in a variety of ways. Typically, several parents started talking with one another in the waiting room of the treatment center, or after an educational session provided by the hospital staff. For example, in a small city in the upper midwest, parents attending an annual pediatric oncology educational meeting began talking with one another during post-meeting coffee and cookies. They compared notes about their children, their experiences with some of the staff members, and the impact this illness was having on their lives. After a while, they remarked pleasurably on the value of this conversation and wondered why they could not have more of them. They decided not to wait for the staff to call the next yearly meeting, and set a time and date to meet again, a month later, in one of their homes. At that next meeting, the three couples once again enjoyed good conversation, and began to plan a larger gathering to which they invited many more of the parents they had just met. They asked the hospital staff to post a notice in the clinic and to inform parents with children in the pediatric oncology service of the next meeting.

Several other groups started when a parent happened to hear about the idea of a self-help or support group from the literature of the Candlelighters Childhood Cancer Foundation. For example, one parent from a southern city reported as follows:

I happened to pick up this newsletter in the clinic waiting room. It was from something called the Candlelighters Childhood Cancer Foundation. At the time I had no idea what that was. I was fascinated by the articles in the newsletter—it was as if they were written about me and my child—so I wrote to them. They sent me a lot of information and suggested I start a local self-help group. They even sent a handbook telling me how to start one. So I did it.

The American Cancer Society also occasionally played an important initiatory role. As a California parent reported,

An American Cancer Society workshop brought it all together. They brought in representatives from support groups all around the Bay area. And we wanted

Case 1. The Share-Care Group

Share-Care is a small, active group, led by parents themselves, focused on meetings where parents share their feelings with one another and try to support and affirm one another.

The Share-Care group was formed two years ago, when three mothers of children with cancer found themselves attending clinic sessions together. They talked with one another in the waiting room, and then decided to get together on a regular basis outside of the clinic and clinic hours. Shortly after starting to meet regularly, in one of the active member's homes, they decided to try to include their husbands in these sessions. They also revisited the waiting room and recruited several other parents to join them at meetings. The original three mothers are still involved, and they have been joined by one father and another mother as part of the core and planning group of five people. There is an active membership—parents who regularly attend meetings—of 12–15 people, representing about ten families.

The five leaders of Share-Care are all "middle-class" folks: they include a real estate agent, two homemakers whose husbands are professionals, a secretary, and an engineer. To date, this leadership cadre has not experienced severe energy drains, although they sometimes talk about the time when one or more of them will have "had enough" and "done enough" and will want to drop out of the group and go on to other things in their lives. The fact that they seem to be quite close friends now appears to weigh against any of them "dropping out" very soon. One member of the core, whose child has relapsed twice and does not have a good prognosis, is especially short on time and energy for group work. However, the other inner-core members go out of their way to keep in touch with her and include her in all group decisions. They also often call her, not on group business, but to ask about her child's progress and her own and her husband's emotional states.

The group meets once a month, after dinner, for about two or three hours. A typical meeting starts with all attending parents stating their names, their child's diagnosis and current status (in-treatment or off-treatment, relapse-free or relapsed, in the hospital or not, "doing well" or not, etc.), and their own current worries or concerns. When any parent indicates that he, she, or their child is in a physical or emotional crisis, or that particular family problems have arisen (e.g., with regard to siblings, grandparents, neighbors, schools, etc.), the group stops and focuses attention on this person. Generally gentle but searching—and caring—questions are asked. Sometimes, questions appear to be intrusive, and either the parent involved or someone else says, "Back off." Sometimes people cry and hold hands with one another during these explorations. Coffee and cookies (or some home-baked cakes) are available at every meeting, and they go fast!

Once every three months or so the core group asks a professional or other expert to attend the group meeting and make a presentation. This represents a recent change, one prompted by some parents saying they were tired of just "sitting and talking," and wanted more structured information and guidance. The leadership

110

cadre decided that a compromise solution was to intersperse "sharing and caring" sessions with educational sessions. The topics of these educational presentations have included information about the latest medical developments in the treatment of childhood cancer, information on how to deal with family and sibling emotional reactions, and the like. Once a year the group plans a social event, with the help of the hospital staff. Then more parents and family members, perhaps as many as 40–50, come to a picnic or a party at the hospital.

The core group has good links with the hospital staff, primarily through the hospital social worker and one of the physicians. The social worker links to the group on his own time, and professionals do not attend group meetings unless they have been specifically asked to make a presentation. Aside from this social worker, the pediatric oncology staff of the hospital does not appear to go out of its way to know about or help the group, but neither are they intrusive about or resistant to the group's efforts. The staff does not openly assist group recruitment efforts, but does not generally resist when group leaders come to the clinic or walk onto the hospital wards to talk with parents. At the same time, the staff does not appear to be unanimous in this regard; one or two of the physicians have been heard to say that they really do not think it is a good idea for these parents to sit around "complaining" to one another.

The Share-Care group does not raise funds, and it has no formal charter or by-laws. Its meager financial resources, held by one of the active core members, come from memorial donations made in the name(s) of children who have died over the years.

Share-Care prints a newsletter twice a year. It is an informally typed and reproduced document, generally running about four pages, which includes parents' writings, articles reprinted from the national Candlelighters Childhood Cancer Foundation newsletter, and occasionally a note from the social worker. It is mailed to the total membership of fifty people who have ever attended a group meeting or a social event.

111

ours to be parent-directed, not under some institutional or agency guidance. We wanted to provide the kind of comfort and healing that comes from being with others of like kind.

Another parent whose child had died of cancer was motivated by a local member of The Compassionate Friends, a self-help organization composed of parents whose children died from various causes. Involvement in a few of those meetings led this parent to form a like group of parents of children with cancer, living and deceased.

Parents' initiatives generally led to conversations with staff members about how parents could work together with the staff. Even parents with considerable experience in community and voluntary organizations needed to connect with the medical staff in order to find the names and addresses of other potential members. Most of the time they found support and assistance, although staff members were usually cautious about providing lists of patients and parents to other parents. In one midwestern town, the local American Cancer Society refused to assist in this process, claiming there was no need for such a group and no professional personnel available to supervise it. In another midwestern city, the hospital staff approved of the idea, but, as a parent reported,

They kept stalling and tried to put stipulations on the group: only parents of kids who were doing well could come, we must have a psychologist at every meeting, and I could only start the group after my child went off treatment so that I could serve as a hopeful model.

This parent decided to bypass the hospital staff and start the group on her own, beginning with the many names and addresses she had already collected by visiting the outpatient clinic and the hospital wards.

Two reports, from parents in small cities in the northeastern and northwestern parts of the country, further illuminate the variety of initiating patterns.

One parent of a recently diagnosed child needed support, so she checked with the nurses at the hospital, but they said that they frowned on parent groups. She also checked with the American Cancer Society, the Cancer Cooperative, and the state Leukemia Society. She received a list of names of other families and started calling. She advertised meetings on the radio, but no one showed up. She tried sending letters to anyone she thought might be interested. A small group started to meet, but one difficult woman kept sabotaging it. So she went to the social worker, who offered her help in dealing with this parent and in getting the group started. She held a new organizational meeting which went well, had a party, and the group was off.

One parent whose daughter died had difficulty coping and thought she needed other people to talk with. She went to a large Candlelighters family support group in a nearby city, which convinced her of the need for a regular group in our town. She met a nurse who said that a psychosocially oriented doctor was soon coming to our city. When he arrived, he called her, and they started working on a local Candlelighters group together.

In a treatment center in a midwestern city, a social worker began the process by sending out letters announcing a meeting to all parents on the clinic's rolls. Then she went to Washington, D.C., to get advice from the staff of the CCCF, and led several sessions with their suggestions in mind. In a number of hospitals, social workers started the organizing process with parents who had come to them for informal counseling assistance. One nurse started a group after she saw the intimate bonds that several bereaved parents had developed with one another through their treatment experiences. She went back ten years in the clinic's patient lists to invite a large number of bereaved parents to a meeting. Out of these sessions came the idea, and then the reality, of a much larger self-help organization for parents of living children as well as parents of children who had died.

Most of the professionals involved in initiating groups, or in facilitating parental initiation, were social workers and nurses. Physicians who started groups generally played legitimating roles, and quickly turned over to social workers and nurses the nitty-gritty details of making contacts, recruiting and sending out notices to parents, and organizing group meetings. For instance, in a medium-sized Iowa city, the pediatric oncology clinic director sent a questionnaire to all parents asking about their needs and desires, and followed it up with a newsletter suggesting that parents who wanted someone to talk to could contact the social worker and the newly emerging parent group. In a northern California community, a physician talked to the parents he saw regularly in clinic and informed them of a date he had set for a group meeting. In an eastern city, a pediatric oncologist who saw a need for parents to have a support group wrote directly to parents, and invited them to a meeting that he co-chaired with several parents. In two Texas and California treatment centers, both chiefs of pediatric oncology called approximately twenty parents and suggested that they get together for a series of support meetings. The parents took it from there.

A few groups were started, or helped along, by physicians or hospital personnel who saw the value of an active support group for their own agendas of fund-raising and expansion of hospital services and facilities. As indicated by a report from a midwestern group,

We wanted a parent support group but it was discouraged by the hospital. At the same time, the hospital had started several research projects but could not fund them. A doctor and two couples who had kids with cancer started a group to raise funds for hospital research. We've been very successful in supporting research, and at the same time we learn from each other about coping mechanisms, etc.

Recruitment and Referral Tactics

Once groups formed, the problems of recruiting new members or of gaining referrals of parents of newly diagnosed children from the hospital staff continued. The above descriptions of group initiations suggest some of the typical procedures that were used in the continuing effort to contact and recruit members. However, medical staff members and parents often used quite different approaches, partly because they had access to different resources and partly because they operated according to different rules.

The official lists of patients and their families typically were only in the staff's hands; they could decide to share that resource with parents directly, to send out notices themselves on behalf of parents and the parents' group, or to refuse to provide access. Professional control of this list and its use for phone calls and letters is standard procedure, as followed by the pediatric oncology social worker who reinitiated the Prof-Care group described in Case 2.[2] Parents, on the other hand, usually had only informal access to the parents they had met in clinic waiting rooms, on hospital wards, or at official meetings: the procedures utilized by the parents in Case 1 are typical. In one instance where a California hospital physician clearly denied parents access to the hospital patient list, active parents took turns visiting the hospital wards in the evenings, dropping in to visit and meet with families in rooms of children with cancer. They were able to tell which rooms to enter by the name of the attending physician, since they knew which physicians were on the pediatric oncology staff. A midwestern group that was un-

Case 2. The Prof-Care Group

Prof-Care is a small group, led by the pediatric oncology social worker at the local hospital, with a primary focus on providing counseling and therapy to help parents share their emotional reactions and solve their emotional problems or difficulties.

Prof-Care was reorganized six months ago. It had existed with a different social worker and a different parent membership three years ago, but died out for apparent lack of interest. The new staff social worker wrote to and called a number of veteran parents, and spoke with parents of newly diagnosed children in the clinic, inviting them to attend a series of meetings. The active membership of this group, in addition to the social worker (and a social work intern who occasionally attends as part of her schooling experience) is composed of 6–8 parents, all mothers. Sessions are held monthly, and the social worker has announced that the group will meet for one year (twelve monthly sessions). It is her plan that at the end of that time there will be little further need for organized sessions, and that she will then organize 8–10 other parents into a new group, with the same short-term therapy agenda.

The social worker is the acknowledged leader of this group, and she plans and organizes the monthly meetings. If she cannot make a meeting during a particular month, the group does not meet. The group does no fund-raising and does not work with other groups in the hospital or community. The social worker does link parents in need to other community services when she thinks it is appropriate or when parents request services; at times, she calls other community agencies and links them to these parents. She also is the group's sole link to the hospital staff and brokers questions that parents have, information the staff wants communicated, or potential problems between parents and the staff.

In a typical meeting the social worker asks everyone to go around and introduce themselves, comment on their child's and family's situations, and state any particular problems or issues they wish to raise. If issues are raised, the social worker responds to them, gently and caringly asking for information and emotional elaboration, promoting insight, and providing direct advice. Sometimes she asks other parents to offer their suggestions, advice, and support. The social worker has a presentation prepared as well, and if no parent places a problem on the agenda, the social worker generally makes a short presentation on a psychosocial issue that is potentially common to these parents and their families (e.g., school problems their child is having, family strains or divisions of labor and energy, dealing with the ill child's fears, dealing with parents' worries about the child's emotional and physical future, dealing with their own emotions, maintaining discipline with the child).

In addition to presiding at group meetings, the staff social worker provides one-on-one counseling during office hours. This is part of her staff role, and parents only pay for this if it is not otherwise covered through their insurance plans.

able to obtain official access to a list of families worked closely with a mid-level staff member to use the hospital's computer system very late one evening. The staff member, operating covertly, pressed the appropriate buttons and the computer printed out a list of the several hundred families whose children had been treated at that center over the past several years. The parent group used that list as a basis for their newsletter mailings and announcements of meetings. One parent summarized the potential parent-staff differences on this issue as follows:

Some professionals are against new parents signing up to receive the group newsletter because they do not want parents to make contact with the group. We think the hospital should release names of newly diagnosed families, but the hospital feels it violates confidentiality. The professionals are not our ally in this.

In the Candlelighters Foundation handbook developed for group leaders, Nathanson (1987) warned parent organizers of the possibility of staff resistance to providing parents' names, and stressed the necessity of reassuring professionals about the group's intentions and potential:

It is important to let the professionals who will make referrals understand that the group knows what it is doing. The group should do its homework before it approaches professionals. Assure the professionals that the group is not taking over their roles. They have jobs that the group cannot and will not attempt to do. . . . Assure them that, just as there are times when it is appropriate for them to refer parents to the group, there are also times when it is appropriate for the group to refer parents in need of professional help to them. (p. 54)

Staff members who did wish to aid group recruitment of parents provided names and referrals in a variety of ways. For instance, some staffs told parents of newly diagnosed children about the existence of the group, with or without sharing group information or a brochure. A parent from an East Coast group described this situation:

The doctor's office calls newly diagnosed families. But the doctors do not connect them to the group unless that is okayed by the parents. There is a potential problem that some referrals may drop through the cracks, since some parents may not be prepared to talk right away but are interested later.

As a second option, some staffs vigorously informed parents of newly diagnosed children about the group and emphasized its potential value, encouraging them to try it out, perhaps even giving them the phone number of the group contact person. Several parent group leaders described this process as follows:

The doctor encourages but does not force parents to attend meetings.

The doctors and social workers play an important role. They inform new families of the group, establish parent-to-parent contact if the new family desires, distribute a group information packet, and place them on the mailing list if they wish.

A third staff option encouraged parents to try participation in the group, and indicated that they would give the group the parent's phone number unless the parent actively did *not* wish them to do so.

Fourth, some staffs told parents that the group was a part, albeit an optional part, of the entire treatment system, and gave the parent's name to the group directly. Some examples of these procedures also came from parental reports:

The nurses often—doctors seldom—give the group leaders the names of newly diagnosed families; then either we talk to them at the hospital or write a letter.

The doctors ask "old" parents to speak with the "new" ones. They also work through the group structure: names are passed along and then we contact the parent.

Professionals who serve as the group's facilitators provide a list of newly diagnosed families to the group secretary. Their names are put on a mailing list, they are sent an introductory letter, and by telephone we establish a parent-to-parent link between these newly diagnosed parents and veteran parents.

Finally, in a few treatment centers, a representative of the parent group served as a more or less regular member of the clinic's treatment team, and met parents of newly diagnosed children at the time of diagnosis as part of the treatment staff.[3] Powell (1993) points to the importance of these last two options, arguing that there is a unique and necessary role of the "referent power of veteran members" in the referral process. He suggests that active contact with experiential experts, not mere mention of a self-help group's existence, is required for successful recruitment.

In addition to gathering referrals through the medical staff and recruiting at the treatment center, some groups recruited in the community at large. They prepared public radio and television announcements, placed notices in local newspapers, and played a prominent role in public events like "Children's Cancer Day." Groups that sponsored public fund-raising events, such as bake sales and races, also engaged in public advertising at the same time. These broad public appeals were not very effective recruitment strategies, because there are relatively few parents of children with cancer in the public at large. However, as many group members argued, if they found even one or two needy people in this way, it was worth the effort.

Group Size

Many studies of organizations, whether of large industrial units or of small groups, have been concerned with the effect of group size on interaction, effectiveness, and structure. Membership size is seen as a pivotal issue related to many other factors of groups' operations and activities.[4] Table 5.1 indicates that many of the self-help groups studied were small: 50% (25 groups) had under 20 people attending meetings and a mailing or contact list under 100. Another 18% (9 groups) were quite large, with over 30 people attending regular meetings, and over 100 people on the mailing list. Thirty-two percent (16 groups) had a small "active core" of members (under 20 people actively involved) and a relatively large mailing list (over 100). This active-core pattern, with a relatively small number of active and committed members, a larger member of somewhat active members, and a large nominal membership is quite common among issue-focused voluntary organizations.

Group Age

The longevity of an organization has also been seen as a key indicator of its success that influences many of its internal processes. However, an alternate approach has been proposed in Miles' discussion of temporary organizations (1964). Although formal organizations are most commonly conceived as permanent entities, limited-duration groups are especially common among local voluntary organizations. Such a group may have immediate or short-term goals with the conscious or unconscious intention of disbanding when those goals are achieved; or it could be formed by people who share a similar situation or emotional connection at about the same time. If recruitment is not successful or new members are not effectively integrated, such a group may disband when the founding members have gotten what they need from the group and are ready to move on to other concerns. Such disbanding may be seen as evidence of success attained, not necessarily as failure to sustain existence. Table 5.1 indicates that most of these self-help groups (62%) had been in existence for less than three years, with only 10% of the groups in existence for more than five years.

Formality of Organizational Structures and Procedures

Some degree of structural formalization occurs in all organizations, even in voluntary associations, since people coming together seeking mutual goals must regularize their interaction and define their roles.[5] In large and formal organizations, procedures and structures are regularized and often codified, and new entrants are socialized and directed to them upon entry. In small and less formal organizations, such as local voluntary organizations like self-help groups, operating policies are often a matter of unwritten (even unspoken) group norms which may or may not be clearly conveyed to new members. These policies and structures are nonetheless real and potent in guiding the organization; however, their informal nature means that they must often be inferred from actions, positions, or attitudes on the part of members and leaders.

Table 5.1 indicates that 32% of the fifty self-help groups had formal organizational structures and processes, as defined by the existence of a formal charter, officers, by-laws, and a committee structure; 24% were somewhat formal in their operations, having some but not all of these features; and another 44% operated quite informally. More than half of the self-help groups had formally elected officers, and somewhat fewer than 50% had official charters, by-laws, and a tax-exempt status. A sample of a standard set of by-laws for local self-help groups appears in Figure 5.1.

One example of a relatively high degree of formal organization came from a midwestern group:

Our officers are selected yearly—no one can serve for more than two years. We have a charter, by-laws, tax-exempt status, and a regular newsletter.

Case 3 presents information on a group that was very formally organized. Parents in this group argued that their executive committee,

Figure 5.1. Sample by-laws (from Nathanson, 1986, pp. 85–87)

Article I—Name & Purpose

Section 1. This organization shall be known as Hometown Parents.
Section 2. The purpose of Hometown Parents shall be:

    a   to provide encouragement, hope, and help to children with chronic illness and their families through support services and education;

    b   to promote public and professional recognition of, research in, and application of such research to the special needs of these children and their families and to the control and cure of childhood chronic illness; and

    c   to affiliate through sharing of these purposes with others in the Chronic Childhood Illness Foundation network.

Article II—Membership

Section 1   Members of families with children who have or have had chronic illness and any other person who shares the purposes and goals of Hometown Parents shall be eligible for membership. Only family members of children with chronic illness, including adult survivors of childhood chronic illness, shall have voting membership, be eligible to hold office, or to serve on the Executive Committee.

Section 2   Any member may be expelled for actions detrimental to the goals of Hometown Parents if Executive Committee recommendation for expulsion is approved by a three-fourths vote of members at regular meeting.

Article III—Officers

Section 1   The Officers shall be a President, Vice President, Treasurer, and Secretary, all of whom shall be elected for one-year terms. In addition to the usual responsibilities and authorities of these Officers, the Secretary shall prepare an annual report of activities, and the Treasurer, an annual financial report.

Section 2   The elected Officers and the Committee Chairpersons shall be designated as the Executive Committee, which shall meet periodically. A majority of the Executive Committee shall constitute a quorum. The Executive Committee shall have full power to act for the Hometown Parents when such action is required between membership meetings. Any such action shall be subject to revision by a majority of the members voting at a regular meeting.

Section 3   A vacancy in any Office or on the Executive Committee shall be filled for the remainder of the term by an interim appointment by the Executive Committee.

Section 4   An Officer may be removed from the Office upon recommendation of the Executive Committee and a three-fourths vote of members voting at a regular meeting.

Figure 5.1. Sample by-laws (from Nathanson, 1986, pp. 85–87) (*continued*)

Article IV—Elections

Section 1   Elections of Officers shall be held at the annual meeting.

Section 2   Nominations for Officers shall be made by a Nominating Committee appointed by the Executive Committee. Nominations may also be made from the floor by any voting member.

Section 3   A majority of members voting shall decide all elections. In the case of a tie, the President, or the Presiding Officer, shall cast the deciding ballot.

Article V—Meetings

Section 1   An annual business meeting and any other meetings shall be held at times and places designated by the Executive Committee.

Section 2   A meeting shall be called at least fourteen days in advance, with written notice of the time, place, and the scheduled business to be considered at all meetings.

Article VI—Committees

Section 1   The Executive Committee may establish committees for various purposes. Committee Chairpersons shall be appointed by the President with the advice and consent of the Executive Committee. All committees and chairs shall terminate at the annual meeting upon the election of new Officers, but may be reappointed.

Article VII—Amendments

Section 1   Amendments to these By-laws may be proposed by the Executive Committee or by petition of ten voting members. An amendment must be adopted by a two-thirds vote of the members voting at any regularly or specially called meeting, provided that prior notice has been included in the call of the meeting.

multiple committee structure, and businesslike meetings were necessary for their efforts to sustain a wide variety of activities and raise and distribute funds.

Other groups that were more informally organized, such as the one in Case 1, justified their operating structures or lack thereof as follows:

Structure can be a burden at times. The chairmanship can come to mean too much, and then people won't volunteer to do it. The group should imitate a family in it's function and style and emotional support system.

Case 3. The Living with Childhood Cancer Group

Living with Childhood Cancer is a large group, led primarily by parents themselves, but with significant professional involvement, and with many multifaceted activities.

The Living with Childhood Cancer group was founded ten years ago. Four parents and a social worker at the hospital got together to initiate this effort in their large cancer treatment center. Some of the founding parents still come to group meetings, but the social worker has moved on, and new sets of parents have taken over the leadership and direction of the group. The group appears to have successfully dealt with issues of leadership turnover; while there have been some ups and downs in total membership over the years, the group has remained stable and functioning during this entire timespan. It is now led by an elected executive committee of six people, all of whom have distinct roles and responsibilities. The executive committee consists of a business executive, two school teachers, a nurse from the local hospital, a homemaker, and an insurance broker. Each of the officers also heads up a functional committee of members that deal with topics such as fund-raising, monthly meeting agendas, outreach to parents and the community, the newsletter, and other publications. At this time, the publications committee is preparing a manual for parents, a guide that represents suggestions from veteran parents about what new parents need to know, where to find things in the hospital, what community resources are available, what Living with Childhood Cancer can provide, coping tips and advice, and a glossary of important medical terms.

There is an active membership of 30–40 people who attend most monthly meetings. Some of these attending are parents of children who have died, although the majority are parents of children living with cancer. The parents of deceased children appear quite welcome and comfortable in the group, as old friends as well as special contributors to discussions. At times, however, the difference in their perspective and experience seems to make everyone sad . . . and sometimes a bit nervous. Two years ago the executive committee raised the question of whether separate groups for parents of living and parents of deceased children would be a good idea; it was decided that such segregation was inadvisable for everyone, and that both sets of parents had much to learn from one another.

Group meetings are held in the hospital. The quarterly newsletter is sent to a mailing list of 300 parents/families, and about 150 people show up once or twice a year for a summer picnic on the hospital's grounds or a winter holiday party in the hospital. All refreshments and entertainment for these social events are paid for out of the group's own funds.

At a typical meeting the president starts with routine announcements, including notice of any special events occurring in the hospital or community that parents ought to know about or be involved in, such as a march for survivors, a meeting with legislators on funding medical insurance programs, a hospital lecture on childhood cancer, or a local educational or fund-raising event that the group is sponsoring. Then there are committee reports and reports from the treasurer and any other officer who has important input. Committee meetings are held outside of these regular monthly meetings. Generally, there is a semiformal presentation of an educational nature each month. Some of these presentations are made by hospital staff members, but occasionally individual parents or community members with special expertise will talk to the entire group. Once or twice a year the group invites a national representative of the Candlelighters Childhood Cancer Foundation to come and talk. During refreshment time, many small clusters of parents gather to sit and talk with one another on a personal level, and this activity goes on for some time; it has been deliberately built into the monthly meeting time.

In addition to officers and committees, Living with Childhood Cancer has a formal charter and by-laws, and is officially registered with the state and federal government as a tax-exempt public charity. The group took these steps because it raises considerable funds from external community sources, both through bingo games and bake sales, and through well-planned bequest sessions with corporate and community leaders. Funds so gathered are used to purchase wigs and prostheses for children, to pay for parents' meals and in-room TV rentals for children who are hospitalized, to pay for families' trips to specialty treatment centers, and to provide support to poor and indigent families whose children are being treated at the local center. On a regular basis, the group also makes contributions to the staff to support staff members' attendance at national professional meetings. The group is considering initiating a fund-raising program to provide support for new, small research ventures into the psychosocial aspects of childhood cancer that can be conducted at the local hospital. The parents of deceased children seem to be especially active in these fund-raising events and programs.

Living with Childhood Cancer is an active part of the national Candlelighters Childhood Cancer Foundation network. One of their members has been on the Candlelighters national board for several years, and they regularly contribute small amounts of money to the national organization, as well as send articles written by local parents to the Candlelighters Newsletter. Moreover, several of their children are long-term survivors of childhood cancer, and are working to establish the Candlelighters national network of survivors.

Given the multiple activities of this group, leadership involves a good deal of time and energy of the executive committee. The officers and members have discussed several times the advisability of hiring one of themselves as a paid, part- or full-time executive director. The president has traveled to El Paso to see how that group's paid-executive directorship worked, and has talked with other groups that have used this model, but no firm decision has been made in this regard.

Living with Childhood Cancer has good working relationships with the local hospital staff, although they are quite independent of the staff in their daily operations. The nurse from the local hospital who was elected to the group's executive committee provides some direct liaison, but many other parents also meet and talk on a regular basis with hospital staff members about group activities. The staff appears to know what's going on in the group, and often is ready to make public appearances to aid fund-raising events or to make presentations at group meetings. Occasionally, conflicts have arisen between individual parents and staff members, and group officers have stepped in to resolve these matters. In addition, every once in a while the officers of the group have presented grievances, or requests for new service or staffing policies, to the hospital staff; most of these conflicts appear to have been addressed in a congenial and timely manner, due both to the skill of group leaders and the good will of hospital staff members.

Officers are selected informally. We drew up by-laws and set policies, but found that it met our needs better to run the group informally. People volunteer to do things, and we never have any problem getting jobs filled.

One parent leader of a group that was in transition from a quite informal to a more formal status indicated the choices many groups faced.

We decided to have a loosely knit organization, with someone to start the meeting, keep track of money, and record what we do. Officers were selected after the first six months. We have no dues, just pass the hat. The mailing list is screened, but we would not say no to anyone. Minutes are mailed to people who were at the meeting. We have no charter, are working on some sample by-laws, and will try to get a tax-exempt status because we want to do fund-raising.

In about half of these groups, the meeting agenda was established ahead of time, either by a parent leadership core or by the social service staff working with the group. That did not mean that the agenda could not be altered, or that there was no time for informal conversation; a major agenda item for almost all groups was some unstructured and open-ended conversation. For the other half of the groups, however, no explicit meeting agenda was ever in place; people just came and talked about what was on their minds.

Table 5.2 indicates several statistically significant relationships between the degree of formalization and group activities in the fifty-group study (study #2). More formally organized self-help groups conducted emotional sharing sessions significantly less often and were involved with fund-raising and business meetings significantly more often. The latter findings reiterate earlier discussions and make good sense, given the necessity of a high degree of formal organization and fiscal accountability for groups raising funds from public sources. Moreover, there were clear trends, although they did not reach an acceptable level of statistical significance, for more formally organized groups also to be more involved in efforts to create changes in the medical system and to conduct hospital visitation programs.

In his early work, Katz (1981) hypothesized a "natural history" of self-help groups; he anticipated that these groups would be transformed from informal structures to formal organizations over time. Although not shown in Table 5.2, there was in our sample of groups a statistically significant correlation ($r = .35$, $p < .01$) between the age of a group and its degree of formalization—the older and longer-lasting the self-help

Table 5.2. Degree of self-help group formalization related to group activities
(*N* = 50)

Group activity	Degree of formalization (%)			Chi-square
	High (*n* = 17)	Medium (*n* = 11)	Low (*n* = 22)	
Information and education	77	100	77	NS
Emotional support	47	73	91	*
Business	94	64	27	*
Fund-raising	94	91	32	*
Social events	88	82	82	NS
Changes	59	27	27	NS
Hospital visitation	55	55	23	NS
Networking	94	91	73	NS

*Chi-square statistic significant at *p* < .05 level.

group, the more likely it was to have a more formal organization. This finding may affirm Katz's hypothesis; on the other hand, it may be that groups that were more formally organized lasted longer, rather than that they altered their level of formalization over time.

Groups and Subgroups

Some self-help groups established subgroups or suborganizations in order to meet the needs of different constituencies, or to deal with the particularities of their physical and institutional location. We have already referred to one such distinction—that existing between emotional support activities and business activities. In some groups, especially smaller ones without much business to conduct, these activities were carried on at the same meeting. In other, larger, groups separate business meetings or separate meetings of the policy and governing apparatus prevailed.

Another subgroup structure was sometimes created to meet the different needs of parents of living children and parents of deceased children. For instance, several self-help groups reported that they were started by bereaved parents, and others reported that they were started by parents of living children; different social networks and recruitment/referral patterns existed for these different sets of parents. In any single location, these two groups of parents had to decide whether they would coexist in one group, coexist in one group with occasionally separate meetings, or form two separate groups. In several cities, and sometimes even in a single treatment center, two clearly demarcated groups existed—one for parents of deceased children, and one for parents of living children. Table 5.1 indicates that most (70%) groups in this study were composed of both parents of living children and parents of deceased children, but that did not mean that they all met together all the time. Numerous groups adopted a procedure whereby all participants sat together at the start of a meeting, introduced themselves, and conducted business. Then they broke into separate subgroups for a period of time in order to talk more intimately amongst themselves. Later, they all got back together for coffee, cookies, and other refreshments. On occasion, parents of deceased children who were part of an integrated group were called upon to share their special experiences and resources with parents of children who were living with cancer. For instance, in one midwestern group the parents of deceased children made a panel presentation to the larger group on "dealing with the terminal phase," including preparing for death and dealing with hospice care and the undertaking establishment. In doing so, they gave public voice to, and promoted discussion of, many of the fears that all these parents had. This program was greatly appreciated, despite the common fears it brought to the surface. Aside from special-request programs of this sort, social occasions were the most likely times for families of living children and of deceased children to meet one another, especially when they included all family members, parents and children as well as siblings and grandparents, and sometimes staff members and their families.

At one joint session in a group meeting in the southeast, a parent whose child was living with cancer but who was rapidly approaching a terminal phase, said,

I am afraid that I will go crazy if my child dies. I worry that I will go nuts, leave my husband, become promiscuous, drink a lot, go off the deep end, and totally fall apart.

Another mother, sitting across the circle, calmly looked her in the eye and said,

You will probably do nothing of the sort. Look at me. My child died one year ago. I had some of the same fears you do; I think many of us do. But you don't have to fall apart, very few of us do. With the help of the rest of us, and your husband and friends, you can make it. You can go on with your life . . . differently, but you go on.

For the first, frightened, parent, stating and facing her greatest fears publicly and hearing them responded to in realistic terms was enormously important. For the second parent, already bereaved, discovering that she could be helpful and responsive to someone who was about to experience what she had experienced already was very rewarding and confirming.

The question of whether and how to form special groups or subgroups for parents of living children and parents of deceased children has been a focus of debate among professionals as well as self-help group members. Two primary arguments in favor of having parents of both living and deceased children as part of the same self-help group have prevailed:

1. Parents of deceased children still have ties to the hospital, to the staff, and to other parents, and might be sadder and lonelier if these ties were cut.
2. Parents of deceased children can help prepare others for the possibility of death, and for the reality that parental life continues after the death of a child.

At least four arguments against such integrated groups have consistently emerged:

1. Parents of newly diagnosed children especially might be frightened by meeting parents of children who had died, and might thus be discouraged from attending other meetings of the group.
2. Parents of deceased children may be at different stages of their lives, and thus not interested in talking about the same issues as are parents of children who are living with cancer.
3. Parents of deceased children may find it too painful to meet and see parents of children who are living.
4. It may be too guilt-provoking and uncomfortable for parents of living children to talk frankly about their hopes or be optimistic in front of parents of children who have died.

Many groups dealt with this dilemma by making sure that they were not perceived *only* as a group of parents of dead and dying children, regardless of the actual makeup of their membership and content of their discussions.

Comparisons between groups that included parents of deceased children and those that excluded these parents demonstrated some interesting patterns. Groups with more formal organizational structures, and those with medium or large fund-raising agendas, were significantly more likely to include parents whose children had died; this was also true of groups with fuller business-oriented agendas and groups that worked more often for change in the medical systems. As noted in Chapter 4, conducting fund-raising activities and having business meetings often went hand in hand. It is likely that these parents of deceased children had more time and energy available for these activities than did parents of children still in treatment. It appears that many parents of deceased children were especially interested in helping to raise funds as an act of memorializing their children—funds for research, for facilities, for services, for families in need—and that their support for this agenda may account for the relationship between group membership characteristics and fund-raising activities. Without children in treatment, these parents also may have felt less vulnerable in their relationships with the medical staff and thus more likely to be involved in change efforts. None of the other aspects of group structure, history, or programmatic priorities were related significantly to the inclusion of parents of deceased children at a statistically significant level.

Other subgroups formed around particular diagnoses. Especially in the case of children with brain tumors, some parents felt that their concerns about neuropsychological effects, schooling issues and cognitive deficits, and their interactions with the pediatric neurosurgery staffs were so unique that they needed to meet separately or to form a separate organization. Similar feelings were sometimes expressed by parents of adolescents with childhood cancer. A few groups did establish separate sessions or subgroups for the patients themselves or their siblings. These youth groups were hard to sustain, and there were only a few reports of their long-term existence. When such groups did meet for a considerable period of time, they were typically led by an especially sensitive parent, social worker, or nurse, and focused not just on emotional sharing, talking, or recreating, but on "product-oriented tasks," such as the creation of a video or booklet for other young people—usually teenagers—with cancer. Separate mothers' groups were maintained in some sites, but there was no evidence in this sample of separate fathers' groups being sustained for any substantial period of time. Occasional meetings to discuss fathers' emotional concerns, or occasional recreational events involving fathers existed on a sporadic basis, but were not sustained.[6]

Sometimes the differences in goals and needs of members led to internal group conflict, and thus some subgroups were formed as a result of struggles over group purpose and direction. Nathanson (1987) warned group leaders of this potential, noting that individual parents' needs differed, and that parents' needs changed as their child's condition changed. The important issue appeared to be for groups to adapt creatively to these changes and to avoid the situation wherein "groups may align into factions. As new members with new ideas challenge old leaders, the group may split and take different positions" (p. 101). The formation of subgroups might have been a creative response to this natural situation, but it needed to be undertaken in a spirit of compassion and cooperation about responding to different needs rather than in a spirit of adversarial or factional development.

Parental Leadership and Group Governance Structures

All stable organizations, whether operating in the public, private, or voluntary sectors, sooner or later establish a relatively clear pattern of leadership and decision-making. Self-help groups are no exception. One of the central questions facing the self-help movement in general, and certainly groups of families of children with cancer, is whether leadership should be vested in professionals—that is, skilled and expert members of the medical or social service staff—or in parents, or in both. The three cases presented earlier in this chapter illustrate this range: in Case 1 leadership rested solely in the hands of parent members; in Case 2 the social work professional led the group; and in Case 3 both parents and professionals exercised leadership, although the primary leadership roles remained in parents' hands.

Even within the context of parent leadership, there are significant debates about the type of parent who is appropriate as a leader for a self-help group. For instance, some scholars and self-help group members have argued that leadership should be vested, insofar as possible, in parents whose children are living and doing well in treatment. It has been suggested that they are likely to be better models of "success" for others, and thus better recruiters. Moreover, it has been argued that parents in this situation can provide more energy for group tasks than can parents of children who are in medical crisis. Parents of children who are "not doing well" may be facing such great demands on their time and energy in the near future that they may be risky leadership bets. In addition, parents of children who have relapsed or who have died may be seen as frightening rather than liberating models by others. All debates of this sort aside, it often was difficult to find people prepared and able to take major leadership roles in local self-help groups. The task usually fell to whomever was willing and able—regardless of their child's situation.

Some groups we studied were led by charismatic and energetic individuals—in many cases the original founders who carried on over several years or even a decade. Such was the case in a group in a mid-southern state. The original founder was dominating as well as charming; he ran the meetings, decided on the agenda, represented the group to the medical staff, and conducted all group maintenance functions personally. One result was that there was no room for others to exercise leadership. When this founder died, the group fell apart. This was not an uncommon result, as Nathanson (1987) warned:

One real danger in parent support groups is that founding leaders tend to remain in power too long through their own drive and investment or through the reluctance of others to assume the load. This can make the group unresponsive or closed to new members, needs or goals. A limit on the amount of power and the length of time one leader may serve increases a group's success. (p. 72)

Other groups were run by a small group of founders or veteran members, a pattern that had certain advantages. For instance, members of several groups reported satisfaction with this arrangement:

The group is run by a small core; others do not want the responsibility. The small group of parents who are taking charge always decides on the agenda of the meeting ahead of time.

Leadership stays with a small group. Prior to last year there were no elections, no officers, just a core group running things.

On occasion, small parent cores that ran groups became relatively impenetrable, and a clique developed that created feelings of resentment or alienation. As a parent from a southern group reported:

Six parents and a nurse who have been in since the beginning are currently still the most active members. I would like to see some new people in that core and break up the clique. New parents feel isolated.

One result of such cliquishness was internal conflict that led to struggles for leadership and control, and internal factions that battled for the loyalty of members and the content of group meetings. Such leadership struggles on occasion led to hard feelings, to people leaving to form their own groups, or to the demise of a group.

In a number of other groups, especially large and diverse ones, leadership shifted effectively and peacefully as elections were held. New people, perhaps with new and different ideas, were integrated into leadership roles and offices. In a few local self-help groups, sufficient resources were generated to hire a parent member as a paid executive secretary or director. This was the case in groups in El Paso, Texas, and Las Vegas, Nevada. In several other locations, the hospital or clinic hired a parent group leader to act as patient representative or advocate on the staff of the medical organization.[7] Such arrangements provided constant and consistent leadership to a group and suggested a relatively formal level of internal organization. In both cases of a director paid by the group, the director was accountable to an elected board of parents. In both cases of a hospital-paid representative, it was not always clear to whom the parent in the role of patient representative was really accountable—the parent group or the hospital administration. Predictably, conflict around the definition and scope of this role was common.

Leadership Transitions

Regardless of the particular type or structure of parent leadership, the question of leadership transition was a vital matter. When not planned for and not handled well, leadership transition problems became transition problems for entire groups, leading to struggle and even termination of some groups. For groups with a long history, leadership transitions commonly occurred in about the fourth or fifth year of their existence. At approximately that stage in many groups' development, original founders seemed to have tired of their role. Perhaps their children with cancer died, perhaps their children had come off treatment, or perhaps the parents had had enough of the leadership role and were just "burnt out." However it happened, as established leaders prepared to or were pressed to cycle out of this role, new people had to be found. The outcome of the search or struggle for new leadership was often successful, as several parents in different groups reported:

Two parents from the beginning of the group run the meetings, but leadership is shifting away from these founders.

Some of the original parents, who were all parents of deceased children, and some newer parents of living children, are currently the most active.

Leadership recently shifted from the original group to a fairly small group that is now getting bigger.

In contrast, an unsuccessful example of leadership transition led to termination of a midwestern group. One of the founders of this group, who had been the formal (elected) and informal leader for three years, tired of this role. An effective transition was undertaken to a new leader, who held office for two more years. When this person had to leave the community fairly suddenly, a new parent was elected to the key leadership position. In the midst of this transition, the new leader himself was diagnosed with cancer and was unable to provide leadership resources to the group. With both early leaders unavailable (one due to choice and the other due to physical move), the group floundered, eventually ceasing to sponsor activities.

But even inactive self-help groups were not necessarily permanently dormant. New groups often arose out of the ashes of old groups. In the group in a midwestern city referred to above, the original group "died" when the leadership transition did not occur successfully. Although the group discontinued meetings, newsletters, and regular contacts with the hospital, the original group founders were still called on occasionally by the hospital to meet with parents of newly diagnosed children. Moreover, one of the original founders still maintained an active set of "books," including a bank account and state/federal charters and tax-exempt status. Six years later, when another energetic, creative parent and a committed social worker began to develop another parent group in this same treatment center, arrangements were made to transfer the formal records, bank account, and group name to the new leader and the new group.[8]

Other examples of groups re-forming themselves after earlier termination confirm this "phoenix-like" principle. One report came from a parent active in a group on the west coast.

Ten years ago, the first group of parents of living children and parents of deceased children asked the staff to help them form a support group. They started with monthly information meetings discussing new treatments, and met in the hospital's hematology department. They disbanded after two years because some people had moved on, and the others lacked hospital support. A second group formed more informally three years ago. We had support of the hospital because of our Ronald McDonald House efforts. A group of parents who had lost young children, between the ages of six months and two years, decided among themselves to become friends, and that a group was necessary to provide all of the things they missed. The hospital actually made a mailing to all parents announcing that we were starting a group.

A second example came from a southeastern group.

There was a group long ago; the Patient Education staff organized it, and it met after clinic appointments. It did not work well, partly because parents were eager to leave the clinic right away. Recently, some parents became more interested in starting a group again. The social worker knew about Candlelighters and parent groups, and personally contacted some parents who had gotten together informally but had not organized anything. They wished that there was some kind of a group, and she helped them start it.

These experiences emphasize the importance of not assessing the value or success of self-help groups on the basis of the typical criteria of size and longevity utilized to evaluate formal and bureaucratic organizations. Long the hallmarks of organizational success, they are not necessarily appropriate for assessing self-help groups. Some self-help groups can best be characterized as the "temporary systems" (Miles, 1964) discussed earlier. It is far from a disaster if a self-help group dissolves, and a group is not necessarily successful merely by virtue of its long-standing existence. When goals designed for a particular set of members have been fulfilled, the group may well have achieved its purpose and be well advised to cease operations. Certainly, dissolving a group at that point may make more efficient and compassionate use of human resources than maintaining a failing bureaucracy or a dysfunctional community. Good things can happen for parents in brief periods as well as lengthy ones, and in small groups as well as large ones. Moreover, as we have seen, even evidence of the "death" of a group may be premature. Some groups that have ceased activities may be resurrected years later, and others may simply disappear from view, substituting private and informal networks for public and formal meetings and activities.

Leadership Development

Maintaining effective leadership was often a challenge for local groups. In response, the national networking agency and clearinghouse of self-help groups for families of children with cancer (CCCF) has taken the lead in providing leadership development activities for local groups. These activities were designed to provide information and skill-development opportunities to parents who were in the position of group leadership, or who anticipated being in such leadership positions in the future. They have been accomplished through the work of a staff member who established liaison with and helped suggest programs to local groups, as well as a *group newsletter* informing all group leaders of the activities, operating styles, and problems of other groups. In addition, members of the national board of the Foundation, themselves typically leaders of local groups, often consult and problem-solve with other local leaders.

CCCF also developed and conducted a weekend workshop for group leaders throughout the state of California (Ayers and Chesler, 1987). In a pre-workshop survey, group leaders identified the greatest problems faced by their groups to be participation and parent involvement, contacting parents of newly diagnosed children, increasing interest and attendance, getting people who attend to participate in group operations and leadership, fund-raising, and overcoming energy loss due to travel distance. The general design for the leaders' workshop focused on the following issues:

- What are the common stresses/needs of families of children with cancer?
- What kind(s) of self-help groups and group activities do these needs suggest?
- How does one lead a group?
- What organizational structures seem to work?
- How can one facilitate parent-group/professional-staff collaboration?
- How may groups reach out to resources available in their community?
- How can we help each other?

After an introductory session where people identified their own personal situations as parents of children with cancer, and their group situations, particular sessions explored the above concerns. The style of work was primarily participatory rather than didactic: brief lectures, group discussions, situational problem solving, role-play scenarios, and practice in both leading sessions and modeling leadership skills were utilized as learning activities. In addition, the experience and expertise of workshop participants provided a basis for sharing effective ideas and practices with others; participants shared the difficulties they faced and the lessons they had learned in their own self-help groups. At the conclusion of the workshop, participants identified four types of knowledge gained from the program experience: (1) group activities for parents and children, (2) ways of being helpful to bereaved families, (3) how to start a group, and (4) leading a group.

Groups' Relationships with the Health Care System

In addition to understanding the internal structure of these self-help groups, it also is important to understand their relationship with the external environment in which they operate. There are several important aspects of the external environment, including the groups' relations with professionals in the local health care system or treatment center. We referred earlier to the crucial distinction between parental or professional leadership in self-help groups. Moreover, the three cases presented in this chapter and in Figure 1.1 (in Chapter 1) suggested the existence of a continuum from professionally led and professionally dependent support groups to parent-led (or non–professionally led or experientially led) self-help groups, on the basis of the primary importance of the role of the leadership person or cadre (Mellor et al., 1984). While we eschew what are often unrealistically exclusive definitions and distinctions, we do recognize this basic leadership distinction and the continuum so presented. Clearly, self-help and mutual support may occur even in a professionally run group; but, just as clearly, that may be quite different from the experience people have in a group run by peer-members.

The fifty groups in this study were divided into three types, based upon several criteria reflecting the level of professional involvement and leadership in the group. Fifty-two percent of these groups ($n = 26$) were run by parents, and were relatively *independent* of professional involvement or control. Another 26% of the groups ($n = 13$) in this sample were run by *professionals*, and 22% ($n = 11$) were characterized by a *shared* pattern of professional *and* parent leadership.[9]

Some comments by the parents we talked with indicated the nature of the independent groups—groups run solely by parents:

Two parents run the meetings. The nurse and doctor come to some meetings to lend support but keep a low profile.

Parents run the meetings and are the most active. Professionals may attend but do not plan anything.

A parent leads the group and semi-facilitates the meetings. She talks with other parents and then decides on the agenda. This is an issue of our control. We did not want to be worked on, processed, experimented with by professionals.

We (parents) broke away from the American Cancer Society and ran the organization. We did not want to be providing support to each other with onlookers—professionals, doctors, ACS staff—attending the meetings.

These excerpts, and the group presented in Case 1, reflect groups that approached one of the extreme ends of the continuum presented in Figure 1.1 (Mellor et al., 1984). They were run by parents, which meant that parents occupied all the governance or decision-making roles, and planned and ran the meetings. As the first two quotations indicate, staff members may have attended some meetings, but they did not play key roles in the operations of the group and its activities. These groups were not antiprofessional in structure and ideology, but they were proexperiential and often took an aprofessional stance.

Parents characterized the professionally led groups quite differently, as follows:

The group is run completely by professionals. A nurse practitioner runs the group with a male psychiatric social worker.

There are no parents who make up the core of this group. The nurse and social worker are co-facilitators; their role is direction, conversation, long-term cohesion, guidance. They do not plan or introduce topics, but come up with ideas or have thoughts in mind in case of a lull.

A doctor is the leader. He and his nurse run the meetings; leadership stays with them. The doctor sets the agenda ahead of time.

These groups were not merely supervised by professionals; the staff set the agenda, recruited and determined the membership, made key decisions, and ran the meetings. In this context they may better be considered mutual support or professional support groups, rather than self-help groups. They occupy the other extreme end of the continuum in Figure 1.1, and are illustrated by the group in Case 2.

The shared leadership groups operated with a variety of interactive and collaborative relationships between parent leaders and professionals:

Parents and one social worker are co-chairs and run the meetings; they are the leaders. Parents are most active. Initially the social worker brought an agenda to meetings, but not anymore.

Parents and the social worker are currently the most active. The parent is the president and runs most of the meetings. The social worker wants to be a resource person—to step back and yet be there if the parents needed something from her or from the hospital.

A core of the Board runs the meetings: two parents of children on treatment, three parents of deceased children, the doctor, and the nurse.

These shared-leadership groups, reflected to a certain extent in Case 3, appear to present efforts at parent-professional coalitions. Parents held most of the key leadership positions and played the dominant roles in planning and running meetings, but professionals were often active as well. Although they operated autonomously from the medical institution, these groups involved staff members in meaningful internal roles and in external liaison relationships.

How Did These Differences in Leadership Patterns Affect the Self-Help Groups?

Table 5.3 demonstrates a series of significant and important relationships between these three patterns of parental-professional leadership and other key variables pertaining to self-help groups' internal structures, operations, and activities. For example, the data in Table 5.3 indicate that there was a significant relationship between how the group was initiated and its later leadership structure. Groups that were initiated solely by parents appeared to remain independent of professional leadership or to evolve into shared-leadership groups. Of those groups that were initiated by professionals, about half continued to be led by professionals. The ones that were initiated by social work professionals appeared to continue with professional direction, while those initiated by doctors often made a transition to independent or shared leadership status. This may be explained by the different initiation and involvement patterns of these two groups of professionals. Doctors started and sanctioned groups with letters or verbal suggestions, but typically re-

Table 5.3. Self-help group characteristics by type of group leadership pattern

Group characteristic		Group leadership pattern (%)			
		Total (n = 50)	Prof. (n = 13)	Independ. (n = 26)	Shared (n = 11)
Structure					
Initiator*	Parent	42	0	62	45
	Professional	46	92	27	36
	Mix	12	8	11	18
Formalized structure*	High (incorporated, differentiated)	34	0	42	55
	Intermediate (semiformal)	22	0	32	27
	Low (informal gatherings)	44	100	27	18
Size*	Large (large attendance and mailing list)	18	0	23	27
	Active core (small attendance, large mailing list)	32	16	31	55
	Small (small attendance and mailing list)	50	84	46	18
Age*	Stage 1 (3 yr or less)	62	84	61	36
	Stage 2 (3–5 yr)	28	8	27	55
	Stage 3 (over 5 yr)	10	8	12	9
Operations					
Retain parents after child dies*	Yes	70	31	81	91
	No	30	69	19	9
Budget size*	Small	62	100	54	36
	Medium	22	0	27	36
	Large	16	0	19	27
Activities					
Emotional support at meeting*	Yes	72	92	65	64
	No	28	8	35	36
Information and education: speakers, movies, etc.	Yes	82	69	92	73
	No	18	31	8	27
Business: organizational maintenance, commit-tee reports, etc.*	Yes	58	8	77	73
	No	42	92	23	27

Table 5.3. Self-help group characteristics by type of group leadership pattern (*continued*)

Group characteristic		Group leadership pattern (%)			
		Total (*n* = 50)	Prof. (*n* = 13)	Independ. (*n* = 26)	Shared (*n* = 11)
Fund-raising	Yes	66	15	85	82
for organizational	No	34	85	15	18
maintenance, service,					
or large projects*					
Social: parties,	Yes	84	69	88	91
picnics, holiday	No	16	31	12	9
events for children					
and parents					
Efforts to change	Yes	42	23	42	45
medical system to	No	58	77	58	55
meet needs of					
families*					
One-to-one network:	Yes	84	62	96	82
contact among	No	16	38	4	18
parents outside					
meetings (telephone,					
personal)					
Number of above	1–4	40	69	23	45
activities that	5–7	60	31	77	55
the group offers*					

*Indicates a statistically significant relationship at the $p < .05$ level or beyond, using the chi-square analysis.

moved themselves from active participation in the group's structure or activities, unless called upon for guidance. Social workers, on the other hand, often perceived leading the group as part of their professional role obligations; their initiation efforts were much more likely to extend beyond legitimation and recruitment, expanding over time to include active group leadership.

Separate analyses comparing the two categories of parent-led groups (independent and shared-leadership types) with the professionally led groups revealed that the professionally led groups were significantly less formally organized, and were significantly more likely to emphasize emotional support activities, even to the exclusion of some other activities engaged in by the parent-led groups. Moreover, the professionally led groups significantly less often engaged in proactive functions such as promoting changes in the system of medical care. Also, the professionally led groups were significantly more likely to be smaller, to be of shorter duration, and not to involve parents of deceased children.[10] Support groups led by parents themselves, or by parent-professional partnerships, were likely to be more formally organized, to be larger, to have had a longer period of existence, and to have had a wider variety of activities.

Professionally led groups' greater prevalence of formalized emotional support activities may be explained in terms of the availability or dominance of leadership that defined the needs of families of children with cancer in these ways—with a primary focus on regular sharing and ventilating of feelings. These groups certainly were responsive to parents' emotional needs, or they would not have existed, but it appears they were primarily responsive to a narrow set of needs of a relatively small portion of the population of parents of children with cancer. Professional access and dominance also may explain the nearly total reliance on medical system referrals in professionally led groups, and the lack of a formalized structure of operations. Indeed, there was no reason for these professionally led groups to have developed more formal structures; the professional staff was there to do such organizational work for them. These groups also were likely to be too dependent upon the staff to openly challenge individual medical staff members or the organization of care.

The more diverse and often more task-oriented activities of both types of the parent-led groups probably reflected the wider range of needs and priorities parents themselves saw and wished to act upon—a need to have an impact on the fight against childhood cancer, a need to improve the medical system's services and responsiveness, a need to reach out to and assist other parents in times of crisis, a need to socialize and have fun together, a desire to raise funds, and to deal as well with intense emotional issues. The shared-leadership groups generally were similar in structure to the independent groups, but were somewhat more likely to have had an established active core, to have existed for a longer duration, and to have had larger budgets. Thus, they appeared to be able to benefit from their independence from professional control—and the consequent encouragement of parental autonomy and empowerment—but at the same time benefit from their good access to the personal and institutional resources that professionals provided.

Where and When Did Groups Meet?

Table 5.4 indicates that over one-half (52%) of the fifty groups studied met in the local treatment center. The location and timing of group meetings were largely dependent upon the local geography of the "catchment area" the group defined as its base of operations. For instance, in a large metropolitan area, with several hospitals treating childhood cancer, several definitions of "catchment populations" prevailed. In New York City, where several different groups existed, most concerned themselves with parents whose children were being treated at "their own" individual hospital. The same was true for several groups operating in and around the Los Angeles metropolitan area. The Chicagoland Candlelighters, however, considered the entire metropolitan area their bailiwick. They established regional subgroups and meeting locations based on parents' residential patterns and the distance they had to travel to get to meetings, but were organized across hospitals on a citywide basis. In St. Louis, an area-wide group established a "spoke" design. The central area group printed a newsletter for all the groups in

Table 5.4. Diversity in self-help group external structures and operations (N = 50)

External structure		Percentage of groups
Meeting location	Treatment center	52
	Community center	36
	Home	12
Horizontal links	None	18
	Few to other childhood cancer groups	34
	To many other cancer groups	26
	To several community agencies	22
Vertical links	None	22
	On Candlelighters Foundation list	22
	Use Candlelighters name	56

the area, and its governing board was composed of representatives from several independent groups located throughout the metropolitan area. However, each of the local groups was independent of the central hub, except for their relationship with the newsletter. Several other groups across the nation experimented with a statewide apparatus, but this design was not sustained over time. For instance, in Oregon, a state-wide self-help group located in Portland for many years "supported" and "coordinated" the activities of local groups in other parts of the state. However, this arrangement always was fraught with tension and dis-agreements between local groups and the state group about issues such as autonomy and control of finances. By and large, the trend appeared to be for localization and autonomy at every step.

In smaller cities, it was most likely that only a single group existed. Sometimes these groups met in the hospital. In some situations, how-ever, groups deliberately met elsewhere. As one parent noted,

Now we meet alternative months at a church and at the hospital. The issue is one of people not wanting to go back to the hospital versus the convenience of everyone knowing where it is, easy parking, etc.

Many parents indicated that they would have preferred that their meet-ings, especially the informal sessions, had not been held at the same hospital that reminded them so vividly of their treatment experiences.

Groups that formed to serve parents living in widely dispersed rural areas faced quite different problems in selecting meeting places, or in having meetings at all. For instance, central and easily accessible loca-tions were quite difficult to find in the reaches of western Texas or the mountain states. As suggested earlier, in these settings extended tele-phone networks often substituted for regular meetings.

The most common meeting schedule was once a month (64% of the groups reported this pattern). Several groups met every two weeks, and a few reported meeting every other month or even quarterly. However, the scheduling of meetings was somewhat dependent upon the type of group or the type of activities involved. The groups that met most often were most likely to be engaged in substantial emotional sharing and dialogue; such an intimate activity focus literally demanded constant contact and feedback. The groups that were oriented toward educa-tional and social events were most likely to meet every other month.

Some groups, with a differentiated sense of their focus and structure for specific functions and agendas, held various kinds of meetings at different intervals. For example, a parent in a large group in New York State reported as follows:

We have a meeting with a speaker every other month. Then we have a business meeting, to plan activities, once a month. And then the governing board meets four times a year to discuss policy and long-range plans. Committees meet anytime.

Another group reported from the northwestern coast:

We meet as a small support group once a week at the hospital. Then the Candle-lighters group has a formal meeting once every other month.

Finally, a Texas group reported the following:

We have a general parents' group that meets monthly for about three hours. A group of mothers whose children are in the hospital or in treatment meets three times a week. We have a business meeting monthly.

The diversity in groups' meeting schedules and sites was as great as the diversity in their operations and activities.

Groups' Horizontal Links to Local Community Agencies

Another aspect of groups' relations with their external environment involved their links with other local community agencies concerned with the problems of families of children with cancer. A number of self-help groups actively sought connections with other local voluntary organizations or social service agencies in the local community. Table 5.4 indicates that almost half of these fifty groups (twenty-four groups, or 48%) had established working relationships with several other cancer-related groups or community agencies, while the other half had few or no external links. The sole statistically significant relationships between such horizontal community linkage and group activities involved fund-raising and business activities. Groups that had more local community contacts generally were engaged in more fund-raising; as we have already reported, groups that did more fund-raising needed to conduct business at meetings.[11] Obviously, these community contacts represented fund-raising targets and facilitated groups' fund-raising activities.

One particular community agency of special interest and relevance for these self-help groups for parents of children with cancer was the American Cancer Society's (ACS) local units and divisions. Of the fifty groups in this sample, 36% indicated that they had had no contact, or no "helpful" contact, with local ACS personnel or offices. In some cases, this occurred because group members had never contacted ACS personnel, or vice versa. This was especially likely for small, community-based groups which were not linked to a local medical center or hospital. However, several groups located near or at major medical centers also reported no sustained or helpful contact with the American Cancer Society, even when a medical social worker or pediatric nurse familiar with the ACS staff worked actively with the group. In some cases this was the result of a conscious decision of ACS personnel not to link to or work with a local parent group, and in other cases it was a result of the ACS unit's lack of knowledge (perhaps a mutual lack of knowledge) about a local group's existence or needs. This may also be an outgrowth of the general priority within the American Cancer Society to focus on issues relevant to adult oncology, and the relatively low incidence of pediatric cancer cases compared to adult cancer cases.

The remaining 64% of the groups indicated some helpful contact with ACS offices and personnel. ACS assistance sometimes was provided in the form of direct services to individual children and their families. Included in such services were transportation aid, wigs and prostheses, and information about disease, treatments, social services, and medical referrals. These services were not provided to the self-help group, *per se*, but to group members, or to individual needy families identified by group members. Direct assistance to groups from the ACS was reported by 52% (twenty-six) of the groups. They included arranged or sponsored speakers, offices for meetings, printing and distribution of group newsletters and brochures, and various forms of administrative liaison. In providing most of these services, the ACS offices evidently absorbed such effort within their existing budgets and staff arrangements; there was no evidence of ACS offices directly providing local groups with funds. In addition, five of the fifty groups reported that the local or state ACS reached out to include self-help group representatives in special ACS-sponsored programs aimed at publicizing camps for children with cancer, educating school personnel, or otherwise engaging in public education or fundraising activities. In fact, some groups, and many individual parents and children who were group members, were active in helping ACS fund-raising campaigns be successful. Seven groups also reported that ACS staff members had helped the local self-help group get and stay organized, either by providing patient referrals on a reliable and consistent basis or by lending personnel for the training of group members in leadership skills. Finally, three groups reported that ACS had invited group representatives to sit on state or local ACS committees, thus including active parents in the organizational activities of ACS.

On the negative side, eight groups (16%)—including some that had also reported helpful contact and services—reported tension or resistance in their relationship with ACS. In several cases, the focus of this resistance was seen by group members as the ACS staff's desire to control or "guide" the content of self-help group meetings and newsletters. Thus, it became important for these groups to determine "whose group it was"; in several cases, parent groups refused offers of ACS assistance that were tied to such control. Another basis for tension in several locales was disagreement over the timing and nature of ACS or group fund-raising, and concern about competition for local donors and programs. Relatively few self-help groups attempted to raise funds that seriously competed with local ACS efforts, but this tension occasionally existed, nevertheless. In several other cases, the reasons for ACS unwillingness to assist with program development, referrals, or newsletter distribution were unclear, and could not be accurately identified as either due to resistance or lack of connection.

Relationships between local self-help groups and local ACS offices generally were facilitated and sometimes were complicated by the relationship between the national ACS and the national clearinghouse of self-help groups for parents of children with cancer, the Candlelighters Childhood Cancer Foundation. In an agreement that spans more than twenty years, the national ACS has helped fund the national Candlelighters' office and activities. Nevertheless, local ACS offices and local self-help group members (who may or may not be formally affiliated with CCCF) have, on occasion, struggled with one another in coming to a common understanding of the details of this arrangement and their working relationships.

Groups' Vertical Links to CCCF

Figure 5.2 provides a brief description of the national Candlelighters Childhood Cancer Foundation, and some suggestions regarding the relationship between the national organization and local parent groups. Table 5.4 indicates the degree to which there were links between the local self-help groups and the national CCCF. These vertical links were defined as "high" for over half ($n = 28$, 56%) of the groups, those who clearly identified themselves as part of a national movement, who utilized the Candlelighters name for their own group, and who participated in national meetings or contributed to the national newsletter. Such vertical links were virtually nonexistent on a formal level, or "low" for 22% of the groups ($n = 11$). Almost all of the fifty groups received the Candlelighters newsletters, but those with "low" links neither utilized the Candlelighters name nor self-consciously saw themselves as part of a national movement or network.[12]

Independent self-help groups, those led by parents themselves, tended to have the strongest vertical links (adopting the Candlelighters name), and the professionally led groups the least (often not knowing about CCCF). Similarly, the groups with no vertical link tended to be small, young, and to have a low degree of formalization. There appeared to be a pattern in these self-help groups of parents of children with cancer in which an organizational norm fostering independent, member-led, support-oriented groups was associated with participation in a national network of such groups. The professionally led groups were much less likely to be connected horizontally or vertically to a national or local community network.

The Candlelighters Childhood Cancer Foundation was renamed as such in 1976; it was originally founded as the Candlelighters Foundation in 1970.[13] Its programs include a library that is accessible to parents via an information hotline; newsletters and materials for professionals, parents, and children with cancer; an ombudsman program that serves members with legal questions concerning insurance, employment and education discrimination, and unproven treatments; a network and speakers program involving long-term survivors of childhood cancer; leadership-development workshops for group members and leaders; liaison with professional medical and social service organizations in the pediatric oncology field; and an active research program (of which the

Figure 5.2. How the local/national Candlelighters' relationship works
(Nathanson, 1986, pp. 76–77)

The Candlelighters Childhood Cancer Foundation, founded in 1976, is the organizational, liaison, educational, and service arm of an international network of over two hundred support groups of parents of children with cancer.

Most groups of parents of children with cancer are in this Candlelighters Childhood Cancer Foundation network. Many are called Candlelighters, but not all use this name. (The name "Candlelighters" and the identifying "burning candle" logo are registered with the U.S. Office of Trademarks and may not be used without the permission of the Candlelighters Childhood Cancer Foundation.) Some groups in the network adopt acronyms (LODAT—Living One Day at a Time), incorporate the name of their treatment center (Hopkins Oncology Parents), or of their geographic area (San Diegans Against Cancer).

The Candlelighters Childhood Cancer Foundation services are free to groups. Individual groups pay no dues, and the Foundation issues no directives for groups to follow. However, it is expected that groups in the network share and act upon the Foundation belief in the benefit of parent mutual support systems in the service of children with cancer and their families.

Sample Local/National Organizational Relationship

The Candlelighters Childhood Cancer Foundation Board of Directors is made up of parents selected from local groups, paid staff directors (who are parents), and a few representatives of the professional community who have demonstrated their commitment to the beliefs and goals of the Foundation. Efforts are made to balance the board in respect to geographic area, professional discipline, gender, type, and outcome of child's disease.

The Foundation staff under the direction of and with assistance from the board helps new groups form; refers families to groups in the network; links existing groups; provides problem-solving assistance, training, and referral services to groups; serves as an information clearinghouse for the groups, families, educators, medical and psychosocial professionals; conducts surveys of patients/family needs; promotes the development and production of quality education materials; maintains liaison with support, professional, and parent organizations; works for changes in the medical care and educational systems and in public policy; produces publications for parents, professionals, children with cancer, and their brothers and sisters.

The national affiliation between the Candlelighters Childhood Cancer Foundation and the American Cancer Society, which funds the major portion of the Foundation's activities, in no way binds the local parent groups. The Foundation works with the local parent groups and the American Cancer Society to encourage cooperation in developing and funding programs for young cancer patients, their families, medical care teams, treatment centers, educational systems, and communities.

work reported in this volume is part). Its newsletter and materials are distributed to over 40,000 parents, professionals, patients, and others concerned with childhood cancer.[14] CCCF deliberately has not tried to establish formal "chapter" or formal affiliation arrangements with local groups. Instead, an informal process of local group affiliation with the national Foundation exists, with CCCF retaining the copyright on the use of the name "Candlelighters." Thus, the Foundation has tried to preserve the indigenous, bottom-up, and locally democratic nature of self-help by operating as a spokesperson, clearinghouse, and network organization for parents and parent self-help groups throughout the United States (and with links to groups in thirty other countries). It links groups to one another, provides them with information and advice, but makes no effort to control or direct the 400 local groups in its network.

Parental Criteria for Effectiveness of Group Operations

The contribution of specific group activities to parents' reports of group effectiveness or ineffectiveness were discussed in Chapter 4. But what about parents' views of general group operations? Members' most potent concerns about group operations centered on what it was that kept the group functioning successfully, and how they could operate better. Twenty-nine percent of all the individuals surveyed in the fifty groups reported that the group they were involved with was "very effective," while another 39% reported that it was "pretty effective." Only 8% reported that their group was "ineffective" (2%) or "somewhat ineffective" (6%). This is what we might expect from a survey of members themselves; if they did not think their group was relatively effective, they probably would not have been members. Parent members commented on specific reasons for groups' effectiveness and ineffectiveness. Group maintenance, or group-building activities, allowed the organization to survive, sustain itself, develop the capacity for leadership and autonomy, and grow in membership. Although inappropriate activities were cited as reasons for groups' ineffectiveness by 43% of the sample, the majority of the responses related to ineffectiveness dealt with organizational operations, with the functioning and attendance of the group, with its leaders, and with the relationship between the self-help group and the hospital.

For instance, a lack of leader commitment or clarity was viewed as a serious problem. At times, parents reported that parent or professional leaders made decisions about group directions and activities with little input from, or against the wishes of, the members. For instance,

There was a difficult period at the beginning. They had a difficult time defining goals. The president wanted the focus of the group to be research and religion. Others didn't, and he left.

There's too much business. They are shutting people off. The old leaders push the agenda off feelings and back to fund-raising.

Other common organizational problems involved the recruitment and retention of members, and publicizing the group.

Sometimes only one person comes to meetings.

People drift in and out, but many haven't stayed long.

Further, in some groups members raised special concerns about the low level of participation of minority and lower-income families.

Members reported that their groups' relationship with the hospital and health care professionals often affected survival and effectiveness. The development of successful relationships with the staff and institution required careful work. One parent leader spoke of being successful because she was

non-threatening, no competition to medical and social services staff. The group leader is potential competition until she establishes a unique and non-threatening role.

Another group invited professionals to lead a series of emotional support sessions as an adjunct to the lay/member-led organization.

We had good professionals and could see advantages to having them there. They raised good points, did not constrain, moved the group, used silence, expected work. People felt commitment . . . to someone we knew and trusted and had faith in.

Our exploration of the structure and operations of self-help groups for parents of children with cancer in this chapter has ranged from issues of recruitment and group maintenance to patterns of group leadership and group involvement in wider communities of relevance. In Chapters 6 and 7 we turn to an individual level of analysis and to explorations of members' (and nonmembers') views of and experiences in these groups.

Part 3

Patterns of Participation
and Outcomes:
Crossing the Bridges

In this section we present empirical findings related to an individual-level analysis of parents' choices to become involved in these self-help groups for parents of children with cancer, or their choices not to become involved, and of members' experiences in these groups.

In Chapter 6 we examine the characteristics of parents who participated in these self-help groups, and explore the reasons why they elected to become involved. In addition, we utilize a sample of parents of children with cancer who did not become involved in these groups to explore how these members and nonmembers differed, and to examine the latter population's reasons for noninvolvement.

In Chapter 7 we explore participants' reports of the benefits they felt they gained from their participation in these self-help groups, and compare participants' and nonparticipants' reports of their current coping adequacy and outcomes.

6

Self-Help Group Participation

Who Joins and Why

This chapter examines the characteristics of parents of children with cancer who joined self-help groups and compares them with parents who chose not to join local groups. We explore the reasons why many parents of children with cancer chose to become involved in a group, as well as why many others chose not to become involved. Underlying these explorations is the realization that self-help groups, a significant resource for some people, are not attractive or useful for everyone. The unique culture of self-help will *not* appeal to *all* parents experiencing the common crisis of childhood cancer, nor will the activities and operations of particular groups be attractive and useful for all parents' unique needs and styles. In presenting the perspectives of those parents who did not choose to become involved in a self-help group, we further illuminate how and why groups work for those who did become members.

In Chapter 3 we described some of the procedures used to generate a comparative study of parents of children with cancer who did or did not elect to become self-help group members. Members in eight groups (Study #3) were identified via lists maintained by group leaders (parents or hospital staff members), and interviewed and given self-administered questionnaires by project staff—usually at group meetings and sometimes in clinics. Nonmembers were identified through hospital records and generally were contacted, interviewed, and provided with questionnaires in clinics. The analysis of these data in this chapter proceeds as follows: (1) we first examine the relationships between parents' demographic characteristics, children's medical status, and self-help group membership; (2) we then examine the associations between parents' reports of their use of varied coping strategies and their self-help group membership; (3) we then discuss the associations between parents' reports of their receipt of social support and self-help group membership; and (4) finally, in an extended discussion, we present some parents' own reasons for deciding to join a local self-help group and the reasons other parents elected not to join these groups.

Group Members' Demographic Characteristics and Children's Medical Status

Research on self-help groups has attempted continually to construct the "profile" of a typical self-help group member. Most of the research, especially that which examines self-help groups in the medical arena, reports most members to be female and relatively well educated.[1] However, some recent work focusing on groups composed of people from politically or economically disenfranchised social strata has generated somewhat different results, suggesting greater diversity in gender and educational backgrounds.[2]

Table 6.1 indicates that parent self-help group members in our eight-group study were not significantly different in their overall demographic status from nonmembers. On the average, parents of children with cancer participating in the self-help groups were between thirty-five and forty years old and female; they were married, with modest family incomes, and lived relatively close to the medical center where their child was treated. Although these profiles did not significantly differentiate group members from nonmembers, the two populations did differ significantly in educational level; the proportion of self-help group members who had attended some college or who were college graduates was much greater than the proportion of nonmembers with similar educational backgrounds. Perhaps advanced education reinforced or prepared people for the predominantly verbal style of interaction so common in these groups. Or, given the prevailing evidence that people with greater education participate more actively in many sorts of voluntary groups (Bauman, Garvey, and Siegel, 1992), perhaps this finding reflects that greater activism and community participation.

With regard to their children's medical status, self-help group members were significantly more likely than nonmembers to be parents of children diagnosed with cancer less recently; almost three-quarters

Table 6.1. Parents' backgrounds and children's medical status by self-help group membership

Parents' backgrounds	Percent of members	Percent of nonmembers	Percent of significance
Marital status			NS
Single/divorced (*n* = 15)	60.0	40.0	
Married (*n* = 84)	64.3	35.7	
Age			NS
Less than 36 (*n* = 32)	56.2	43.8	
36–41 (*n* = 34)	64.7	35.3	
42–63 (*n* = 27)	74.1	25.9	
Education			*
High school graduation or less (*n* = 18)	44.4	55.6	
Some college (*n* = 36)	58.3	41.7	
College graduation or more (*n* = 39)	79.5	20.5	
Family income			NS
Less than 10,000 (*n* = 9)	33.3	66.7	
$10,000–$20,000 (*n* = 19)	78.9	21.1	
$20,000–$40,000 (*n* = 23)	56.5	43.5	
$40,000–$60,000 (*n* = 25)	58.8	41.2	
More than $60,000 (*n* = 25)	76.0	24.0	
Gender			NS
Female (*n* = 84)	61.9	38.1	
Male (*n* = 9)	88.9	11.1	
Distance from home to medical center			
Less than 25 miles	70.5	29.5	
More than 25 miles	55.6	44.4	NS
Time since child's diagnosis			*
Less than 2 years (*n* = 28)	46.4	53.6	
More than 2 years (*n* = 65)	72.3	27.7	

*Difference is statistically significant at the .05 level or better, using a chi-square test of independence.

NS: No significant difference between members' and nonmembers' responses.

(72.3%) of the members' children had been diagnosed more than two years ago, compared with about one-quarter (27.7%) of the children of nonmembers. It would appear from these data that it took parents some time to adjust to the nature and demands of the illness and treatment, and perhaps to get over the initial shock, before they decided to seek out and become involved in a group. In a prior study (Chesler, Barbarin, and Lebo-Stein, 1984), the relationship between time elapsed since diagnosis and self-help group involvement was found to be curvilinear, with involvement low in the first two years, increasing after two years, and decreasing after four years. Thus, some time after their children had "recovered," or had died, parental involvement fell off once again. While curvilinearity could not be tested with the current dataset, both the earlier study and this more recent investigation suggest that some time generally passes after diagnosis before most parents engage in self-help group activities.

These data regarding who participated in self-help groups for parents of children with cancer affirm our observations, and those of many other group activists and leaders, that active membership is composed primarily of females. Informal observation also indicates that very few people of color—African-American, Latino or Asian-American—were represented in most of these groups. However, there are some childhood cancer self-help groups populated by significant members of Latino and/or African-American parents, especially in those hospitals and cities with a high concentration of Latino or African-American children in treatment.[3] Generally, men/fathers are involved in every group, but they rarely constitute a major proportion of any group's members. The challenge of targeting and serving the mutual support needs of persons of color, fathers, and other groups of parents of children with cancer whose voices have not been fully heard remains to be met.

Self-Help Group Participation and Coping Strategies

When a person's normal external and internal resources are challenged by the excessive demands of a situation, unique coping mechanisms are required (Lazarus and Folkman, 1984). As we discussed in Chapter 2, parents of children with cancer faced unique demands and challenges, and thus had to develop or maintain coping strategies specific to the situation. Individual parents' coping responses to their child's diagnosis and treatment varied considerably. Some employed passive strategies, electing not to acknowledge or deal directly with the challenges they faced. They complied with the medical regimens required, but generally avoided asking questions or thinking about the situation any more than absolutely necessary. Others responded to the crisis actively, gaining mastery and building skills geared toward responding to or anticipating specific problems. This included participating in the management of medical routines, reorganizing household chores and tasks, and working directly with their child's school and classroom. Active coping strategies were used by many parents, especially those who sought information about their child's illness, control over their lives, or both.[4] One parent illustrated his use of an information-seeking coping strategy as follows:

I desperately needed to learn and keep up to date on children's cancer, to obtain the technical medical information I needed.

Some parents coped by seeking help from their friends and families, as reported by one mother:

I was afraid of going it alone. I was a single parent at the time of diagnosis, and I needed to talk with people.

On the other hand, other parents chose to cope by being alone; they went for long walks and drives or prayed and thought and read a lot by themselves.

Some of these individual strategies, especially the active and publicly oriented types, seem consonant with self-help group participation, while others do not appear to be reinforced easily or directly by the mutually supportive, open, public, and collective setting of a parent group. For example, parents who share their feelings with others, seek help and information from friends, and focus on solving problems are likely to be supported in their coping efforts by the self-help group culture. In contrast, those who avoid thinking about their problems, try to be alone, and keep feelings to themselves may not be as comfortable in or as well served by a group setting. However, analysis of parents' responses from the eight-group sample indicates no significant differences in the preferred coping strategies of self-help group members and nonmembers (see Appendix A for details of coping items and scale construction). Thus, the member and nonmember portions of this sample did not differ in their use of varied coping strategies, such as seeking help, sharing feelings with others, being active, being passive or being alone. Moreover, regardless of self-help group involvement, parents reported using a wide variety of these strategies; no one pattern of coping appeared to dominate this sample. The absence of a dominant coping posture among members argues for the lack of a self-selection bias on active coping in the sample and for a more structural rather than personality-oriented view of the conscious choices made by those members who *do* become active in self-help groups (Chesney, 1989).

Self-Help Group Participation and Social Support

Many parents dealt with the stresses and crises of childhood cancer by trying to get help and support from others in their local environment. However, analysis of parents' reports of their receipt of various types of social support, and their receipt of support from various sources, showed only one statistically significant relationship with their self-help group membership (see Appendix A for the details of support items and scale construction). The only *type* of social support received that was significantly related to parents' self-help group membership involved nonmembers' reports that they received significantly more practical medical support than did members: emotional support, support for taking action, and support with family tasks and relationships did not discriminate members from nonmembers. Moreover, none of the scales of *sources* of social support significantly distinguished members from nonmembers, not help from community members, family members, friends or medical professionals. Although it did not reach an acceptable level of statistical significance, there was a strong trend for nonmembers to report receiving more support from medical professionals than did self-help group members.

Why might nonmembers of these self-help groups have reported receiving more help of a practical medical type, and more help from medical professionals, than did members (or conversely, why might members of these self-help groups have reported receiving less practical medical support and less support from medical professionals than did nonmembers)? Perhaps members' feelings of a lack of support and help from the medical staff was one of the factors that led them to join a self-help group, or perhaps their need for medical help was greater than that of nonmembers, so that regardless of what they actually received, they felt that they received less. Thus, we might assume that people who felt they received more support from the medical staff—perhaps sufficient help for their needs—had no need to join a self-help group, and no need for the additional kinds of help and support that might have been available therein. It also is possible that this causal chain may have been reversed, and that parents who were actively involved in the self-help group over time felt they received less practical medical help than they needed, especially from the medical staff. This interpretation makes sense if we assume that the self-help group experience encouraged parents to identify and articulate their needs for help, perhaps at a more complete and vigorous level than could nonmembers, and to identify and evaluate the help they received from the medical and professional staff more critically—with less satisfaction—than did nonmembers.

Reasons for Group Participation

Parents had a wide variety of motivations and agendas for becoming involved in these self-help groups. For some, the search for knowledge and information brought them to the self-help group; they viewed the group as an arena for potential learning (Kieffer, 1983–84) and problem solving (Suler, 1984). As several parents said when asked why they joined the group, the search for information sometimes centered on medical issues and sometimes on coping or lifestyle issues. Thus, at times medical experts were the appropriate educators, and at other times "peers" or "experiential educators" were the appropriate sources of information. Several parents reported directly that one reason for joining a local self-help group was to gain information.

I wanted to find out more information about leukemia and the hospital medical staff.

To learn as much as possible about cancer from others who are also experiencing the same things.

To learn to live with my leukemic child's needs—physical and emotional—and mine too.

In addition to gaining information from the medical staff and experiential knowledge from other (expert) parents, some parents reported that they joined local groups in order to receive support and affirmation. The search for support at a difficult time, perhaps when existing support resources were not functioning (Lynam, 1987) or were not perceived as most useful (Morrow, Carpenter, and Hoagland, 1984), motivated many parents of children with cancer to become group members.

We felt our friends and family really didn't understand our difficulties completely.

I was looking for support from someone other than the medical staff.

I joined for the help they provide and the support of others.

Quite explicitly, new sources (and types) of support were being sought by parents, as indicated by these excerpts. As suggested in Chapter 1 (see Table 1.1), the kinds of support and affirmation potentially forthcoming from peers in a self-help group setting were different from both the expert (but often distant and nonmutual) technical help available from the professional staff and the well-intentioned (but often misinformed and awkward) lay support available from friends and other family members.

The desire to get help in coping with some of the practical issues raised by the experience of childhood cancer also brought some parents to self-help groups.

We needed help in coping with the stresses of hospitalization and treatment of our son.

I was in *shock*, and I needed to know how others were coping.

These comments reflect parents' needs for help in learning about new coping skills—skills focused not (or not solely) on generic coping strategies, but on the specific emotional and practical tasks they faced in dealing with the stresses of childhood cancer.[5]

A number of parents indicated that the major reason they joined a group was to connect with other people having the same or similar experience. The desire to reduce social and intellectual isolation and to find the common ground of shared life experiences was repeated often.

I needed to be around people who share a common thing with me and know exactly how I'm hurting and the specific struggles I'll be going through.

Because I felt a strong need to meet others with the same problems, to reduce my feeling of isolation and of going through this alone.

We wanted to talk with other parents in similar situations.

Sometimes this search for connection and shared experience with others took the form of a desire to find out or confirm whether one's experiences and reactions were "normal."

I wanted to see if others were going through the same things my son was; whether his situations were normal or not.

Another major reason parents gave for joining a local self-help group was to provide help to others, to "give back" some of the help and support they had received from other parents.

After my son passed away I wanted to help the other parents for all they did for me while he was alive.

I wanted to establish a place to help parents that could not afford professional help and to have speakers educate other parents—and me. Also, I wanted to help those who could not attend by sending a newsletter to inform them about social activities, fund-raisers, or educational materials.

I joined because I wished they had one when we were going through treatments and I wanted to help.

These efforts to help others reflect a sense of competence and empowerment in being able to rise above one's own situation and ease others' struggles. At the same time, parents expressing this motivation seldom were naive about their altruism; most recognized and articulated the gains they themselves experienced in reaching out to and assisting others.[6]

Finally, some parents indicated that they joined for unspecifiable reasons—reasons that were stimulated by the actions of friends or by intriguing and appealing information they received.

Several friends encouraged me to go to the first meeting.

They sent a newsletter, and it sounded like something I needed.

The topic of a certain meeting's presentation interested me, and I felt that after being invited so many times I could at least attend one meeting.

The doctor said it would help, and a member came by the hospital to see us.

My husband forced the issue.

Despite the diversity and perhaps vagueness of this latter set of responses, most of the above excerpts indicate that joining a self-help group involved a fairly active, conscious choice that may have been based on a desire to satisfy a variety of personal needs, a search for personal spiritual development (Wuthnow, 1994), the attractiveness of perceived or actual group activities and orientation, or the appeal of existing group membership characteristics (Powell, 1985). Some parents' initial—even "accidental"—encounters with a self-help group resulted in a person/group "fit" that evolved into long-term involvement (Luke, Roberts, and Rappaport, 1993). At any rate, parents of children with cancer who availed themselves of these groups made the choice to spend their precious time and energy in certain ways, and to explore the unique resources of a group of supportive others with whom they shared a common crisis. Moreover, the several reasons these members cited for deciding to join and attend regular meetings of the local self-help group mirror the five major themes of self-help groups first explicated in Chapter 1 and repeated in Chapter 2 (see Table 2.2) and Chapter 4 (see Table 4.1). They include the availability of other parents and activities that provided the following:

- Experiential knowledge
- Shared life experiences
- Support and affirmation
- New coping skills for dealing with stress
- Collective empowerment and activist opportunities

Why Did Some Parents *Not* Join Self-Help Groups?

Research on self-help groups often has addressed the question of why some people joined such groups, but seldom has been able to answer the question of why others in a similar situation did not. Partly this is due to a lack of interest in answering this research question; but even for scholars and practitioners who are interested in this issue, it has been difficult to address. To do so adequately requires a sample of non-members that has been controlled in ways that render it completely comparable to a sample of members.[7]

We explore the issue of group nonparticipation or nonmembership in four ways:

1. We report members' answers to questions of why they thought others like them did not join a group.
2. We examine members' and nonmembers' reports of what they perceived went on in group sessions, in order to understand whether nonmembers accurately understood the nature of group activities, and thus whether or not their choices were informed accurately and realistically.
3. We examine members' and nonmembers' evaluation of group activities and their assessments of possible benefits and drawbacks to group involvement.
4. We discuss members' and nonmembers' reports of why they did not go to group meetings—at all or as often as they might have.

We first asked parents who were members of these groups why they thought other parents had not joined. One important reason they suggested dealt with the logistics of travel and distance from the hospital.

Distance, the treatment center covers a wide area.

It is a far distance to the meetings for some people.

Table 6.1 suggests that distance from the medical center (a stand-in for probable distance from the central meeting place of the group) was not an important or significant factor distinguishing members from nonmembers, but perhaps a greater range on the variable of distance, or a measure of the subjective experience of distance ("felt distance") rather than actual mileage, might have altered these results. It certainly was true that groups in rural areas, where great distances separated people, had a hard time holding well-attended meetings.

A second reason suggested by members was a lack of parent information about the group's existence and the nature of its operations.

Parents aren't informed about what the group offers. No one has told them there are parent groups, so they go through it by themselves.

Some people wait to be asked, and we fall short of getting to them and asking them.

The discussion in Chapter 5 of recruitment and referral tactics and problems is highlighted by the above remarks. It makes sense that parents who are not informed about a group's existence, who do not know what a group does, or who are not contacted by group members in ways that are appealing, would be less likely to join.

A third reason mentioned by parent members was the possibility of some parents having different coping strategies, ones not involving public discussion, examination, or sharing of feelings.

They have a fear of getting involved, of talking about it, of discussing cancer openly, of meeting parents of deceased children, of getting close.

It is hard for some people to admit need and accept help.

Some people are not outgoing or necessarily organizational.

Different people handle things differently. They have different reactions to an illness or a loss of their child. Some choose to put it all behind them, and some see it as a potentially positive aspect of their lives and want to focus on it.

Some people get lost in a big group and don't feel they can open up.

These perceptions by members directly address issues of coping styles or strategies, and suggest that members felt that nonmembers may have preferred to deny or get distance from their feelings, and may not have wanted to cope in public or to share their feelings in public. However, analysis of data from parent members and nonmembers discussed earlier in this chapter did not support these perceptions. Members and nonmembers in this study population did *not* appear to differ with regard to their coping strategies, at least not with regard to their generic strategies and not at a statistically significant level. However, parents' responses to the structured items regarding coping strategies may not have characterized fully their actual coping strategies, and this must remain an open question.[8]

Further elaboration of the issue of coping strategy was offered by several members who singled out men as having special difficulty in sharing their feelings, and thus as especially unlikely to find the self-help group a comfortable environment.

Men tough it out for a fear of breaking down.

The men don't want to show their emotions. They never show their emotions at a meeting but will get together at the bar and share emotions. Other men will help with fund-raising but don't seek emotional support from the group. Maybe they seek it out from their friends.

And two women who were active in a group reflected on their husbands' unwillingness to join—and perhaps on men in general—as follows:

To get a husband to sit down and talk is difficult.

My husband is just not a joiner.

These potential gender differences in expressing emotions in public certainly have been a major theme in recent research on gender relations, and may be reflected in the generally low number of men in attendance at many groups' meetings.[9]

Parents in one northwestern urban group spoke especially clearly about targeting the recruitment of special populations of parents of children with cancer, as well as about the need for assisting people who needed new social support resources in times of crisis. Their typical summer decrease in attendance at group meetings prompted the leadership core to think about ways to bring new parents and families into the group in the fall. In the early fall they sponsored a free day at an otherwise costly small amusement park, in hopes of recruiting new members. In fact, a record number of parents showed up for the first fall meeting—parents, that is, not couples. There was a noticeable absence of partners, not uncommon to these groups, but also a prevailing theme of lack of support on the homefront. More stories of marital strain and lack of family support were forthcoming at this informal social event than at any time in recent memory in the group. New members were so open about the fact that they desperately needed the special environment of mutual support and common experience the group could provide that oldtimers and leaders worried about the folks who were not there—the spouses and partners of these new people. The upshot of this concern was the formation of a subgroup for fathers and another subgroup for mothers, and the provision of childcare to facilitate both parents' attendance at meetings. These new subgroup sessions, held in addition to regular meetings, were a big success, largely because of the timely way in which the group identified the motives for participation of at least some of the new "recruits."

A fourth major reason members offered to explain why other parents of children with cancer did not join a self-help group involved the great emotional strain of the illness and treatment. They suggested that at certain times (e.g., diagnosis, relapse) there simply might not have been enough emotional energy for group participation. As several members noted,

At diagnosis, there is too much overload. There was security in ignoring, withdrawing . . . it's too painful.

There is no energy to be active when your kid is seriously ill. When you need the help the most, you can't get out to get it. When a child is so ill, there is no time for group sessions.

My life had been intruded upon. I didn't want any more interference. I didn't want to sit and talk with anyone, not even anyone who wanted to help me. When my child was in the hospital I had nothing left to give anyone else. It was taking everything I had to care for her. You can only concentrate on your child, and I didn't want help or intrusion . . . or to offer help then.

As Table 6.1 indicates, parent members were significantly more likely (72.3%) than nonmembers (27.7%) to have had their child diagnosed more than two years prior to our study. Thus, members were more likely to have passed through some of the times of most extreme stress—the diagnosis and beginnings of treatment. Figure 6.1 shows this time frame, depicting the stresses of childhood cancer discussed in Chapter 2. It indicates, with information drawn from the averaged responses of a subsample of parents ($n = 26$), how for most of them the intensity of various stresses, and thus overall stress, peaked at and shortly after diagnosis and the beginning of treatment, and tended to decrease in the months (and years) following. Certain almost "normal" events, such as major checkups, side effects, or the decision to successfully go off treatment, led to occasional re-escalation and peaks of stress. When children relapsed, experienced surgery or other relatively unique events (indicated by the dotted stress lines), this led to greater parental anxiety and higher levels of reported stress. For parents whose children did not relapse, however, stress continued over time, but at a decreasing level. Figure 6.1 is not strictly a time-line, since the events along the horizontal axis are not time periods, but significant events in parents' encounters with their children's illness and treatment.[10]

A fifth major reason members suggested for parental noninvolvement focused on groups' track records and abilities in reaching out to other parents to involve them.

Figure 6.1. Stress events and intensity, over time (N = 26)

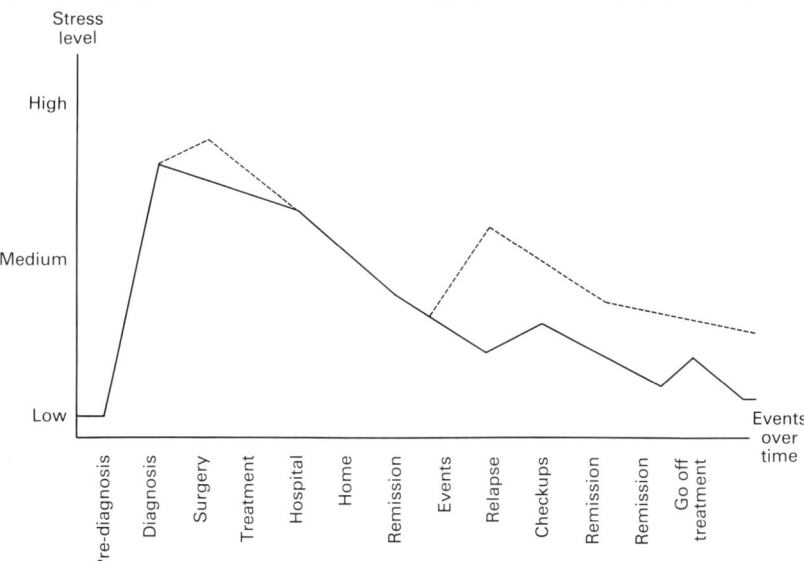

Note: The lines are averages of the height of stress indicated by parents. The solid lines represent most parents' experiences with the *most* common stresses, and the dotted lines indicate *less* common stresses.

Parents of newly diagnosed children have a hard time breaking into the veterans' group.

Perhaps this group is cliquish, and this might keep people out.

I've seen a lot of people stop coming to meetings, and it's because nothing is being offered, nothing is shared, we spend all our time on administrative matters.

There is a gap between black and white in the community, and it's in here too.

Really affluent parents don't come because maybe they're not treated at this clinic.

Thus, the way the local group went about its business, its openness to new members, its appeal to parents of diverse class and racial backgrounds, and its ability to offer useful activities and programs, also were seen as potential reasons for others not to join. Some of the data reported in Chapter 5 indicated concerns about ineffective groups that echo the above themes: concerns about groups dominated by cliques of veteran leaders and groups that spent too much time on administrative matters. Moreover, in the context of a society geographically and socially separated by race and class, it was obviously hard for self-help groups to overcome or transcend these dilemmas of social privilege or advantage/disadvantage and inclusion/exclusion. Thus, it is reasonable to expect that many local groups were not able to create environments totally conducive or attractive to parents of different social backgrounds. Although childhood cancer itself treats race, gender, and class as irrelevant, the social organization of health care, as well as local support systems, are not so egalitarian.

This approach to answering the question of why more parents of children with cancer did not join self-help groups resulted in the identification of five potential factors:

1. Logistics of distance to meetings
2. Some parents' lack of information about the group and its meetings and activities
3. Some parents' coping strategies that emphasized denial of feelings or the reality of life-threatening situations, privacy, or discomfort about dealing with emotional issues and sharing feelings in public
4. The physical and emotional strain of dealing with the illness, especially at times of high stress and shortly after diagnosis
5. Groups that did not welcome a wide range of parents, that did not operate effectively, or that did not reach out and recruit effectively.

In another approach to understanding parents' choices about group involvement, we asked both members and nonmembers to indicate the extent to which they perceived the local self-help group as engaging in various activities (of course, on cannot expect nonmembers to report accurately the activities of a group with which they were not involved). Our purpose in asking this question of nonmembers as well as members was to assess the degree to which members and nonmembers perceived the operations and activities of local groups in the same ways. If nonmembers did not see groups doing the things that members reported the groups were doing, we could explain nonparticipation on the basis of these "inaccurate" perceptions. On the other hand, if nonmembers and members perceived groups' activities in similar ways, we could be more assured that nonmembers' choices not to join the groups were based on accurate information. Table 6.2 lists a number of activities of local groups, and indicates that there are not statistically significant differences between members' and nonmembers' perceptions of the extent to which groups engaged in these activities. Perhaps information and referral patterns to self-help groups have become more consistent within local treatment centers, and as a result patients and families now have more uniform information about what local groups do or might do. Whatever the real reasons for nonmembers' decisions not to join local groups, these decisions were based on relatively accurate information, accurate at least to the extent that they conformed to members' perceptions of groups' activities.

Table 6.2. Perceptions of frequency of self-help group activities by membership (*N* = 102)

		Mean frequency		
Activity		Members (*n* = 65)	Nonmembers (*n* = 37)	Difference
a.	Talk about the stresses on the family	3.45	3.59	NS
b.	Talk about very personal feelings	3.05	3.26	NS
c.	Discuss recent advances in treatment	3.14	3.12	NS
d.	Learn how to deal with emotional issues	3.32	3.18	NS
e.	Give feedback to doctors or nurses	2.60	2.53	NS
f.	Plan to change things in hospital/ clinic	2.07	2.03	NS
g.	Raise money for the hospital	1.90	1.91	NS
h.	Plan to get together socially	3.12	2.94	NS
i.	Visit other parents at home	2.34	2.26	NS
j.	Contribute funds for needy families	2.56	2.41	NS
k.	Plan group activities	3.33	3.09	NS
l.	Discuss how to recruit new members	2.50	2.56	NS
m.	Pressing for change in social policies that affect us	2.13	2.41	NS

Notes: The means are derived from views expressed on a 4-point scale: 4 = a lot, 3 = sometimes, 2 = a little, 1 = never.

NS: No significant difference between members' and nonmembers' responses.

In addition to assessing members' and nonmembers' information about group activities and operations, we also sought to assess the evaluative judgments they made about these groups and their potential benefits and drawbacks. Several important statistically significant differences did occur in parents' evaluations of groups, presented in Table 6.3. Members' and nonmembers' assessments of groups differed in several important ways. First, nonmembers were significantly more likely than members to evaluate groups' as having a "negative" capacity to increase parental stress (to fail to reduce emotional stress, to fail to decrease parents' loneliness, and at less than a statistically significant level

Table 6.3. Parents' views of self-help groups by membership

View		Mean views about groups		
		Members	Nonmembers	Significance
a.	Groups will lead to questioning medical authority	2.71	2.94	NS
b.	Groups will increase the emotional stress on parents	1.80	2.50	*
c.	Groups will encourage nontraditional treatment choices	1.98	2.36	*
d.	Groups help people feel less lonely	4.42	3.96	*
e.	Groups will make parents sad	2.13	2.29	NS
f.	Groups will increase parental misinformation	1.82	2.26	*
g.	Groups will reduce parents' emotional stress	4.14	3.48	*
h.	Groups will encourage inappropriate coping patterns	1.76	2.38	*
i.	Groups will encourage parental anger	1.98	2.27	NS
j.	Groups will encourage attacks on professionals	1.70	1.92	NS
k.	Groups will invade parental privacy	1.77	2.21	NS
l.	Groups give parents hints about how to solve problems	4.18	3.76	*

Notes: Means derived from views rated on a 5-point scale: 5 = definitely agree, 1 = definitely disagree
NS: No significant difference between members' and nonmembers' responses.
* Difference is statistically significant at the .05 level or beyond, using the F-test of means in a one-way, single-factor analysis of variance.

to encourage parental anger, to invade parental privacy). Moreover, nonmembers were significantly more likely than members to assess groups as likely to increase misinformation and to fail to provide help in solving problems. Finally, nonmembers were significantly more likely than members to assess groups as encouraging nontraditional treatments and inappropriate coping (and at less than a statistically significant level to encourage treatment comparisons). Parents who were members of these groups obviously assessed their groups more positively on these dimensions. These differential, albeit generalized, judgments about groups begin to provide real insight into nonmembers' choices. To the extent that some parents saw groups providing nonhelpful—or worse, inappropriate—help, or as increasing rather than decreasing emotional stress, or as providing misinformation rather than helpful information, it was reasonable for them to avoid group involvement.

As a final inquiry into parents' decision to join or not to join self-help groups, we asked nonmembers directly to indicate some of the reasons they did not attend group meetings, and asked members why they did not attend group meetings more often. As Table 6.4 indicates, nonmembers gave many more responses to this question than did members (the 65 members provided a total of 52 reasons, while the 37 nonmembers provided 68 reasons). Table 6.4 also indicates that parents who were

Table 6.4. Reasons parents don't go to (more) meetings (N = 102)

Reason	Percent of members	Percent of nonmembers
Too emotional	2	12
Conflicts with other things	12	12
Not relevant	17	10
Logistics	13	18
Time or energy	37	26
Private person	0	12
No problems	15	3
Other stories too painful	4	7
Total reasons	100%	100%

Note: Because of the opportunity for multiple responses, the total number of reasons (52 from members; 68 from nonmembers) is greater than the total number of respondents (65 members; 37 nonmembers).

group members reported that they sometimes did not attend meetings primarily because of time and energy drains, logistic problems with meetings, conflicts with other events, or because certain meetings were not relevant for them at the time. Parents who were not group members also emphasized time and energy drains, logistics and conflicts, but in addition they indicated the priority of other reasons for not attending: being a private person, and feeling that the group was too emotional. The particular combination of perceiving self-help groups as being too emotional or increasing emotional stress and identifying oneself as a "private person" is a powerful deterrent to participation.

We also assessed whether joining a self-help group was in some way an extension of people's general willingness (or unwillingness) to join groups and organizations of all sorts, and was not necessarily specific to self-help groups or their childhood cancer situation. Thus, we posed a variety of questions to members and nonmembers regarding the extent to which a person should be involved in civic or social issues and their own actual involvement in such issues and organizations. Members and nonmembers did not differ significantly in their ratings of the importance of citizen involvement in national, local, or medical issues. However, members were significantly more likely (71.4%) than were nonmembers (32.4%) to be involved in human-service-oriented voluntary activities, and also were significantly more likely (82%) to be active in a wide variety of voluntary and civic organizations (e.g., unions, social groups, cooperatives) than were nonmembers (45.9%). These findings suggest that self-help group members may have been more inclined toward general voluntary and civic action than were nonmembers.[11]

Conclusions About Parents' Decisions to Join a Group

These approaches to the question of why some parents of children with cancer joined local self-help groups and others did not result in several different, and sometimes contradictory, answers. Among the dominant and repetitive or reliable answers were the following:

1. Information about groups' existence and programs. Members suggested a lack of such information as a reason others might not have joined, but non-members surveyed did appear to know what local groups were doing, or at least they agreed with members' perceptions of group activities (see Table 6.2). It is possible, however, that medical staff members failed to inform

some parents about a group's existence, and that this basic lack of information still was a factor for some parents in some medical settings.

2. Distance from the hospital or group meeting place. Although members also suggested this explanation, and some nonmembers did refer to it as a relevant factor, Table 6.1 did not confirm that it differentiated members from nonmembers. It is possible that a subjective sense of distance, in terms of travel time, energy, logistic impediments, and the comfort of varied meeting places, was more relevant than mileage per se.

3. Time and energy (physical and emotional) available. Members indicated that lack of time and energy sometimes led to their missing meetings, and this factor also was indicated as important by parents who had decided not to join a local group. They both suggested that the strain of dealing with the illness may have wearied some parents enough that they had no energy left for group meetings (perhaps this is another aspect of the concept of "subjective distance"). Time and energy may have been especially precious at times of diagnosis or during a medical crisis, and some data in Table 6.1 indicated that parents were more likely to be in a group two years after diagnosis, rather than shortly thereafter, when their shock and stress may have eased somewhat—or when they may have become more accustomed to the continuing stresses of childhood cancer.

4. Way of coping with stress. Members suggested that a pattern of denial of stress, or of coping with stress in private, so that there was not a felt need for or comfort in group activities, helped explain nonparticipation. Analyses of closed-ended survey questions regarding the use of various coping strategies failed to indicate differences between members and nonmembers in this regard, but both members and nonmembers suggested in their open-ended responses the relevance of this factor in their discussions of why some people might not or did not join a local self-help group. This factor seems especially relevant for helping to explain why more men did not join local groups.

5. Some groups did not extend a welcome to a wide range of potential members. Group members suggested that poor leadership, cliques, an overemphasis on administrative issues, and a failure to overcome societal patterns of race and class separation might explain why more parents did not join local groups.

6. Activities that met parents' needs. Depending upon the activities emphasized in a particular local group (e.g., fund-raising, social events, intense emotional discussions or informational sessions), some members suggested that the group's inability to meet some parents' needs was one reason they did not attend more meetings and why others might not attend any at all. More active members obviously felt—and reported—that their needs for

information, support, and so on were being met by group activities and programs.

7. Perceptions of goals or potential outcomes of groups. Many parents who were not members of groups indicated, in Table 6.3, that they were more concerned than were members that self-help groups were likely to increase rather then decrease parental stress, be too emotional, increase misinformation and inappropriate coping patterns, and encourage nontraditional treatment choices.

We could not, with the available data, "test" all of these explanations, nor analyze their respective power and relevance in contributing to parents' choices. We also could not resolve instances where different ways of approaching the issue (e.g., structured survey questions v. open-ended responses, asking members' views v. asking nonmembers' views) led to different explanations. By triangulating the responses gained from different approaches, however, and by combining different forms of information, we have been able to identify these seven potential reasons for parental participation or nonparticipation. In addition, this list provides some interesting starting points for further inquiry and for better planning of local groups' recruitment and programming efforts.[12]

In Chapter 7 we continue this individual-level inquiry, examining some of the reported outcomes of self-help group membership, and how parents of children with cancer felt they benefited from their involvement in these groups.

7

How People Benefit
from Self-Help Groups
The Outcomes of Participation

In this chapter we examine parents' reports of the benefits they derived from self-help group membership. Within the context of their stresses and struggles with the deep and troubled waters of childhood cancer, many parents talked about how communication and communion with others eased their pain and increased their skills and options. Individual members provided rich and revealing evidence of positive life changes and new skills and resources they attributed to self-help group participation. In an attempt to understand the sources of these positive reports, we compare self-help group members' and nonmembers' reported outcomes of their experiences in dealing with childhood cancer. Members who were active leaders of these groups shared additional insights regarding how their roles in these self-help groups benefited them especially.

Benefits of Group Membership

In response to the stresses and demands of childhood cancer, parents were challenged to develop and use new resources and abilities. Many of these new responses have been identified by parents themselves as deriving from their experience in a self-help group; in a sense, they represent the benefits of self-help group involvement. Table 7.1 indicates parents' mean reports of a number of perceived self-help group benefits. The five major types of benefits categorized in this table match the major themes of self-help involvement:

1. Sharing life experiences with others in a similar situation
2. Gaining new practical coping skills
3. Gaining experiential knowledge and information
4. Getting emotional support and affirmation
5. Feeling empowered and adopting an activist role.[1]

Shared Life Experiences

The highest-ranked set of benefits shown in Table 7.1 were associated with being able to meet and talk with other parents. As some parents elaborated,

The pain may not be necessarily diminished but somehow more bearable when the lonely struggle and alienation of social isolation is replaced by the comfort of knowing that others share and experience it too.

Mutual support made it easier, talking to others dealing with the same problems—(ones) sometimes even the family couldn't deal with.

One of the most crucial aspects of adjustment and adaptation to the continuing crisis of childhood cancer was the opportunity for disclosure and self-acknowledgement provided by the mutual support group.[2] Through public sharing and disclosure parents engaged in a process of social comparison and, for some, identification with a larger group and transformation of their own social identity. As they shared life experiences and feelings, they subtly compared themselves with others. They compared diagnoses and treatments of their children, their own personal and familial reactions, and their future options. As they discovered the existence of a larger group of other parents with whom they shared similar and vital life experiences, many parents began to identify themselves as "part of a larger group," and some began to adopt a new social identity as a parent of a child with cancer, as a member of a widespread family or community of suffering with special interests and needs.

The activity of one group located in the suburbs of a major eastern city provided an example of the benefits of sharing feelings and exploring new social identities. This parent population was much more homogeneous financially and occupationally than most groups. Most of the mothers did not work outside of the home. Most of the fathers worked in highly paid, high-stress urban settings, and generally found little sup-

Table 7.1. Benefits of self-help group participation (members only, $N = 65$)

Reported benefit	Mean
Shared life experiences	
Meeting others with similar problems	3.70
Talking about my child	3.66
Feeling part of a larger group	3.45
New coping skills	
Coping with my child's problems	3.68
Getting help from other parents	3.45
Being helpful to other parents	3.52
Coping with public attitudes	3.25
Learning to cope differently	3.23
Coping with problems in my family	3.09
Dealing with my child's school	3.00
Experiential knowledge	
Understanding the treatments	3.54
Getting information about cancer	3.49
Learning my "rights" as a parent	3.22
Learning who's on the staff	3.08
Emotional support and affirrnation	
Expressing and learning compassion	3.52
Feeling freer to express feelings	3.46
Being supported/approved of	3.35
Developing self-confidence	3.00
Feeling a spiritual uplift	2.74
Feeling empowered and adopting an activist role	
Developing self-confidence	3.00
Getting help from the medical staff	2.92
Being an active part of the medical care system	2.83
Learning to be a leader	2.72
Changing things in the hospital	2.22

Note: Means were derived from a 4-point scale: 4 = much benefit, 3 = some benefit, 2 = little benefit, 1 = no benefit.

port in the work setting to help them after their child's diagnosis. It was nearly impossible for them to get even minimal time off from work to attend treatments or discussions with their children's doctors. They reported that their co-workers generally were not supportive of or interested in hearing about their struggles as fathers of children with cancer.

In the industry in which they worked, largely Fortune 500 companies, there was a low level of workplace support and almost no assistance for the new demands of their role as fathers in crisis. As a result, most men chose to protect their jobs and financial status by keeping feelings about decreasing control over their lives to themselves, and consequently continued with their heavy work schedules, thereby missing time with their ill children. A few jeopardized—and some, in fact, lost—their jobs by taking time off to be with their child and family. When individual parents, especially individual fathers, got together in the group, they began to discuss their new social status as fathers of children with cancer. They began to view this new status as a major, self-defining one, and one that required new responses—at home and in the workplace. Most importantly, they formed a subcommittee to compare and develop strategies for presenting the conflicts of family and work roles to their co-workers and supervisors. The experiences they shared in the self-help group gave them the information and support that led them to adopt and act on their new social role.

In fact, many parents often *were* profoundly different after their child's diagnosis, and the self-help group often provided benefits that resulted in members' greater understanding of and ability to respond to their newly acquired social situations as parents of children with cancer. The unique experience of caring for and advocating for their own child was recognized in the self-help group more immediately and fully than by others in the community, workplace, or society at large. Through self-help group contact with others in a similar situation, parents were often able to overcome their sense of estrangement and confusion, and once again feel part of a community—now a new community. A new identity—albeit grounded in crisis—helped reduce the isolation and powerlessness many parents felt.[3]

New Coping Skills

A second highly ranked set of benefits of group participation centered around parents' ability to cope differently, especially with their child's problems, with the external community, and with the opportunity to be helpful to other parents. The new demands of a child's illness put unique strains on parents' skills, and many group activities facilitated the development of new skills geared to meeting that challenge. Hearing what occurred in other families, recognizing how others adapted their skills to their child's needs, and—in the worst case—learning how parents dealt with the death of a child, helped many parents feel better about and respond more effectively to their own situations. Several parents reported such benefits in the form of practical coping skills that were generated by self-help group membership:

I felt I would never figure out how to deal with this! Other folks told me what they did, how they coped. That helped a lot.

One woman talked about losing her child and how she was there for all of us to hear her and know she was still whole. Did that mean that I could really think positively and make it through that too? I needed to follow what she said.

Things are all different after the diagnosis. You need to change how you look at each day. I would not have believed that would work for me, but the group said it would—and they were right.

Self-help group members in a southern city were challenged to learn new ways of coping from each other by the example of a brave young man who dealt in his own way with his illness. After experiencing several rounds of unsuccessful treatment for his cancer, a young man who was the son of active group members implored his parents to respect his desire to terminate and avoid more aggressive treatment, and seek hospice assistance for the process of dying. His parents looked to their fellow group members to help them understand his refusal of what they felt was potentially life-sustaining, although risky and painful, therapy. None of the other parents had themselves faced such a coping challenge, yet they were able to talk with this family about their own strategies for coping with their families' needs and decisions. In the face of such an acute call for help, the group was able to pool its resources and enable this family to find its own way of coping, strengthened by collective wisdom and support. In the end, these parents elected to support their son's wishes, and the group members continued to provide support to the entire family through the terminal period of this young man's life.

Many parents were at once givers and receivers of help in the self-help group setting, and benefited from both processes simultaneously. Those who helped were helped themselves as they used the group arena to display both the resources they had to offer and their own continued need for assistance. Several parents reported evidence of this benefit as follows:

The group which I am working with gives me something positive to do. I feel that I am helping someone down the road and changing things in a positive and constructive manner.

I talked a lot and hope I helped other people by being there.

In the process of helping others, many parents discovered that they had information, skill, compassion, and even energy beyond their earlier self-assessments. Some discovered that even in the midst of a personal crisis they had spare resources, that they could reach out to and care about others. Perhaps these acts of helping others helped distract some parents from their own pain and anxiety. Perhaps they helped parents respond to some of the stresses of social isolation and existential loneliness or confusion.[4] Whatever roles mutual support and help-giving played in people's lives, much of this reciprocal helping proceeded on a communal rather than exchange basis (Clark, 1983), without the expectation of "payback" so common in friends' and neighbors' good works.[5] It also often led to the development of lasting and intimate social bonds.

Gaining Experiential Knowledge

In response to their child's diagnosis and treatment, parents needed much new information. They needed to understand as much as possible about their child's present and future health status, treatment regimen, access to hospital personnel and resources, and psychosocial responses. As Table 7.1 demonstrates, parents felt that the self-help group provided them with informational benefits by serving as a clearinghouse for needed information and by promoting the sharing of life experiences. In this social setting, parents not only received technical information about the illness and treatments that resolved some of their anxieties, but also confirmation that many of their questions were valid and that their fears were reasonable; thus, knowledge that others had similar questions and concerns was enormously comforting. As several parents reported,

Information other parents shared made it easier to deal with the system, to understand treatments and drugs better. I even learned to ask questions of the staff.

I was able to absorb more information in the group over time than you can learn from the staff at the time of diagnosis. You don't always know what you need to learn.

Regardless of the breadth and detail of knowledge provided by members of the medical staff, there were some things that parents could learn only (or perhaps best) from their peers. For example, physicians seldom were experts on children's toilet training, yet parents who had dealt with young children whose bowel control had regressed as a function of chemotherapeutically induced diarrhea or constipation had crucial experiential knowledge to pass on to other parents currently experiencing this difficult problem. In similar fashion, veteran parents often had experiential wisdom about how to maintain some reasonable nutritional levels in children whose appetites had been ravaged by treatments (e.g., How many vitamin pills can you stick into a Twinkie and not spoil the taste? How do you slip crushed vitamins or pills into a chocolate milkshake?). This sort of experiential expertise represents a unique wisdom created and shared by parents. It echoes one of the core themes of self-help: new knowledge, special knowledge, knowledge by people with firsthand experience, and knowledge that is created by the acts of collective sharing that occur in a group.

It also was important for parents to get information about the workings of the medical care system—information gleaned from the experiences of other parents. This knowledge enabled parents to identify key actors and to maximize their own and their child's interactions with the medical system. Information about their own and their children's rights also enhanced some parents' sense of control and direction. For instance, parents of newly diagnosed children picked up valuable clues about the personalities and styles of the medical staff from veteran self-help group members. In one group, parents who had received somewhat contradictory information about the probability of their child's survival from two different doctors on the staff, were relieved when they were informed that other parents knew very well that one of the physicians was "chronically depressed and pessimistic." Group members felt that this physician was competent and caring, but consistently presented them with the most negative interpretations and prognoses— perhaps as a way of dealing with his own emotional pain. In another group situation, it was helpful when several parents consoled a mother of a newly diagnosed child with the information that they, too, had experienced a given staff member as unable to "talk nicely" to mothers; members reported that this physician regularly bypassed, ignored, or put down mothers as he addressed himself primarily to fathers. These examples of parental experiential wisdom in the form of sharing information about staff members' styles and of (re)interpreting staff members' behaviors occurred regularly in many self-help groups.

Another example of parents' unique contributions to each others' knowledge bases comes from a support group in the southwest. This group drew its members from several hospitals serving as treatment centers for the many parents whose primary language was Spanish, not English. This language difference posed difficulties for some parents who spoke only Spanish, and additional difficulties for the caring, hard-working, but monolingual (in English) staff who was constantly trying to disseminate knowledge and information to parents of newly diagnosed children. The self-help group gathered and developed bilingual resources—pamphlets, videos, and translators—in the clinic. In addition, they scheduled presentations by parents, for the staff and other parents, about various cultural groups' lifestyles and preferences, including festivals and holidays. The membership of the self-help group grew substantially, as did the volume of requests for written Spanish-language information about treatment and community resources. One year later, when the inevitable needs-assessment was conducted by administrators of two of the local hospitals, the self-help group was identified by parents as one of the major sources of information—so much so that one of the hospitals began supporting the group overtly and enthusiastically, in contrast to their prior passive posture. Better-informed parents helped to make the hospital administration better informed about the group, resulting in more information being made available to more parents.

Getting Emotional Support and Affirmation

Table 7.1 also indicates that self-help group membership resulted in emotional benefits that may not have been available elsewhere. Thus, private realities (hopes and fears, struggles with their own and others' emotions) could be expressed and explored publicly. In their own special setting, parents publicly shared their fears and hopes, supported and approved of one another, vented strong emotions, and validated some of their "strange" or "crazy" responses.[6] For example, some parents needed a forum for expressing their feelings of isolation and disbelief, especially shortly after their child's diagnosis; others sometimes questioned their own mental health, and wanted a safe place to voice that concern; still others reported feeling guilty or awkward about wanting some respite from the pressures of caring for their ill child and a chance to rest or laugh or cry by themselves. Some parents used the group setting to vent their "horror stories" with parents who understood and could sympathize with their feelings of terror or anger. It often was difficult to do any of these things with friends and family members, but other members of the self-help group understood these needs, and often were willing to provide respite care and "swap stories." These reported benefits provide evidence of peers' responses to the unique emotional challenges of childhood cancer; in the self-help group parents who needed emotional suport were given a stage and found a voice and a responsive audience.

The essence of the emotional support and affirmation that many parents found beneficial in the self-help group environment involved others hearing what each parent said, and each parent hearing what others had to say. Experiencing what others like oneself went through and feeling what they felt often led to gaining confidence in one's own feelings, reactions, and decisions. For some, the group environment and supportive atmosphere was uplifting spiritually as well. The result, for many, was that they felt supported and approved of by people who really knew what was going on for them and their child.[7] As several parents reported,

The group meetings give me hope. We support each other like pillars; we hold each other up through the hard times.

When I see someone else who is going through the same thing I am, and they can handle it, then I can conquer it too.

Most of the parents in one self-help group in a midwestern city came with their children for treatment to a large, university-affiliated medical center. The staff there had tried repeatedly to recruit parents to the group from nearby farm communities, not just from the local city. One evening open-house for prospective parent group members was especially effective in making the emotional benefits of self-help group participation clear to all. It was held at the new Ronald McDonald House that was part of the medical complex. The promise of refreshments, information about new therapies, and games for children lured many nongroup members to the wintry evening event. The children enjoyed themselves, while the parents from the self-help group circulated with a quiet determination throughout the room, encouraging newcomers to come listen to stories told by "oldtimers." An informal version of the regular group meeting was held, so that new parents could more readily feel a part of things. No attempt was made to make them share experiences; but as the veterans' stories flowed, new attendees started to chime in. Invitations to attend the next regular meeting were made, and sign-up sheets were passed, but nothing much happened. Suddenly, one woman who had previously identified herself as one of the longest-standing members spoke clearly and dramatically. She stated that so many new faces made her think vividly about when she finally found a niche in the group at a crisis point in her child's treatment, and quietly she began to cry. One by one, obviously moved by familiar emotions and pain, each of the new parents got up to sign the sheet to be contacted for the next meeting. The voice of parental experience sounded enough like their own—no longer alone, but still special and in need—that all identified the potential emotional benefits ahead for them as group members.

Feeling Empowered and Adopting an Activist Role

Although activism-related benefits of self-help group involvement were not ranked as highly as others in Table 7.1, many parents indicated that they gained confidence and benefited from groups' efforts to be part of the medical care system, and even to play a role in improving clinic or hospital procedures and policies. Active engagement in the external social environment affecting oneself and one's child, as contrasted with the internal psychological benefits of gaining skills and expressing feelings, is another framework for the positive effects of group membership on parents. Several parents indicated these benefits, both for themselves and for others, as follows:

I have become more assertive with the medical staff as a result of being in the group. When my three-year-old had to receive a spinal tap, I told the nurse I wanted to stay in the room. The nurse replied, "It isn't going to be pretty," but I insisted, and I was right. My daughter was calmer when I could hold her.

I feel good about helping to alleviate financial strain for some in our area and keep the group going.

I feel better when I see improvements in the system, which are always needed.

A parent group affiliated with a northeastern urban hospital viewed itself as an integral part of both the hospital and the community, a vision ultimately realized through their interactions with these social systems. The hospital catchment population included both urban and rural patients, and the parents in both areas got to know each other at group meetings. As it turned out, many of the self-help group members had a vision of the kind of impact they could have on their childrens' care center—the area urban hospital. Those visions ranged from vague notions of parent rights to specific roles for parent advocates. The group lobbied for and got a paid staff role for a parent-advocate position sanctioned by and supported by the hospital—a new commitment on the part of physicians and administrators. The parent group became a regular and institutionalized part of the hospital community through the group-level advocacy they successfully promoted.

These five categories of benefits continue to echo the principal reasons parents gave for joining a local group (see Chapter 6) and the five core themes of self-help groups outlined in Chapter 1. They include the sharing of life experiences with other parents, giving and getting skills in coping with the stress of childhood cancer, gaining experiential knowledge, getting emotional support and affirmation, and developing a sense of empowerment and a stance of activism.

Parental "Outcomes" of the Childhood Cancer Experience

Several research studies have reported that parents of children with cancer often state that they coped well with their child's illness and its aftermath.[8] In fact, a substantial number of parents reported that their lives changed for the better as a result of their experience with childhood cancer—or perhaps as a result of the ways in which they dealt with this experience. In order to understand the possible connections between such reports and self-help group participation, we first examined parents' reports of their coping adequacy and the life changes that they experienced. Parents' views of themselves and of their social and emotional situations since their child's diagnosis can be indicators of internal and external adjustments, or life changes, and some of these may have been facilitated by group membership. In fact, researchers and clinicians, in attempts to evaluate the outcomes of self-help group membership, commonly ask about tangible evidence of cognitive and social benefits.

We explored the question of outcomes of self-help group participation in several ways. First, we asked parents, "In general, how well have you handled your child's illness?" Table 7.2 indicates that 56% of the sample of 112 parents (in Study #3) reported that they felt they handled their child's illness "very well," 44% checked the "fairly well" option on the questionnaire, and none checked "not well at all."[9] A second series of questions asked parents to indicate the extent to which their lives had

Table 7.2. Outcome measures of coping adequacy and life changes

A. Outcome measures ($N = 112$)	
1. Coping adequacy: "How well did you handle your child's illness?"	Percent reporting
Very well	56
Fairly well	44
Not well	0
2. Life changes	Scale means
a. Mental health	+.14
b. Activism	+.54
c. Life satisfaction	+.29
d. Physical health	−.09

B. Parents' reports of their coping adequacy by reported life changes ($N = 112$)			
Reported life changes	Scale means		Difference
	Handled very well	Handled fairly well	
a. Mental health	+.32	−.07	*
b. Activism	+.63	+.42	*
c. Life satisfaction	+.37	+.20	
d. Physical health	−.18	−.02	

Note: The means were determined from responses coded on a three-point scale, ranging from changes for the "worse" (−1) through "same" (0) to "better" (+1).
 * Significant at the $p < .05$ level, using a one-way, single-factor analysis of variance.

changed, had gotten "worse," "better," or "stayed the same" since their child's illness.[10] Table 7.2 also indicates that the aggregate sample of parents reported that their lives had improved relatively since their child's experience with cancer—mean scores on three of the four scales are positive, indicating movement in a "better" or positive direction of life change. Only changes in the assessment of one's physical health changed relatively—and slightly—in a negative direction. Table 7.2 indicates that parents who reported that they handled their child's illness "very well" more often reported life changes for the better, significantly so with regard to changes in their mental health and activism. Thus, in this sample there is consistency (or reliability) in these two outcome measures—self-assessed coping adequacy and reported life changes.[11]

How, then, should we interpret these findings about positive coping outcomes, in general and with regard to the specific life changes assessed?[12] We could attribute these life-change scores to differences in parents' feelings from the nadir of shock and despair of the immediate post-diagnostic period and the early stages of their child's illness to the current time, and not to a generally positive comparison of their situations prior to the diagnosis and when the data were collected. After all, Figure 6.1 indicated that parents' reports of their stress levels were highest right at and after diagnosis. We also could treat parents' responses to both sets of these outcome questions—coping adequacy and life changes—as examples of "denial"—of parents' unwillingness to admit to themselves or to others that they were not able to cope with such a difficult situation. Or perhaps parents of children with cancer deliberately presented themselves as "up," as on top of a situation; by feeling and acting as if they coped well, they may also have become convinced of their successful coping. At the same time, they may have tried to convince others of their success, thereby avoiding the pity of others and the stigma of weakness.[13]

Perhaps, too, parents altered their self-anchored definition of coping, and meant by "coping well" under these extraordinary circumstances simply that their heads had been above water, and that they were still alive, well, and doing what was necessary (for self, for child, for family) despite great trauma. What else could they have done? The very life and health of their child and family demanded that they be able to care for their child, respond to other family members and generally cope with the situation. Some parents may have seen themselves as having grown relative to the crisis at hand, growth defined in this sense as "a better capacity to fulfill the vital roles one is expected to play" (Wuthnow, 1994, p. 210) as the parent of an ill child. A final option is to accept these findings at face value, as indicating a new and positive sense of self and strength gained in the process of dealing with a parent's worst nightmare. In this sense, the demands of dealing with their child's cancer may have provided some parents with the opportunity (or forced them) to learn new skills, become aware of and master new feelings, gain new insights into themselves, and behave differently. These various interpretations are not necessarily exclusive of one another, but the fact that this generally positive message about coping was confirmed in this sample through several different methods of inquiry, and by several other studies and researchers, should provide increased confidence in its validity.[14] Of course, these findings should not be taken to mean that it was "good" for parents to have a child diagnosed with cancer, or that any parent was happy with that situation.

We explored coping adequacy and life changes further by investigating what parents meant when they reported that they coped "very well" or "fairly well" with the childhood cancer experience. For instance, we asked parents directly what it was that they handled well or less well. Their open-ended answers, categorized in Table 7.3, identified five ma-

Table 7.3. Parents' open-ended responses to what they handled well and handled less well (N = 166)

| | | Coping adequacy | | |
	Coping task	Well (n = 92) %	Less well (n = 74) %	Total responses (n = 166) %
1.	Managing my own emotions	29	38	34
2.	Dealing with family and lifestyle issues	22	27	24
3.	Dealing with medical treatment issues	21	15	18
4.	Dealing with my child's emotions	15	7	11
5.	Dealing with medical routines	11	12	11
6.	Everything/nothing	2	1	2
	Total	100	100	100

Note: Some respondents provided more than one response.

jor categories of coping tasks that represent the content of the issues parents felt they had to deal with, and thus the context of parents' responses to the question of how well they coped. The data indicate that parents felt they coped relatively well with medical treatment issues and their child's emotions (more "well" than "less well" responses), and relatively less well with their own emotions and family lifestyle issues (proportionately more "less well" than "well" responses).

For example, with specific regard to the *management of their own emotions,* several parents said, in a positive vein,

I've accepted her illness and am 99% convinced that we will be able to control it.

It was important to be optimistic and keep positive thoughts.

On the other hand, a less-positive perspective was provided by parents who said,

The fear of relapse, at times, is almost unbearable.

Dealing with my anger and frustration was hard when I watched her suffer physically as well as emotionally. I resent the fact that my daughter has given up most of her ten years and socialization. You can never give that back to her.

The necessity of *maintaining a relatively normal lifestyle,* and dealing with other family members' reactions, occupied a significant amount of parents' time and energy. It both stressed and defined their coping capacities. Several parents mentioned their "successes" in this regard:

I kept family life normal and positive after the diagnosis.

I shared my thoughts and feelings openly with my family.

Parents also reported negative outcomes in dealing with these issues:

I had marital problems . . . lack of communication on my husband's part.

I had trouble dealing with my relatives, and sometimes I was too tired to deal with my other children.

As Table 7.3 indicates, when it came to the issue of maintaining family life and managing family members' reactions, parents indicated proportionately more examples of not coping well than of coping well.

In contrast, *coping with the medical aspects of treatment* was reported by parents as a task they more often handled well.

I handled the treatment well . . . chemotherapy, surgery, radiation, and the physical and medical consequences.

However, for some, this too was a depressing situation:

When my son had ill side-effects from the medicine and treatment, and got sick, that was probably the most depressing for me.

Dealing with one's child's emotions was also an issue that parents more often reported handling well as opposed to less well.

I kept the child's life as normal as possible.

I was good at being a friend, a loving mommy, a more devoted caretaker to his needs, a nurse, etc.

This was true in general, despite the fact that dealing with emotionally distressed children was hard.

Her crying and not smiling upset me. She never cried before she got cancer.

Talking about death with my ill child was hard.

Evidently these are the key issues parents had to handle in coping with their child's illness. Parents' extended comments about these issues add considerable depth and meaning to the structured questions about their coping outcomes. Managing their feelings and emotional reactions, their child's emotional reactions, and their social relationships with other family members obviously occupied center stage, and provided the greatest challenges. In addition, parents had to find ways to manage the practical and technical aspects of medical treatment, including their relationships with the hospital or clinic staff and varied routines as well as logistical arrangements. More effective or less effective coping with these issues defined much of parents' reports of their general coping adequacy.

The Relationship Between Self-Help Group Participation and Outcomes

If parents of children with cancer did cope relatively effectively with this experience, including some who reported significant personal growth, what might have been the role of self-help groups in this process? Table 7.4 indicates a positive and statistically significant set of relationships between self-help group membership and the outcome measures of coping adequacy and life changes. Parents who were members of local self-help groups were significantly more likely than nonmembers to report that they coped "very well" (Table 7.4) and to report significantly more positive life changes with respect to their mental health and activism, and less negative changes in their physical health (Table 7.4). No set of findings could more dramatically reinforce our contention of an association between self-help group membership and real psychosocial as well as practical benefits for parents of children with cancer.

The bridge evidently worked—it helped members more successfully cross the troubled waters of childhood cancer. Not only did group members self-assess their own coping as more adequate in general than did nonmembers, but members also viewed changes in their own mental health and activism more positively and were better able to deal with challenges to their physical health. However, it is clear that we have made a choice of interpretive frameworks in arguing that it is self-help group membership that leads to these more positive coping outcomes. It also is possible to argue in a reverse direction, that people who were coping more positively self-selected themselves into self-help groups. Moreover, one could argue that parents who became self-help group

Table 7.4. Coping outcomes by self-help group membership ($N = 102$)

	Members ($n = 65$)	Nonmembers ($n = 37$)	Difference
A. Coping adequacy			
Very well	42	13	*
Fairly well	23	24	
B. Mean life changes (scale)			
Mental health	+.26	−.04	*
Activism	+.68	+.22	*
Physical health	−.03	−.27	*
Satisfaction	+.35	+.35	NS

* Difference is statistically significant at the .05 level or beyond, using the chi-square test of distribution in A, or the *F*-test of means in a one-way, single-factor analysis of variance in B.

members reported positive coping outcomes as a way of justifying or rationalizing the time and energy they put into group activities, and as a way of resolving their cognitive dissonance or tension about such investments. We chose the interpretive frame we did on several bases: (1) its consistency with our general theoretical and applied approach of examining the social role and utility of self-help groups; (2) the evidence that parents' reports of several of the prior categories of self-help group benefits were also positively related to reports of coping outcomes, especially to activism (Chesney, 1989); and (3) parents' own reports of the causal connection between their self-help group participation and positive outcomes, as presented below.[15]

Parents who were members reported, in their own words, some of the ways in which they felt that their self-help group involvement was related to gains in their mental health.

The group gave me the realization that it was all right to feel panic in the beginning and a complete and utter sense of loss of control.

The other people there are testimony enough that life goes on.

They know how it feels and how your life changes, and thus can help.

With regard to increased activism, parents remarked,

The group meetings made it easier for me to deal with the system. I took the chance to ask questions of the staff.

The group gave me the impetus to start a petition to make a change on the pediatric floor.

In addition to these findings, more empirical as well as theoretical support is appearing in the literature for the argument that participation in self-help groups and other voluntary organizational activities can increase psychological feelings of well-being and empowerment.[16]

In order to pursue further the possibility that other factors besides self-help group membership might have helped create these positive outcomes, we used an iterative (user-defined, stepwise) multiple regression procedure to analyze the interactive influence of parental coping strategies, social support mechanisms, demographic factors, and group membership on reported life changes. Membership alone significantly explained these outcome differences between members and nonmem-

bers.[17] How did self-help groups help create these outcomes? In order
to explore that question, we reexamined the reports of self-help group
members *only*, for only they directly experienced the groups' influences. Analyses revealed little direct association between parents' perceptions of particular group activities and their reports of life changes,
but substantial significant association between perceived benefits and
these outcome measures. Correlations exploring the relationships between parents' reports of the benefits they received from group involvement and their reported life changes indicated that the strongest link
between benefits and life changes occurred with regard to positive
changes in activism. Not surprisingly, given the physical and emotional
stresses of childhood cancer, the weakest relationships occurred with
respect to the outcome of changes in parents' reported health. Regardless of the benefits of peer support, group involvement could not overcome the negative impact of parenting a child with cancer on one's physical health.

Some additional, although quite general, answers to the "how
groups help" question can be found in case study reports of group activities and sessions. For example, reports from a group in one midwestern
town provided a striking example. Most members in attendance at an
early spring evening self-help group meeting were dressed in casual
clothing. One couple arrived slightly late, he in a dark suit and she in a
Sunday-best dress. They were local farmers who had driven a fair distance from an event earlier that evening—the funeral of their young
adult daughter. Their reason for coming was stated clearly as an effort to
thank other parents for their years of support and affirmation. They gave
immensely moving testimony to the ways in which the self-help group
had facilitated their adjustment throughout the process of dealing with
their child's cancer (from diagnosis through treatment, remission, and
relapse, to death). In their own words, to a rapt group audience, they
told of the role of the group in helping them find a place of comfort,
friendship, and intimacy, and of increasing their feelings of mastery
over their daughter's treatment, illness, and inevitable death. They had
joined the group with reservations about its usefulness and yet returned
that night to pledge their continued attendance to help others in the
same situation. Many members cried and held each other, and reached
out to hug the bereaved couple.

In another midwestern setting, a parent group struggled with the local hospital's long-standing policy of not letting them have access to the lists of names of other parents with children diagnosed with cancer. The group was historically reluctant to challenge that policy, but became mobilized by the recent discrimination their young adult and teenage children, who were surviving their cancer, were encountering during job searches. The group's commitment to an organized effort grew as the stories shared about discriminatory experiences grew in number and intensity. They decided to challenge the hospital's patient access policy, in an effort to reach all parents and inform them of their childrens' employment and educational rights. The hospital eventually responded with unprecedented compliance, releasing the lists for use by the group. The self-help group's activist efforts to contact parents who were not members resulted in three vital outcomes—recruitment of new members, organized efforts at the nearby state capital for legislative reform on insurance and employment discrimination issues, and feelings of individual competence and activism on the part of individual group members.

Parental Intervention in Medical Care

Another potential outcome of parents' experiences with childhood cancer, and thus of their involvement in self-help groups for parents of children with cancer, was their active participation in the medical care process. This participatory role, closely related to personal activism and efforts to change the local medical system, took its most vigorous form when some parents intervened upon perceiving that medical "mistakes" (errors of omission or commission) were being made. Fifty-seven percent of the parents in this sample of members and nonmembers of the eight groups (in study #3) reported that they intervened in the medical care process. The major categories of such intervention included (1) parent as patient expert (3% of reported instances), (2) parent as interpersonal negotiator (13% of reported instances), (3) parent as IV monitor (17% of reported instances), (4) parent as procedural historian (30% of reported instances), and (5) parent as rescuer (37% of reported instances).

The first three categories of intervention (patient expert, interpersonal negotiator, and IV monitor) reflect relatively minor medical events, although they no doubt were disconcerting and uncomfortable for parents and children. The latter two categories of intervention (procedural historian and rescuer) may have represented quite serious situations. For instance, parents who acted as procedural historians questioned or reminded the staff about treatment plans or procedures, correcting errors or preventing them from taking place.

Twice technicians were going to draw blood from a vein when my child had a catheter for that purpose, until I stopped them.

I stepped in to prevent administration of a bone marrow and spinal tap which weren't due for two more weeks.

At one point when his counts were very low he had to share a bathroom with a child who we discovered had pneumonia. His doctor wouldn't do anything, so I went to the administration and he shortly had a private room.

In other situations, parental actions to prevent seriously inappropriate procedures included rescuing the child from the administration of a wrong drug or dangerous situation. As several parents reported,

Many medications were in pill form, and once she was given the wrong pill at the wrong time. Perhaps more mistakes could have happened, but I checked everything that went on.

When in the hospital, a nurse started to administer a second dose of an anti-nausea drug approximately 15 minutes after my son was administered the first dose of the same drug. I questioned her and she checked his record again and discontinued the second dose. This could have been very dangerous for him.

My child's condition took a dire change, and immediate tests had to be administered—it was a life-and-death situation. I was with the child and immediately called and had to demand the treatment. This occurred on two occasions.

Parents who were involved in the self-help group were significantly more likely (75%) to have reported intervening than were those parents who were not involved (25%); repeating the afore-mentioned association between "activism" and self-help group participation. Perhaps participation in a support group of "veterans" facilitated or supported parents' adoption of an active, informed, and monitoring role. In almost all of the self-help groups studied, parents shared and compared their experiences with and reactions to the medical institution, and to its staff and treatment procedures. They also often discussed how important it was for parents to monitor the treatment process. After all, in the midst of vast and busy medical bureaucracies, and faced with constantly rotating or changing staff members, parents often were the only consistent and ultimately knowledgeable actors in the treatment situation. Thus, the need for parents to be informed and active was a constant emphasis in these groups. Of course, it also is possible that the direction of causality was reversed, and that parents who intervened were then more likely to have sought peer support for this behavior by becoming active in the local parent group. Whichever way it worked, the self-help groups supported such intervention, as one parent noted:

You have to be aware and watch what a staff person is doing. The Candlelighters group (the name of the self-help group in this locale) in this city tries to educate the parents about these issues.

Benefits of Self-Help Group Leadership Roles

One of the ways in which self-help groups may be even more beneficial for some parents is through their own adoption of leadership roles in a group. Beyond membership status, group service and involvement at the leadership level can be rewarding—a fuller immersion into the culture of the group, an increased opportunity to facilitate the group experience for others, a chance to "pay back" others who have given help, and a chance to learn and practice new social and organizational skills.[18] Thus, not only did some parents of children with cancer join self-help groups while others did not, parents also varied in the degree to which they participated in these local groups. Some parents came to group meetings as "regular" members, not really involved at any level beyond attendance at meetings and occasional participation in special group events. Other parents became more active, serving as group leaders, meeting planners, project or event organizers, or membership recruiters. At the institutional level, some group leaders became active lobbyists for the group with medical, social service, and community resource systems. Still other parent leaders represented and advocated for the group at an external political level, interfacing with city officials and legislative systems to bring about needed change.

In the study of fifty self-help groups (Study #2), over 68% of the parents reported having taken some type of leadership role during the course of their group involvement (Yoak, Chesney, Schwartz, 1985).

Moreover, in the study of eight groups (Study #3), nearly half of the parents who were self-help group members reported taking the role of active leaders at some point. The widespread involvement of members as group leaders clearly demonstrates the democratic and participatory nature of these local voluntary organizations. Parents' own comments regarding their reasons for taking on group leadership roles, amidst the strains of coping with a child with cancer, indicated the personal as well as organizational value of such involvement. For instance, several parent-leaders noted how they benefited from their decision to accept a leadership role.

The group was my idea, and I benefited from it as much as the other parents.

Being now in an active, giving role in Candlelighters helps me to use my skills in writing and public speaking, which makes me feel good about myself.

In giving support, I always end up getting as much as I give.

Other parents' comments focused on their contributions to others' welfare.

I felt a definite need to effect changes in hospital rules and regulations concerning personal relationships with other parents of patients.

I wanted to pay back some of what was there for me in the way of financial support. Help make conditions better for all of us by being willing to be a mouthpiece.

Crazy, huh? Real interest, I guess. I wanted to make the quality of life better for all involved with a child diagnosed with a life-threatening illness. It's work, fun, challenging, and personally satisfying.

I think its very important to keep the group going. Its an opportunity to help others right at our doorstep. The most effective help comes from someone "who has been there." I felt the group was so important that I had to invest myself in its continuation.

Their motivations for leadership varied. They included a desire to help improve the quality and character of medical and social service, to help others, to "give back" what help they received, to be of positive service, and to use their skills to gain help themselves.

Not only was self-help group membership related positively to personal outcomes, as indicated earlier in this chapter, but so was leadership status within the local groups. Group leaders, overall, were significantly more likely to have reported that they "coped very well," to have experienced more positive changes in their lives, and to have intervened more often than did active but nonleader group members, or than did nonmembers. It is likely that group support for these positive changes in mental health, activism, and especially intervention was yet another benefit of membership and leadership for these parents. Of course, as noted earlier, it also is possible that parents who already had taken active stances and had made positive life changes were more likely to join the self-help group.[19]

These data still do not indicate that all self-help groups will be beneficial for all members, or that all parents of children with cancer can or want to join them. However, it is clear from the various analyses reported in this chapter that self-help group membership was associated with positive outcomes for parents, that more positive outcomes were reported by members than by nonmembers, and that more positive outcomes were reported by leaders than by regular members. We might think of self-help involvement as being a continuum, from no involvement on the part of nonmembers, to involved members, to members who also played leadership roles. The more active parents were, the more they put into these groups, and the more they got out of them.[20]

Part 4

Working with the Medical System: Bridging Parents and Professionals

In this section we examine some of the issues that typically arise in the organizational relationships between self-help groups for families of children with cancer and medical care institutions and staffs.

In Chapter 8 we focus on the roles that members of the professional medical staff (physicians, nurses, social workers) played with regard to self-help groups, and present self-help group members' views of these roles.

In Chapter 9 we focus specifically on the inherent conflicts that arise in such interorganizational relationships, and the ways in which self-help groups and medical institutions can work together to resolve or manage these conflicts.

8

Roles of Professionals in Self-Help Groups

There is substantial agreement among professionals, self-help group activists, and scholars that under certain circumstances human service professionals can be very helpful to self-help groups and their members. However, the tremendous variety of self-help groups creates great variation in the attitudes of members toward professionals, in the attitudes of professionals toward groups and their members, and in the options available to professionals. Moreover, formal service agencies and institutions vary considerably in their commitments to self-help groups. They often establish the "rules of engagement" between self-help members and individual professionals and staff members, as well as the range of acceptable roles professionals may play. In this chapter we concentrate on the potential and actual roles played by individual medical and human service professionals in these groups, and in Chapter 9 we explore the relations between childhood cancer self-help groups and medical organizations. Since most of the literature on the roles of professionals in self-help groups is written by and for human service professionals and scholars, we must be wary of the assumptions and potential biases that limit both their discussion of these roles and the options available for implementation.

Most discussions of professionals' roles in self-help groups do not examine or articulate clearly the problems or tensions in these relationships, but focus on generating solutions—often prematurely and simplistically. For groups led by human service professionals, the issues are fairly straightforward; although we review such options below, there is not much disagreement about their focus. However, the situation is different in relatively autonomous or independent self-help groups. If such groups are to be member-led, and not professionally led or supervised, what are appropriate roles for professionals? If the forms of medical information, psychosocial help, social networking, and general advice provided by these groups represent alternatives to the services normally provided by professionals, what are the implications for professionals' identities, expertise, and careers, let alone roles? Is there any validity to the argument that definitionally dismisses all professionally led groups as not being "true" self-help groups?

The Importance of Professionals for Self-Help Groups

Whether the focus is on group initiation, member recruitment and referral, group maintenance, institutional liaison, or member needs and growth, parents of children with cancer generally agree that professionals can be very useful to self-help groups. This view may not be common in all types of self-help groups (e.g., members of avowedly antipsychiatry groups, or groups of people pursuing different lifestyles), but parents of children with cancer in all our studies appreciated those members of the professional staff who seemed both genuine and competent in their relations with them. As several parents noted, for instance,

We had good professionals and could see the advantages to having them there. They raised good points, did not constrain us, moved the group, used silence, expected work. People felt commitment to someone we knew and trusted and had faith in.

Without staff support our group would have had a much harder time getting this far.

They support us because we can discuss specific problems with them to get ideas of how to deal better. They give us access to anyone in the system and to get information. They help make certain aspects of the group more successful, helping with contacts and referrals. I feel that it is very important for the group's real success to have the interest of key medical personnel, but they do not necessarily have to be active in the group's meetings unless asked for a specific purpose.

Thus, the question is not whether professionals are important for these groups and their members, but what the nature of their importance is:

What specific resources do they have to offer? How might those resources best be delivered? How can these resources be delivered in ways that support and empower groups rather than compete with or control them? What should be the nature of the ongoing relationship between parent groups and members of the professional medical or social service staff?

Physicians, nurses, and social workers—in addition to other professionals such as child life workers, health educators, and clinical nurse practitioners—have access to certain resources that are crucial to self-help group survival and effectiveness. Among these resources are specialized *information* about the disease and its treatment, about how to handle difficult social and emotional issues, about the workings of the hospital and its staff, and about community services. To provide this information in ways that lay people can understand readily, professionals write articles for group newsletters, present lectures, and lead discussions and panels at group meetings. In addition, human service professionals may have special expertise and information about family and personal coping strategies, and can share this information personally or through written materials. Several parents commented on the utility of these resources in the self-help group setting.

The medical professionals seem to have more time for answering questions in our group than they do privately at the hospital.

They contribute a better understanding of treatments and hospital procedures . . . better communication.

Providing information about cancer and about the hospital.

Another resource professionals generally have that is critical for self-help groups is access to hospital *services and personnel:* the ability to arrange for meeting rooms, mailing lists, financial support in the form of stamps and mailings of newsletters and notices, a postal address, and linkages to medical personnel who may speak at group meetings. Some specific comments from parents about the value of these services follow:

I am sure they have been able to get their hands on information needed and to direct us in finding much needed resources, both financial and emotional.

They provide us with excellent background and leadership when we need and ask for it.

Further, professionals generally have control of the *referral* process. It is primarily through staff contacts and referrals that parents of newly diagnosed children learn of the group, and that the group itself gains access to the names and addresses of these parents. Several self-help group members indicated the value of professional assistance in this process.

The group knows promptly of new families and their needs from the social worker.

The past year has brought us closer to the hospital, and the doctors, nurses, etc., as we have invited them to meetings. We have seen more calls from nurses about patients and one actual request for intervention with a family dealing with relapse. New families appreciate and accept the group more readily now that we have this cooperative working relationship with the staff.

Parents who were active in these self-help groups recognized that professionals making referrals often had to strike a balance between overt advocacy and gentle suggestion regarding group involvement, a balance that respected both parents' needs and their freedom of choice or privacy.

Support groups are hard to get going. You need the professional touch. Professionals get people to a meeting—grab them. Parents won't talk to a parent "off the street" at first.

Most parents feel totally helpless, so a group referral by a professional can give them the idea that they need to take some control, make decisions.

Balancing this referral process sometimes presented dilemmas for staff members; for instance, several physicians who appreciated the role of parent groups had the following comments:

Sometimes I might *not* refer a parent. It's their choice, not mine. They can get information even if they don't want to attend the group.

Let people make that decision. You can't legislate people into a group.

They (the self-help group) have taken over much of the planning for new patients; but on the other hand, I have a new referral source for other parents.

These excerpts from conversations with physicians illustrate some of the value dilemmas and role conflicts many professionals face in their work with self-help groups.

Parents' efforts to *deal with the emotional stresses* of childhood cancer in the context of a self-help group may invite professionals to present lectures and discussions or guide group counseling sessions. Staff members also may encourage parents' efforts to provide emotional support to one another, and may even train group members in how to co-counsel and respond to others' emotional needs.

Finally, medical professionals can (or can decide not to) *legitimize* a group and its activities in the eyes of the medical staff, the community, and the constituency of parents of children with cancer. Although staff members cannot literally prevent parents from meeting and talking together, they can make it easier (or more difficult) for parents to find, rely on, and support one another. When parents are fearful or cautious about joining a group of "nonexperts," professionals can help allay their fears by assuring them that the self-help group is a credible and valuable source of support. Several comments from group members exemplified the importance of this resource:

They give the group credibility.

The group feels more secure now that the doctors are giving us credit as a valuable resource and are beginning to recommend us to new patients.

We are now allowed to talk to parents inside of our hospital about their children's medical problems.

These are not the only resources medical professionals may possess and may or may not deliver to a group, but they are among the most essential ones. Specific professionals may have other resources, depending upon their own training, skill, and personal or organizational mission. For instance, professionals may help groups become formally organized and plan programs, may help link the group to local community resources, and may educate the rest of the staff about the group. When conflict occurs between the group (or some members) and the hospital (or some staff members), informed and committed professionals may intervene to reduce such conflict and create better understanding and collaboration. Similarly, specific groups may need or utilize some of these resources and not others. With this discussion as a starting point, we can examine some of the barriers and options open to these professionals and to local parent self-help groups.

Differences Between Professionals and Parents

The necessity of discussing "appropriate" roles for professionals in parent self-help groups stems from the obvious reality that professionals and parents of children with cancer are not members of the same interest groups or constituencies. They may work together, and they may on occasion share each others' realities and visit each others' worlds, but they do not stand on the same shoreline and do not inhabit the same realms of status, suffering, and struggle. Table 8.1 lists some important differences that were outlined briefly in Chapter 1 (see Table 1.1) and that frame this discussion.

One important difference stems from their fundamental functions in the struggle with childhood cancer: professionals are the providers of service and parents and their children are the recipients. Moreover, given the high medical and psychosocial stakes of the crisis of childhood cancer, professionals are the relatively powerful providers of potentially life-saving services, while parents are representatives of the class of relatively powerless and dependent recipients of services. Since much of their interaction takes place in and near the medical system, in which professionals are the "home team" and parents the "visitors," professionals are the higher-status party in this relationship.

Table 8.1. Major differences between parents of children with cancer and professionals working with these parents and children

Difference	Parent	Professional
Function and status	Service recipient Relatively powerless	Service provider Relatively powerful
Knowledge base	Experiential wisdom Personal Particular	Academic expertise Technical General
Interests and accountabilty	Child Particular child Child and family	Career or profession Children in general Medical community
Mindset	Affective intensity	Affective distance
Job and family concerns	Family internal to illness Job external to illness	Family external to illness Job internal to illness

The power and status differentials embodied in the high-stakes medical scene are enormous.

A second important difference concerns the knowledge and skill bases that parents and professionals bring with them to their interaction with one another. As prerequisites for obtaining the credentials defining them as professionals, staff members receive specialized training about the realities of childhood cancer. Of course, the particular nature of this specialized information and their consequent skills depend upon the particular professional role involved: physicians obviously receive different kinds of knowledge and perform different tasks than do nurses or social workers. However, all professionals have a technical basis of information and knowledge, one that is rooted in a general understanding of the disease process and its physical and psychosocial manifestations, prognoses, and treatments. Parents, at least at the beginning of their struggle with childhood cancer, lack such general background knowledge of the disease and its medical and psychosocial realities and treatments, but over time many become quite well-informed on these matters. In addition, parents do have highly personal and specialized lay knowledge and expertise regarding their own children and their medical histories, life-styles, emotional status, personal vulnerabilities, family involvements, and social and school orientations.[1] These different forms of knowledge sometimes rival one another for primacy, as in the case of decisions about whether to apply formal rules and procedures in particular cases. The perception that professionals' knowledge about cancer is "old" knowledge, while parents' knowledge generally has been "newly gained," and that in the context of the medical system these two forms of knowledge are accorded very different legitimacy and relevance, means that the struggles between expertise and experience are usually uneven. Case 4 involves a successful strategy to define a special vehicle for parental expertise and influence within the medical setting, the parent advocate group (see box).

Professionals are typically highly committed to their roles, their careers, and to the institution employing them, and therefore to the clinical caseload in general; parents are committed primarily to the particular case of their own child. Professionals are formally accountable to their colleagues and supervisors within the professional medical community, parents to themselves and their other family members, and sometimes to close friends. Each party's concerns about childhood can-

Case 4. The Parent Advocate Group

This group was founded four years ago, with a primary focus on providing emotional support and educational resources to parents of children with cancer. One of its officers now serves as a regular member of the hospital's psychosocial staff, in a half-time position that is paid for by the hospital.

The group has three elected officers and an executive director; the latter is the parent who also serves as a member of the hospital's pediatric oncology staff. The officers run the monthly meetings of this group. Meetings generally have a specific agenda that includes a presentation on a topic of interest to group members. In addition, substantial time is set aside during each meeting for parents to go around the room and talk about their individual situations, asking for and giving aid and support during this process.

The Parent Advocate Group started out, like many others, with a desire to create settings in which parents could talk with one another and learn more about their own and their children's physical and psychosocial situations and futures. Over time, one of the veteran parents became quite close to several members of the hospital staff, and was seen by them and by other parents as a useful resource in times of stress and need. This parent began to feel that she was spending a lot of time in this capacity, and that perhaps her work should be recognized and institutionalized on a more formal basis. The group petitioned the staff to create a role that would enable this (or some other) skilled parent to be a regular member of the hospital's staff, and thus to formalize the liaison between the parent group and the staff and legitimize the special expertise this parent was providing to both parents and staff. Lengthy discussions ensued, both between the pediatric oncology staff and the group, and within the hospital staff at large. In addition, consultations were held with physicians in Rhode Island, Rochester, and Kansas hospitals, where such a position had been developed earlier. Not all the staff members thought this was a good idea, but finally it was decided to test this position on a three-year basis.

The parent-advocate sits in on all staff meetings, is part of staff rounds, and also attends all group meetings. She "represents" parents' views and needs directly to the staff, communicates staff concerns to the parents, and tries to influence the staff when appropriate. Parents and staff seem quite pleased with the added communication and expertise that this role provides. Occasionally, however, both parents and staff ask "Whose side is she on?" because disputes between parents and individual staff members sometimes place this person in a double-bind and stretch her loyalties.

It is worth noting that the creation of this role has not substituted for good communication between individual staff members and individual parents; if anything, more parents and staff members seem comfortable talking with one another, secure in the knowledge that a resource exists to help them overcome and work through any communication difficulties.

cer derive from different sources as well: professionals' interests derive from their voluntary inclinations, training, licensing, and on-the-job experience; parents' concerns derive from their involuntary experience as creators and caretakers of their child who is now seriously ill. Case 4 also illustrates alternative ways of dealing with this difference between parents' and professionals' interests and accountability.

Their training and role obligations generally create in professionals an emotional and cognitive mindset and role of affective distance and caution.[2] On the other hand, parents come to this scene with intense affect and deep concern. The very emotional intensity of the psychosocial situation surrounding as life-threatening an illness as childhood cancer reinforces these alternative emotional stances and approaches. None of the above discussion is intended to suggest that professionals do not feel deeply about their craft, or about individual children—only that their orientations and commitments in these regards are fundamentally different from those of parents of children with cancer. Likewise, parents are not unconcerned about the entire population of children with cancer, and about certain professionals' lives and health as well, but the basis of their concerns and priorities is quite different.

A fourth major difference between providers and consumers involves the nature of job and family concerns, those vital components of many social situations. For professionals, their job is in the situation at hand—to deal with the illness and with children and parents. For parents, their job is outside the situation of their child's treatment for cancer; in fact, their job demands may conflict seriously with the demands of the illness and treatment situation. For professionals, their family is outside this situation, and most professionals struggle to keep substantial emotional, if not physical, distance between their job and their family. Thus, for professionals, being with their families often is a form of relief and refuge from the intensity of the situation of children with cancer. For parents, on the other hand, the family is seldom a refuge, since it is very much a part of the situation of illness. Despite the social support that may be forthcoming from family members, the complexity and intensity of family life also can be very stressful for parents in these circumstances, and can affect (and be affected by) parents' responses to the illness and its treatment.

The Situation of Social Workers

The professionals who are most often assigned or elect to work on a sustained basis with self-help groups are social workers, so we concentrate here on their roles in particular. As the primary links between medical staff and self-help groups, social workers' roles and role dilemmas highlight many of the foregoing conflicts and tensions between these stakeholders. Figure 8.1 presents a series of problems or dilemmas that social workers reported facing in their working relationships

Figure 8.1. Problems that social workers face in working with organized parent groups

Professional role/responsibility issues

Concern about not having the right skills (or enough of them)
Avoiding telling (or being manipulated into telling) parents what's right
Feeling responsible for parents' emotional safety
Dealing with rumors or fads about treatment
Dealing with intrusive or manipulative parents (who may hurt others)
Watching out for parents who get overlooked
Feeling like the expert in psychosocial care
Feeling responsible for what group does

Personal feelings in involvement with patients/parents

Feeling close with some and distance (or dislike) with others
Time and energy demands
Need to feel appreciated (get strokes) and supported
Lack of clarity about how open to be personally
Specific questions about going to funerals, parties, socials
Feelings of not doing enough
High emotional stress

Institutional support issues

Lack of clarity about own role
Staff disinterest in or worry about groups
Difference between parents' needs and the medical staff's desires
Turf conflicts with other staff members
Feelings about the character (quality) of formal medical or psychosocial care
Low status on staff
Lack of staff information about parents' needs and experiences
Staff hesitancy to share with each other

with parent self-help groups. These reports come from personal interviews with social workers in the several studies we conducted, as well as from informal discussions at professional meetings and conferences.

The first set of important problems social workers reported concerned the definition of their own roles and responsibilities. The dynamics of counseling parents in highly emotional and threatening situations are indeed difficult. Anyone working in such situations could be expected to have a normal level of anxiety about their utility and the most effective ways to use their helping skills and their craft. In addition, many social workers were not trained to work with organized parent self-help groups. The interpersonal counseling orientation of most medical social workers provided them with skills in working with individuals, and perhaps with small, therapy-oriented groups, but not necessarily with independent and collective organizations of parents. Such work often called for community organizing or organization-building skills, rather than skills in interpersonal practice. Thus, despite their intentions, some social workers who wanted to help active parent self-help groups simply did not know how to do so and did not have the relevant skills in group recruitment, programming, leadership development, constituency mobilization, community outreach, or conflict management. They were often confused about what was an appropriate group agenda, in dealing with their feelings about protecting or feeling responsible for group members, and in negotiating the interface between the group and the medical staff. Further, once they "knew" how they felt and what "should" happen in these regards, many did not have the skills to act appropriately.

A second set of reported problems involved professionals' own personal feelings about themselves and others. Social workers working a full day in the hospital and then also working with an organized self-help group often felt stressed in their roles, and had little energy for difficult group situations. In situations where "caring" was a precious commodity, overstressed social workers sometimes felt that they had no more to give. In addition, they themselves felt "uncared for" by parents with whom they had become quite intimate. The burn-out rate is high in pediatric oncology services. Social workers experienced severe strain when they perceived parents as being demanding rather than supportive, and when their own home and family life was compromised. This was especially likely when well-meaning professionals became the target for parental ventilation regarding negative experiences with the medical system, or when they experienced rejection or distance from self-help group leaders.

These first two sets of issues were compounded by reports of the lack of support and reward many social workers received from the hospital for their performance in the group-liaison role. Support from the medical system for professional aid and assistance to parent self-help groups was often ambivalent or unclear. For instance, at one midwestern hospital, the administration assigned a social worker to work especially with the Candlelighters group, but according to a parent leader in this group, things changed quickly:

They hired him to help us, and we had such high hopes. But now they are not nearly as supportive of his helping us. They think all of the staff spend too much time in the clinic.

As the social worker himself commented,

Things started out great. The physicians lobbied for this position. But now there is a money crunch, and they are unwilling to pay for work in the oncology clinic. They have already stopped support of staff in other clinics.

Two other social workers from other treatment centers also commented on the lack of hospital support for their group role—a lack that bordered on what these professionals saw as hostility:

The hospital doesn't recognize this group. They compete against them— schedule their run one week before the group's marathon.

Meetings are on our own time. That was made clear by the administration.

Although it is obvious that these institutional constraints, in active or passive form, did stop some professionals from working with the self-help groups, it did not stop all of them. As several social workers reported,

I didn't ask if I could do this project. I just did it, and no one protested.

The Social Work Department is changing. We are unsure about our future. But we won't let that be a barrier to working with the group.

Still others felt supported and positively rewarded for their work with the local self-help group:

There is much more administrative support for work in the clinic. Shift staff expect overtime pay, and that is viewed negatively. In the clinic, the policy is that overtime to work with the group is okay—you can get paid for it.

I feel supported most of the time from the pediatric oncology team, but at first it was hard—I had to break ground with them.

In some institutions physicians and clinic chiefs were active and vigorous supporters of parent self-help groups, and one of the ways they demonstrated this support was through their assignment of social workers to work with local groups. For the most part, however, time spent with self-help groups was off-job time, uncompensated time, and time not viewed as critical by the medical staff. Sometimes, professionals working with such groups were negatively sanctioned for such activities, or blamed when the self-help group did something the medical staff perceived as contrary to their interests or their conceptions of parents' interests. This was especially true when medical staff members felt they knew best and wished to determine or direct the activities of a group, and discovered that they—or their designated social work representative—could not guarantee such control.[3] These limited visions of parent self-help groups and the consequent constraints on professionals' roles in these groups are another result of the "counternormative" nature of self-help. Traditional professional protocols and role behaviors were often at least minimally in conflict with the culture and orientation of self-help groups.

The above difficulties helped create unclear expectations on the part of social workers regarding the roles they could and should play with self-help groups for families of children with cancer. Well-meaning professionals were often uncertain whether to lead or to follow, to do for a group or to let or encourage a group to do for itself, to be a group member or not, to be quite open with the group on matters involving the medical staff or not, to spend time and energy with the group or not, to advocate for the group with the medical staff or not. When there were other, clearer, role requirements and service demands on these staff members, they were likely to gravitate to those tasks instead.

Some Role Options for Professionals Working with Self-Help Groups

How should medical professionals relate to and interact with self-help groups? Earlier in this chapter we discussed some of the resources professionals possessed that might be useful to groups and group members. What ways of delivering these resources, and which roles, relationships, and actions might enhance groups' effectiveness? Which might burden or disrupt groups? Most discussions of these issues are speculative, anecdotal, or exhortative. Few studies have actually asked professionals or group members what professionals actually did in such interactive settings. A few researchers (e.g., Gottlieb, 1982) have expanded our empirical knowledge base with actual data about professionals' behaviors and group members' reactions, but these are exceptions. However, even the material that does exist is instructive: professionals' writings on this issue can be taken to reflect their ideology if not their practice.

The particular roles professionals actually play in self-help groups can be understood best as the results of the interaction among several factors. First, the roles depend upon professionals' understanding of the psychosocial impact of childhood cancer on the child and family. In this regard, it matters greatly whether professionals assume that parents in this situation need therapeutic treatment, or that parents should be approached as a psychologically normal and competent population currently laboring under great stress—and therefore needing substantial support, but not necessarily psychotherapy. Second, these roles reflect what professionals understand to be the special nature of a self-help group, as opposed to a support group, a professionally led support group, a therapy group, a social event, or an audience at a lecture. Despite confusion in the literature, most observers have noted something different about self-help groups, and thus have called for professional roles that are less controlling and more facilitative than traditional group therapy. Third, as Toseland and Hacker (1982) pointed out, professionals' roles can also be understood as reflections of their own repertoire of knowledge and skills, and their agency's standard practices and outlooks. Finally, the desires and needs of self-help group members, as well as the reactions professionals' receive from members in self-help groups, help determine the roles they play.

The professional and academic literature suggests the following roles for professionals working with self-help groups.

1. *Consultation on organizational development.*[4] Although the notion of an organizational consultant is often presented in quite general terms, it focuses on helping a group create a structure, identify internal personnel and resources, and reflect on the process the group is developing as it goes about its business.

2. *Leadership training and skill development.*[5] Typical staff-development functions may involve professionals training leaders in how to manage an organization, how to run a meeting, how to help other members "open up" and share their feelings and concerns, and how to support bereaved parents. In some professionally led groups, or in "parent visitor" programs, such training is a prerequisite to group activity or to parents' assumption of leadership. However, in the more autonomous forms of self-help groups it is provided on a voluntary basis, and not as a leadership-screening device.

3. *Recruitment or referral of new members.*[6] No group can long exist if it cannot replenish membership, and this function is thus a life-or-death issue for many groups. When recruitment assistance is not forthcoming from a professional, a group may mobilize to recruit members through newspapers, posters, and personal contact in treatment centers. Recruitment activity also places the professional in the role of helping the group link to the medical system or to other treatment systems.

4. *Liaison with the larger community.*[7] This role involves the professional, with or without other members, in efforts to educate the public about the existence of the group, generate publicity for group activities, and link the group (and its members) to other community agencies and services.

5. *Help plan the group program.*[8] In some groups professionals help plan the program and the agenda for meetings, including the mix of educational or business meetings and the topics for speeches or group discussions. In addition, professionals are sometimes effective links to people who might be good speakers or discussants for the group.

6. *Provision of material support.*[9] Some professionals are a source of tangible goods that a group needs for its own maintenance, such as a meeting site, funds for a newsletter or for refreshments, and clerical assistance in printing information brochures or newsletters.

7. *Referral of members who need special treatment/services.*[10] Professionals may be helpful in identifying or responding to group members who need special help, either from the professionals themselves or from other community services.

8. *Expert with special information or insight.*[11] In this most traditional profes-

sional role, staff members can assist groups who need special technical information about the condition or situation that brings them together, about ways of coping with their situations, and about where to find helpful resources and services.

9. *Legitimation and linkage of the self-help group to the medical or social service system.*[12] As a member of the treatment system, the professional can sometimes play a useful role in convincing others within this system (staff and patients alike) that the group is a legitimate and even positive endeavor. Some professionals have found themselves defending parent activism and group activities to the medical staff, and in the process communicating parental and group needs to other staff members and educating the staff about the group. This role may eventually involve informal sponsorship, presence on a public advisory board, and professional liaison activity. Some observers have suggested that, on occasion, this legitimation or linking role may even require the professional to mediate disputes or conflicts that occur between the group and the medical or treatment staff.[13]

10. *Leadership (or co-leadership) and guidance of the group.*[14] This traditional professional role is performed extensively in hospital-led support or counseling groups, but less often within the context of relatively independent self-help groups. In the latter groups it usually is done on a short-term basis, or in combination or coalition with indigenous leaders. In the context of specific meetings, such leadership may involve facilitation of a discussion group or the processes of a business meeting. Sometimes the leadership provided is symbolic in character, as in membership on a leadership panel, letterhead, or advisory board; at other times it presents itself in the form of informal advice or guidance, or in actual control.[15]

11. *Provision of psychotherapy to individuals in a group setting.* Another traditional role for social workers, conducting therapy or supportive psychological counseling, may occur on a short-term basis in a group setting or on a continuing and permanent basis in a therapist-led support group tied to the hospital, treatment center, or mental health agency.

12. *Protection and safety for individuals in the group.*[16] Some professionals who eschew therapy in the self-help group context make an effort to ensure that, at the very least, no "damage" is done to group members as a result of peer-led conversations and discussions.

13. *Conduct of research or evaluation of the group.*[17] The special skills of professionals may enable them to conduct research on group processes and outcomes, and thus to create procedures for immediate and ongoing evaluation of the group's activities and needs.

14. *Initiation of a group.*[18] Many writers suggest that professionals have been very helpful as initiators of self-help groups, dispelling the notion that such

professionals are necessarily anti-self-help, or that self-help groups are necessarily anti-professional. Most discussions of such initiating activity are followed with reports that professionals gradually stepped, or should step, into the background as member leadership presented itself.

This review of the literature about professionals' roles in self-help groups raises several questions about how specific roles are selected by specific professionals in specific situations. How do staff members decide which roles to perform, and which services or functions a treatment center should try to provide to a group? Are these decisions made on the basis of realistic assessments of clients/patients' needs and the needs of self-help groups? Or are decisions made on the basis of professional ideology about service delivery and the operating assumptions of a treatment system? In an attempt to clarify these postures, and to bring empirical data to bear on the options discussed above, we now turn to an examination of professionals' and members' actual views of professionals' activities in self-help groups for families of children with cancer.

What Do Medical Professionals and Parents Report About Professionals' Roles in Self-Help Groups?

Parents and professionals in our study of the eight self-help groups (Study #3) responded to a set of structured questions inquiring into the roles that professionals played in these groups. Social workers and physicians each made up one-third of the population of professionals responding ($N = 27$), and nurses represented another 15% of those staff members responding to the items listed in Table 8.2. All sixty-five parents responding were active group members. Table 8.2 presents both professionals' and parents' estimates of the frequency of professionals' roles and activities in the eight local self-help groups studied. The roles that both populations reported that professionals most often played included making referrals, providing information about cancer, telling parents where things were in the hospital, maintaining liaison with the medical staff and with public agencies, and advocating for the group's existence.

It is especially interesting to compare professionals' reports of the frequency of their involvement in these roles with the reports of the parent group members. Although parent members agreed with professionals' *ranking* of the roles they reported playing most frequently, they

Table 8.2. Professionals' and parents' reports of professionals' roles in self-help groups

		Frequency of professional roles	
Professional role in group		Percent of professionals reporting always or often ($n = 27$) (% = 100)	Percent of parents reporting always or often ($n = 65$) (% = 100)
a.	Provide information about cancer	81	57
b.	Tell parents where things are in the hospital	77	42
c.	Refer new parents to the group	100	70
d.	Lead the group meetings	19	32
e.	Set the agenda for the group	24	22
f.	Keep discussions "on track"	19	26
g.	Train parents in how to lead the group	8	8
h.	Consult upon request	30	42
i.	Guard against parents getting hurt	31	25
j.	Maintain liaison for parents with medical staff	77	42
k.	Arrange rooms, mailing lists, speakers	46	26
l.	Attend social functions	57	46
m.	Be a referral for parents with serious problems	74	55
n.	Maintain liaison with public agencies/ societies	70	38
o.	Advocate for the group's existence and function	74	50
p.	Teach group members how to cope better	52	42

almost always saw much less *frequency* of activity than did the professionals themselves. For instance, professionals reported that they provided information about cancer and told parents where things were in the hospital almost all of the time (81% and 77%), while parents reported that they did so less often (57% and 42%). In terms of group advocacy, professionals reported quite frequent liaison roles with both the medical staff and with public agencies or societies (77% and 70%), but parents saw professionals doing this much less frequently (42% and 38%). Referrals by professionals, according to their own reports, occurred all of the time (100%); parents also reported professional referrals as quite frequent, but they saw them occurring less often than did professionals (70%). An example of professional involvement where parents' and staffs' estimates varied in opposite directions was the extent to which professionals consulted with parents upon request when there were problems: parents reported that professionals were ready consultants 42% of the time, while professionals reported being available only 30% of the time. Regardless of the direction of the discrepancy between parents' and professionals' reports, several explanations for these findings are possible. Parents are not privy to all settings in which professionals act and advocate, and may not have seen all that professionals did. On the other hand, professionals' estimates of some their own activities may be overstated.

Table 8.2 also indicates that certain types of professional self-help group involvement occurred relatively infrequently, according to both parents and professionals. For example, professionals and parents reported that professionals participated quite minimally in group operational activities—setting its agenda or leading its meetings. Parents' and professionals' reports were also basically in agreement on the issue of whether professionals trained parents to lead the group: it seldom happened. In contrast to discrepant reports of professionals' activities outside the self-help group (e.g., liaison, referral), professional roles specifically in the group or at group meetings were more consistently reported by both parents and professionals. As parents become more inclined to determine the logistic agenda of the group, and as clinical and administrative demands on professionals grow, professional roles such as presiding over meetings and training group leaders may become even less frequent.

The choice of professional roles was made differently by different professionals and in different local self-help groups. In one of the groups we studied there was a very high degree of professional involvement in group maintenance and management activities. This relatively new and small group was affiliated with a medium-sized medical center in a southwestern city, and the professional liaison was a well-respected and effective social worker. The group's major focus was on emotional sharing and support, with many sessions led by the social worker. In contrast, a group composed of members from families treated at a major midwestern medical center had a long-standing core of parent activists and leaders who directed most group activities. In this setting, professional staff members had a mixed history of support and hesitancy toward the parent group, and parents had been clear about their desires to cooperate with professionals but not to be "managed" by them. As a result, while professionals did provide support to the group when asked, they were involved infrequently in group maintenance or management activities.

What Do Group Members Think Professionals Should (and Should Not) Do in/for a Group?

In response to an open-ended inquiry, group members identified the kinds of roles they most wished professionals would perform in their working relationships with self-help groups:

- Referrals of new parents (32%)
- Give information about cancer (30%)
- Listen to the group and consult (23%)
- Be active in some way (20%)
- Maintain liaison with the staff (15%)

We discussed the positive possibilities and the problems involved with professionals' referrals to self-help groups in Chapter 5. Their roles in providing groups with information and in using group meetings to provide individual parents with information were also emphasized. Clearly, these resources were essential for groups' continuing relationships with staffs, and for their own missions and activities. However, some parents, while desiring professional assistance with referrals and information, were still cautious about these relationships.

We'd like their support of the group in terms of informing new patients of our existence, and their willingness to speak with the group on certain subjects. But as a group we're glad not to be under the thumb of professionals.

This concern with preserving a group's autonomy was echoed by many members in many groups.

Although a substantial number of parents approved of professionals consulting with a group and listening to its problems, some were cautious about even this form of professional involvement.

Maybe they should be involved on a consultation basis only. The more they become involved the more they will rule . . . and the less we will.

Thus, the theme of limited professional involvement, and especially of limited professional control (or "rule") of the group, was repeated.

Nonetheless, a substantial proportion of parents expressed a desire for professionals to be active in the group in "some way," even though they were unable to specify what this meant. This general interest often represented both an appreciation of prior professional work, as well as a desire for more contact and assistance.

Be concerned enough to attend meetings and get to know parents in a less stressful situation.

I believe they should all come to several meetings to see what we are about and to find out how we can help them also.

In addition to these positive reactions to professionals' active involvement in parent groups, we also asked parents what they thought professionals should *not* do in self-help groups:

- Control or lead the group or group meetings (23%)
- Set the goals and agenda for the group (21%)
- Be overfamiliar or act like one of us (9%)
- Get too involved in the group (7%)

Parental objection to professional control or leadership of the self-help group was again emphasized, as follows:

Not running the group or leading discussions. They can participate, but not as the group leader.

I think they have tried too hard to lead and pursue an area that is not right for that particular time. Sometimes the professionals tend to make us feel like a case or an object and are unable to really feel for what is going on at the meetings.

Professionals should visit and observe only. This is a place where parents can be in a "sanctuary" situation.

My attitude, right or wrong, is that if parents want it to float they should be the ones to keep it working. If not, the staff shouldn't be expected to run it. Encouragement—yes; forcing or leading—no.

Most of these quite vigorous comments about group leadership came from parents involved in "independent" self-help groups.[19]

Comments from parents in "shared-leadership" groups also re-flected objection to professional control or overinvolvement, but did suggest some useful, albeit limited, roles for professionals in group management.

Not be too heavily involved. I find it nice to get together and talk and complain about the medical staff with other parents. It is a good release of tension, but it is hard to do with some of the staff sitting there.

Professionals feel the group should be structured and certain things shouldn't be talked about. They limit us too much.

Don't try to shield us, especially in the group. It doesn't help to keep the truth about treatment from us—makes us think you're lying to us!

We don't want speakers all of the time—just come and talk to us. We listen to you—listen to us!

Embedded in these excerpts is the repeated assertion of parents' desire to work with professionals, but to maintain their independence and for professionals to value parents' experiential knowledge rather than rou-tinely and automatically to impose their technical expertise. Some pro-fessionals clearly recognized some of the limits on their roles in these groups:

There is too much involvement of psychosocial professionals in the group.

We can give information, talk about options—treatment, coping. But we really are better suited to run a therapy group—parents should run the self-help group. Some of them are professionals themselves.

These quotes from professionals indicate their own awareness that par-ents and professionals can work together as different sets of experts on the same patient-oriented team. Moreover, increased autonomy and responsibility for parents does not preclude self-help group roles for professionals, as long as those roles do not threaten that a group will be "taken over" (Rappaport, 1993).

Comments from parents in professionally led groups seldom fo-cused on issues of control and overinvolvement; in these groups parents generally were pleased that professionals were exerting initiative and directing activities. However, some cautions were raised about the is-sue of role boundaries, once again highlighting the different life situations and experiences that parents and professionals brought to their common endeavor.

> In groups such as these there is so much empathy. Only I and maybe other parents know my love for my child and the fear her illness has caused me. I don't want a professional telling me she knows how I feel. No one who is not a parent does.

Thus, the particular nature of parental views regarding professionals' roles often differed by the type of group with which they were involved. In groups that were founded and led by professionals, those professionals' roles remained quite substantial, and parents involved in such groups generally preferred that professionals play a wide variety of operational and governing, as well as supportive and counseling, roles. Parents involved in shared leadership forms of self-help groups were much more likely to prefer somewhat limited professional involvement that focused on providing information and support, including practical help as a medical and community liaison, but not including an active role in group maintenance and governance. Parents in more independent groups were likely to limit the nature of professional involvement even more severely, perhaps even to excluding them from all but special meetings and occasions.

Meaningful Options Do Exist for Professionals

The voices heard above indicate varied parental and professional views regarding appropriate and preferred roles for professionals in self-help groups. Parents and professionals sometimes differed on these issues, despite significant areas of agreement. The Candlelighters Childhood Cancer Foundation's *Group Handbook* describes many preferred aspects of the relationships between local parent self-help groups and members of the medical staff (Nathanson, 1987). Figure 8.2 presents excerpts from this handbook that specify group-level strategies for creating more effective working relationships with staff members. Obviously, there are advantages to establishing a cooperative working relationship with the medical staff, but the precise nature of this collaboration must vary with the goals and objectives of the group, and the talents as well as values of the parents and professionals involved. Despite the variety of possible roles and role preferences,

Figure 8.2. Working with professionals (from Nathanson, 1987, p. 63)

Service to professionals

Making professionals' jobs easier and helping them to help families promotes group goals as well. If professionals know that the group supports them and their programs, they may feel like partners. Ask how the group can help them. Find out what their needs are and how the group can assist them to have these met.

Remember, professionals who feel good about the group will share this positive feeling with other professionals. Other professionals are more likely to listen to their professional peers than to group members. Professionals who feel they have something to gain from group efforts are more likely to promote the group and to have a vested interest in its success.

Don't forget that professionals, particularly those who work with seriously ill children, have personal needs also. They may be working in understaffed institutions, in crisis situations, in emotionally draining circumstances, with long hours and minimal pay. Acknowledge their dedication and service. Remember their human needs. Something as simple as a birthday card, a wedding or baby gift or shower, and/or a public thank you in the group newsletter, goes a long way in giving professionals deserved recognition. In return, such tributes also create warm feelings about the group.

Sharing credit

Who receives credit for achieving goals is not nearly as important as the achievement. It will create smooth referral and cooperative arrangements if professionals know that the group is grateful to them. Give them credit whenever possible. Thank them in the newsletter. Introduce them as supporters. Let fellow professionals know how helpful they have been. Everyone feels better about working with people who appreciate them. Recognition of their professional cooperation may make it easier for them to promote the group within the treatment center or agency.

It may be necessary to search for something positive to say or even to ignore negative actions or lack of support. But, giving praise or thanks for whatever positive support there is can produce surprising benefits. It can even turn a doubter into a supporter.

---

and frequent confusion and struggle about choices, there do appear to be some consensually agreed-upon options for professionals. Figure 8.3 presents a list of roles and behaviors that both parents and professionals agreed professionals could play in self-help groups and in the medical system to support these groups. Obviously, there is substantial agreement and room for cooperation. Professionals as well as parents can gain insight into their own tasks and possible behavioral options through group involvement and work with one another and

Figure 8.3. Parents' and professionals' agreed-upon role options for professionals in self-help groups

---

At the level of the group

Making resources and contacts available.
Conduct leadership-training programs
- organizational leadership skills
- peer counselling skills

Process parent complaints in ways that empower parents.
Educate parents about the medical care system.
- about the disease
- about stress and coping
- about how the medical system operates and can be altered

Legitimize parents' experiential knowledge as valuable.
Employ a variety of roles.
- partnership with parents
- support for parental action
- separate from parents

At the level of the local medical system

Develop an effective and active referral system.
Emphasize the legitimacy of the group through mailing and outreach.
Educate professionals about the group's value and activity, and help parents educate other professionals.
Provide the group access to hospital resources and vice versa.
Generate publicity for the group in and out of the medical system.
Help the group link to other institutional settings.
- schools and community agencies
- other medical systems
- other groups around the region or nation

---

through open discussion of these issues. The complexities of group-professional collaboration lie in the challenge to balance professionals' level of involvement with the needs and preferences of parents. The best mix of roles and needs will vary by group and by professional, but generally it involves professionals in ways that maximize parents' own sense of competency and empowerment.

9

Consumer-Provider Conflict and the Mobilization of Consumer Activism

Conflict is intrinsic to the organized relations between providers and recipients of health care. When recipients are seriously ill and dependent for a long time on the medical care system, the conflict is likely to be particularly potent and pervasive. The consequences may include patient dissatisfaction, family dysfunction and disempowerment, staff distress, and in some cases inadequate medical care. Self-help groups respond to both consumer-provider conflict and consumer disempowerment by helping to articulate and channel patient and family concerns, create new forms of consumer-staff relations, lessen patient and family dependency upon the staff, and advocate for change in those organizational conditions that create or escalate conflict and distress.

In Chapter 4 we reported that 38% of the fifty local self-help groups formed by and for parents of children with cancer we studied had engaged in efforts to deal with conflict between parents or patients and staff and to change the local medical system. This activity varied by the leadership structure of the group; as demonstrated in Chapter 5, groups that were led by professional staff members were less likely to be engaged in such change-oriented work. The attempts by self-help groups with shared and independent leadership patterns to deal with intrinsic conflicts often led to changes that improved the quality of medical care and the relations between care providers and consumers. Such groups have been described by some observers as part of a social movement.[1] In this chapter we extend the social movement perspective to show how local self-help groups can be treated as social movement organizations

226

that try to mobilize and empower health consumers in the face of great personal stress, disempowerment, and institutional conflict. Thus, we place these self-help groups within the larger context of local voluntary associations or mobilized interest groups, powerful traditions in the American democratic society.

The Background of Conflict in Health Care

The relations between providers of health care services and the consumers of this care are fraught with interpersonal and organizational conflict. The roots of these conflicts have been located in the social psychological or organizational concepts discussed in earlier chapters: the distressed situation of the patient and family members, the sick person role, professionals' roles and status, power asymmetry between care providers and recipients, the bureaucratic organization of care, and differential bases of staff and family experience and expertise.[2] We also can identify the roots of such conflict in the broader political economy of health care in the United States.[3] For instance, the entrepreneurial form and profit motive of modern medicine often compromise the resources (time, energy, funds) that medical staffs and institutions can provide to patients, and may weaken these actors' and agencies' primary commitments to holistic patient and family care. Moreover, state sanctioning of professional competencies places enormous official legitimacy and power in the hands of medical practitioners. At the same time that state action may protect patients against untrained or incompetent practitioners, it also often limits the treatment options open to these patients and families. Class and racial disparities in access to medical care in the United States result in many patients not getting adequate and competent care, and some not receiving care at all. Moreover, the care that is provided is often delivered in ways that fail to be responsive or attentive to distinctive racial, class, and ethnic lifestyles, psychosocial needs, and cultural sensitivities. Finally, the cultural bias toward mind-body dualism in western medicine has led to a focus on biological, radiological, and biochemical treatments for childhood cancer. While this focus is largely responsible for the great advances in successful medical treatment for this family of diseases, it also has diverted attention from a holistic approach to patients' and families' psychological and social situations. Thus, even when good technical medical care is provided, health systems place a low priority on effective psychosocial care, partly because of inadequate insurance reimbursement, and partly because of western medicine's historic insensitivity to psychosocial and interpersonal issues.[4]

Being a patient, especially a cancer patient, and especially a young cancer patient, involves anxiety, discomfort and often pain. Being a parent of a young cancer patient is similarly stressful.[5] A medical crisis usually makes the patient and her close loved ones feel vulnerable and confused about how to express their new needs and concerns. The family with a child in the "sick role" often encounters a loss of its status as a healthy and "normal" family; this loss affects social relationships with intimate friends, with strangers, and with members of the medical staff. Under these circumstances, patients' and parents' needs for emotional support and engagement are escalated and may conflict with the emotional distance and affective neutrality of the professional role, with disappointing consequences for all parties.[6]

Being a patient or the parent of a patient with a serious and chronic illness such as cancer also requires the recognition and semipublic expression of highly personal needs. Every person is somewhat of an expert on his own bodily reactions and medical history, and almost all parents are experts on their children. Professional experts in generalized medical knowledge are not necessarily expert on each patient's bodily history and affliction. Thus, as noted in Chapter 8 (Table 8.1), parents and professionals come to the treatment relationship with quite different sets of expertise and knowledge: one specific and the other general, one experiential and the other academic, one direct and the other vicarious, one based on a need to be cured and the other on a need to cure. These different vantage points, with their different interests and implied roles, may be complementary but are often conflictual.

The status of the professional staff provides them with privileges and obligations that carry enormous power over patients and their family members. The professional role embodies knowledge of patients' illness, the power to label and treat, and state-sanctioned responsibilities for medication and hospitalization.[7] Exercise of these tasks usually creates an asymmetrical power relationship between providers and their patients' parents (Szasz and Hollender, 1956), and patients and their parents usually play a dependent and passive role vis-à-vis service providers. This role structure is often detrimental to high-quality care, and may prevent young patients and their parents from asserting their needs and preferences, and perhaps even from responding effectively to treatment. Patients and their parents who conform to dominant medical norms by taking on the compliant and passive role of "good patients" and "good families," may relinquish self-control and responsibility for their own welfare—inside and outside of the treatment center.[8]

Especially in the case of childhood cancer, these provider-consumer (professional-patient or professional-parent) relationships take place within large, bureaucratized medical systems (Friedson, 1970; Lipsky, 1980). There, patients (depending on their age) and their parents must learn the jargon and culture of organized medicine.[9] Not only do consumers or clients feel awed by unfamiliar rules and language and massive bureaucracies in the health care system, but there even their intimate bodily and physical needs are addressed within a depersonalized context. As distinctions of power and status compound their feelings of vulnerability, many patients and family members feel powerless and alienated, and some resent, resist, or rebel against this kind of care-giving system.[10] Since control of the medical relationship remains in professionals' hands, many young people and many parents of children with cancer avoid overt conflict with medical staffs and organizations by denying their felt needs and internalizing their powerless role. When they do value their own knowledge, do give priority to their own needs or values, or do try to (co)direct the medical relationship, overt conflict may be unavoidable.

The Symptoms of Patient-Provider Conflict

These background conditions of conflict in health care do not always give rise to overt expressed conflict. They are, however, the basis of underlying "structural conflict"—conflict that is inherent in the structure of relationships between medical staffs or institutions and patients or families. Such conflict is not a function of any single person's behavior or good or ill will, but of institutional patterns of role differentiation, power and authority, informational and ideological hegemony, and dominance/dependence relations.[11]

What are the symptoms or indicators of conflict in the organized relations between medical consumers and caregivers or health care systems? The evidence may take multiple forms, some of which may be quite subtle. For example, conflict is often at the root of, or reflected in, sustained patient dissatisfaction, failed communication, or patient non-compliance with medical regimens.[12] It also may be expressed through patient (or patient family) behavior showing passivity, lack of self-confidence, intimidation, or even fear, in relations with the medical staff. In more overt forms, conflict may surface as individual patients, especially young patients and their parents, lodge or press their complaints and concerns. More overt protests also may take the form of letters or phone complaints about the behavior of individual staff members, or public behavior designed to embarrass the staff or the medical institution in the eyes of the community. More subtle forms of protest may occur behind the scenes, in polite discussions between patients (or patient representatives) and the medical staff or in more intense conversations among patients and parents.

Consumers are not the only actors who experience pain and conflict in patient-provider relationships. Physicians and nurses often become distressed when they are unable to effect a cure (Rothenberg, 1967; Vaux, 1977),[13] or when they feel unappreciated by patients and their families. Staff members involved in such conflict with patients may express their anger or hurt by derogating the behavior or character of individual patients, or patients in general. When they express such feelings directly to patients or family members, or leak them in subtle form, open conflict may occur on the ward or in the clinic. In some situations, staff members may challenge the institutional priorities of care (Stone, 1983), and staff-staff or staff-institution conflict results when they advocate parents' or families' interests against unyielding medical bureaucracies and resistant officials.

A number of the conflicts discussed above are reflected in reports by parents of children with cancer regarding their experiences with the health care system. On the one hand, the overwhelming majority of parents in our study of eight local self-help groups reported, in Table 9.1, being "very" or "pretty" satisfied with most aspects of their relationships with medical staffs. They especially respected the technical competence of the staff (reflected in item 1), generally reported good working relationships with staff members (reflected in items 2, 3, and 10), appreciated the information they received (reflected in item 6), and in general appreciated the staff's efforts to heal their children. On the

Table 9.1. Parents' satisfaction with the medical system/staff ($N = 116$)

Aspect of staff or facility	Percentage of parents reporting			
	Very satisfied	Pretty satisfied	Not so satisfied	Dissatisfied
1. Quality of medical care	81	19	0	0
2. Relationship between the medical staff and parents	56	40	4	0
3. Relationship between the medical staff and ill children	62	33	5	0
4. Quality of social work services	49	25	20	7
5. Emotional support for the family in the hospital	41	42	11	6
6. Information on the disease and its treatment	52	38	9	1
7. Hospital liaison with schools	26	44	19	11
8. Help with siblings' problems	23	44	24	10
9. Listen to parents' opinions	39	49	10	2
10. Staff sympathy for my child	56	34	10	0
11. Solve disagreements between parents and staff easily	37	44	17	2

other hand, parents reported less satisfaction with the quality of socio-emotional support they received from the facilities and staffs (items 4 and 5), with staffs' assistance with nonmedical, family-oriented issues (items 7 and 8), and with staffs' responses to parent-staff "disagreements" (item 11).

Chesler and Barbarin (1984b) report that despite generally high satisfaction with the technical aspects of care, a considerable proportion of parents of living children with cancer (60%, or 44 out of a sample of 74) also reported problems in their relations with staff members; 39% reported three or more problems. While any specific problem could reflect conflict between parents and staff members, the most prominent category in their study was "conflict that was hard to resolve," that is, overt conflict.[14] Consider the following parents' comments (Chesler and Barbarin, 1984b, p. 56):

If I confronted the nurses with how I feel about some of them, my child would suffer.

Another doctor became quite incensed over my comments. He came down to our room and called me a "rabble-rouser" and said that if I did not allow whomever was there to work on our child, she should not be treated at the hospital. He said if we didn't like it we could take her someplace else.

Such comments suggested that the status and power differentials between parents and staff often caused parents to fear staff retaliation if they were too assertive, and made it difficult to resolve differences or disagreements except in ways preferred or dictated by the staff. For example, one mother reported that when she questioned the staff about the massive amounts of radiation that were to be administered to her child, her questions were not acknowledged as legitimate. Daunted, but undeterred, she consulted physicians across the country regarding the need for this amount of radiation. Several physicians evidently agreed that such a dosage might be injurious. The parents reported that after they presented this information to their child's physician, he made them feel that they were "stupid, unintelligent lay people, that we were playing with the life of our child." Ultimately, they elected to have their child treated elsewhere.

The depersonalized medical bureaucracy sometimes marched right over parents' needs and feelings. Given the operations of a large bureaucracy and typical professional-client role definitions, it is not surprising that some parents experienced staff inflexibility and insensitivity. The following reports from parents illustrated this issue:

When the hospital expected full deductible before admitting, the financial aspect was difficult.

The interns needed some psychology. They were insensitive, and some were too young to deal with this life experience. They only did short stints in pediatrics. One of them pulled up my 13-year old daughter's shirt to examine her, exposing her breasts to everyone else in the room, and didn't even think about her reaction. The interns were mostly assholes—they couldn't deal with it, they were too immature.

As reported in Chapter 7, many parents were so distressed by the way the staff worked with their child that they felt they had to intervene in the treatment process in order to protect their child and to "correct mistakes." Parents who intervened in the medical care process also were significantly less satisfied with the emotional support they received from the staff, another indication of underlying conflict about the criteria for and delivery of good care. Moreover, the analysis in Chapter 7 indicated that parents involved in a self-help group were more likely to have intervened in their child's treatment process than were nonmembers. Evidently, the peer-oriented and empowering atmosphere of the group helped encourage and support parents to identify and articulate their needs and to think and act more critically with regard to the staff's assistance and operations. Other findings, presented in Table 9.2, indicate that self-help group members reported significantly less satisfaction with several aspects of the emotional support and interpersonal relationships they experienced with the staff than did parents who were not involved in the groups. In particular,

Table 9.2. Parents' satisfaction with the medical system/staff by self-help group membership ($N = 102$)

		Mean assessment of staff		
Satisfaction with aspect of staff or facility		Members ($n = 65$)	Nonmembers ($n = 37$)	Difference
1.	Quality of medical care	3.82	3.81	NS
2.	Relationship between the medical staff and parents	3.40	3.69	*
3.	Relationship between the medical staff and ill children	3.51	3.73	NS
4.	Quality of social work services	2.88	3.58	*
5.	Emotional support for the family in the hospital	3.05	3.39	*
6.	Information on the disease and its treatment	3.24	3.58	*
7.	Hospital liaison with schools	2.57	3.15	*
8.	Help with siblings' problems	2.60	3.08	*
9.	Listen to parents' opinions	3.15	3.33	NS
10.	Staff sympathy for my child	3.52	3.44	NS
11.	Solve disagreements between parents and staff easily	2.96	3.38	*

Note: Responses were rated on a four-point scale: 4 = "very satisfied"; 3 = "pretty satisfied"; 2 = "not so satisfied"; and 1 = "dissatisfied."
   * Difference is statistically significant at $p < .05$, using a one-way, single-factor analysis of variance.

self-help group members reported significantly less satisfaction than did nonmembers with the general quality of social work services, the level of information and support they received, the assistance they received in dealing with siblings' concerns, and potential problems with their child's schooling. The relationship between critical feelings about the staff (or at least about the staff's lack of emotional support) and both intervention and self-help group involvement also may be explained by assuming that parents who felt most neglected or isolated from the staff found the greatest faults in the staff's execution of their duties, and were therefore more likely to intervene and to join the self-help group. Alternatively, in the context of group discussions of their needs and expectations, parents may have decided that they required more psychosocial assistance and should assert themselves vis-à-vis the staff and institution. These parents' active behaviors, in the group and in staff interactions, may have produced negative reactions from the staff, and these reactions then may have created or escalated parents' feelings of conflict and alienation.[15]

The Role of Self-Help Groups in Patient-Provider Conflict

The fundamental dynamic of self-help groups, as in any mutual support system, permits and encourages the transformation of individual concerns and complaints into collective grievances. Individuals' distressed feelings often are shared—compared and contrasted—with others, and through this process of social comparison, they are sometimes translated into formal grievances. This is especially likely when aspects of the medical care system can be identified as helping to create or escalate feelings of distress. For instance, individual parents who were intimidated by the staff or who feared retaliation if they asserted their needs directly were often reluctant to act on their feelings. They often found support and protection in a group setting, especially when the self-help group articulated issues publicly in ways that protected the identity of any individual parent. Since power asymmetry between providers and patients made it difficult for individual parents to express their concerns to the staff in the clinic or hospital wards—on "medical turf"—a neutral or parent-oriented setting, with many parents together, made it easier. Instead of taking individual actions, members of a self-help group could express and pursue their concerns collectively to appropriate members of the medical staff. Thus, self-help groups, like traditional social movement organizations, often facilitated the identification and organized expression of grievances.

There were several tactics that self-help groups (like any group representing the interests of an even temporarily disempowered constituency) utilized to advocate their members' concerns: opening up clogged communication channels, using collaborative problem solving to persuade decision makers of the need for change, developing and exchanging key resources to serve the mutual needs of staffs and parents, pressuring powerholders to make changes, creating coercive challenges or protests to change policies and practices (see Table 9.3). All these tactics required the exercise of some sort of power, and often the surfacing of structural conflict or the escalation of overt conflict to gain attention, engage collaboration, or force new decisions. These are all forms of public advocacy that have been used by various self-help groups of families of children with cancer, and many like organizations.

A common example of the communicative approach occurred when parents in several local groups sought staff collaboration in facilitating the reentry of ill children into their classroom studies and peer groups.

Table 9.3. Change tactics utilized by self-help groups

Tactic	Examples
Communication tactics	
Informing	Presenting the staff with information about patient/ family needs
Requesting	Asking for added staff
	Asking the staff for a parent library
Influencing/Persuading	Convincing the staff to alter clinic procedures
	Sending a delegation to present a complaint
Exchange tactics	
Providing resources	Raising funds to (partially) support a new staff position
	Helping the clinic raise funds for group-approved purposes
Pressure tactics	
Bargaining	Offering to support a staff initiative in return for needed services
Coercing/pressuring	Demonstrating or threatening to protest in public
	Boycotting the clinic

On their own, neither families nor the medical staff were able to solve the problems of school-home-hospital communication, of preparing the ill child's classmates for her new appearance, of arranging for individualized instruction, or of advising teachers on the child's limitations (or nonlimitations). However, several self-help groups sponsored conferences that brought together families, medical personnel, and school staff members to solve jointly the problems they identified and even to make new school policy (see Figure 4.5). Several parent group leaders also reported successful examples of their efforts to communicate their concerns or grievances about medical or psychosocial care directly to the staff.

We got action by pecking away. We mentioned our complaint to the nurse, to other parents, and sometimes to the nursing supervisor. Other parents did the same.

We love the medical staff. We stated a bunch of concerns to the head nurse who, got defensive at first, but after we got over the personal feelings, she was able to do problem solving with us.

Sometimes the communication of grievances produced these positive and collaborative responses, and even changes in the behavior of staff members or the organization of care. At other times communication failed to produce change: then parent groups either ceased their efforts, moved to exchange tactics, or escalated to pressure tactics.

Exchange tactics occurred in a number of communities where self-help groups raised substantial funds to support new school or medical programs, additional staff, or temporary housing facilities (e.g., Ronald McDonald Houses) that they felt were essential for the care of their children. Typically, the medical staff assisted in these fund-raising efforts, and in some cases staff members took or shared lead roles in these campaigns. Self-help groups often employed pressure—as well as exchange—tactics with the medical system to change patient-services systems, staffing patterns, or clinic schedules. In particular, they addressed some of the common conflicts and grievances identified earlier (rescheduling tests, changing rules and hours for visitors, permitting parents to hold their children during some procedures, etc.). One parent group leader discussed a variety of approaches a local group had used, including bargaining and pressure:

We formed a delegation to discuss problems with the medical staff and to make demands: an outpatient lab, children's separate waiting room, etc. The delegation also contacted the hospital director and complained about the lack of physicians on the Oncology staff. Our group provided the hospital with funds for a new staff member's salary for a year, this is "seeding" a position, and if it proves worthwhile the hospital will take over the salary payment.

Another example of a situation that involved pressure as well as communication occurred in a New England hospital, where the staffing pattern of the hospital's emergency service did not include a pediatric oncologist on call. In several instances, parents felt that children with cancer did not receive emergency treatment properly targeted to their immuno-compromised situation—partly because the standard emergency room staff was inexperienced with the atypical treatments needed by their children. Although some individual parents had expressed their concerns, no changes had been made in the hospital's staffing pattern. Finally, the parent self-help group called a meeting, urging the Pediatric Oncology staff to attend. Since the announced purpose of the meeting was to discuss parental grievances, the staff was both interested in coming and cautious about the outcome of such a meeting. At first, the staff sat on one side of the room and the parents, expressing their grievances vigorously, sat on the other side. The staff listened and nervously defended the current staffing pattern—and their inability to change it. Parents represented their case with more information and more passion. The level of overt conflict escalated sharply as voices were raised on all sides. After some time, people moved from their respective sides of the room and mingled with one another; more reasoned, calmer exchanges prevailed. The staff eventually agreed that they had been unaware of many parental grievances, could not continue to defend the emergency room staffing procedure, and would try to place a pediatric oncologist on call for children with cancer who needed emergency room treatment. Parents as well as staff members reported their satisfaction with the outcomes of the meeting, despite a feeling that it had been "hard to take."

Some self-help groups also applied direct coercive pressure to change the medical system. Among the more coercive strategies were representation of parental power to medical authorities, coalitions with other community agencies who wanted to alter the medical system, media campaigns, lobbying efforts with local and state authorities, and public demonstrations or boycotts. One example of a coercive strategy involved a self-help group in the Southwest, where a community-based children's hospital discovered that its Pediatric Oncology clinic was losing money and unilaterally decided to shut down its operations. Parents were informed by mail that their children's treatment would continue at a major children's hospital and cancer center in a neighboring city seventy-five miles away. Parents' expressions of concern were ineffective until the self-help group mobilized support for keeping the clinic open at the local hospital. Some parents affiliated with the self-help group visited local businesspersons and city officials, trying to generate financial and political support for their effort. When they had mobilized their own constituency and had solicited substantial external funds, they called a public meeting. Hospital officials and the local media were invited to a mass meeting and press conference. Parents expressed their concern about the extra expense and stress (and in some cases danger) of travel to the new treatment site. They spoke about the impact of closing the local clinic on the reputation of the city as a modern high-tech locale. They dramatically paraded their sick children on the public stage in a successful appeal for sympathy. Finally, they announced the availability of significant funds to compensate for the current clinic's losses and even to expand its services. The hospital administration was shamed into reversing their decision on the spot; they reopened and expanded the Pediatric Oncology clinic and joined forces with the self-help group to continue to raise funds to support it.

Not all self-help groups for families of children with cancer undertook such dramatic action. Many advocated for change in more subtle ways. Some engaged in little external advocacy, preferring to focus their efforts on support and education of their members. However, they all hoped to increase their members' ability to cope more actively and successfully with their child's illness. As these examples indicate, the range of collective actions that local self-help groups mobilized parents to use in response to conflict they experienced with the medical care system included:

1. Surfacing structural conflict by identifying, collectivizing and articulating parental perceptions and concerns

2. Preparing parents for new roles in conflict situations by enhancing their sense of competence and their skills in creating change
3. Bringing service providers and service recipients together to exchange views and to engage in joint problem solving
4. Escalating behavioral conflict in order to gain the attention and responsiveness of decision makers
5. Advocating changes in the organization and delivery of medical care to patients and families.

Several social movement scholars also have emphasized the ways in which these kinds of group activities utilize conflict in order to surface and clarify differences, heighten individual consciousness and group identity, help correct service inadequacies, tune programs to the real needs of service recipients, and provide a safety valve to reduce the need for more escalated or dysfunctional individual or group reactions.[16]

Self-help groups that are self-sustaining and that do advocate patients'/parents' interest for changes in the medical system—even those that adopt a collaborative posture—typically become direct parties to patient-provider conflicts. This certainly is the case if one of their roles is to help mobilize relatively powerless parents into a knowledgeable, autonomous, organizationally competent, and potentially powerful force. Several scholars have predicted a high level of overt group-system conflict, arguing that self-help groups pose an inherently antiprofessional ideology and style.[17] Some self-help groups may well be antiprofessional, but none of the groups for parents of children with cancer we studied would fit this description. More common was a group emphasis on experiential knowledge rather than technical expertise, and on group autonomy (which may at times appear as an aprofessional or pro-experiential stance) and relative power symmetry with professionals. Thus, although we and other investigators argue that structural conflict between parent self-help groups and the medical system is quite common, overt group-system conflict and antiprofessionalism is neither inevitable nor necessarily high. Wollert et al. (1984) noted that "while conflicts often characterize the interaction of professionals and self-help groups, there are other modes of relating which can avoid these pitfalls" (p. 137). Moreover, when overt conflicts do occur, they are not necessarily negative and dysfunctional for any or all parties. Self-help groups can work collaboratively with agency staffs and institutions on such structural conflicts, and mutual interest and cooperation can prevail.[18] Our own view, and the evidence presented throughout this chapter, is that collaboration and conflict are not mutually exclusive forms of engagement and collective problem solving, and that self-help groups and medical providers need to be prepared to utilize all these tactics—perhaps all at once. At times, self-help groups will serve their members' interests best by escalating conflict as a change tactic (as in most pressuring or coercive approaches), rather than trying to reduce it (as in communicative or purely collaborative approaches). At other times, precisely the reverse will be true. What happens in reality depends more on local needs, resources, and interorganizational dynamics than on vague generalizations.

Interorganizational Conflict: Medical Staffs and Parent Groups

In the attempt to maximize their own resources and usefulness and still collaborate with one another, self-help groups and medical systems have generated tension and conflict as well as consensus and cooperation in their relationships. It is not always easy to combine emotionally sensitive and compassionate relationships, effective technical care, and an efficiently running operation within a single organization, let alone between two apparently different ones. The responses of both parents and professionals confirm the difficulty of resolving these structural and historical conflicts, but they also hint at the possibility of more effective and friendly relationships between self-help groups and medical staffs.

Some staffs and some medical centers have established good working relationships with local self-help groups of parents of children with cancer. Indeed, a number of professionals have reported their view of the utility of these groups for the medical system.

Parents can use these groups to let their concerns about care be known. They could give a physician minutes of their group meeting to read and then give him or her a chance to get back to them. That gives both sides some time to think things over.

The group empowers parents to take a more active role—to tell us what they need.

In addition, some professionals reported their recognition of ways in which they themselves had benefited from the local parent support group.

As a social worker, I find you can learn a lot from parents' group meetings. You can gain insight into how you can help. One psychologist came to a meeting to talk. He said things that were just the wrong things to say. You learn not to say certain things.

Parents are braver in groups. They figure out how to effect change. So professionals get more feedback.

Two professionals articulated the groups' benefits for parents, above all:

If parents know the objectives and the limits of the group, they can get a lot of knowledge—even by comparing kids' treatments.

There just is no substitute for parents talking with other parents. We professionals have to recognize that.

However, not all professional staff members expressed such positive views of local parent groups, and interorganizational conflict between medical staffs or institutions and parents groups were and are common. Why?

One explanation lies in the degree of vulnerability that self-help groups experience in their relations with the medical organization. Like patients and parents of patients, groups are to some extent dependent upon the staff for their existence and success. For instance, gaining access to new members is a constant problem for all voluntary organizations, and local self-help groups must meet and recruit parents of newly diagnosed children. Since the professional staff generally controls the group's access to families of new patients, it may exercise considerable power over this key element in group development and maintenance. When referrals have not been forthcoming from the staff, some groups have bypassed the staff and recruited new patients and their families directly from hospital wards or clinics. While this is legally permissible, it does represent a challenge to some staff practices, a conflict over access mechanisms, and in response some medical staff members have cautioned parents "not to talk to other parents."

Debates or struggles over control of the self-help group's direction and activities are another explanation for potential system-group conflict. Many professionals are quite concerned that groups may practice psychotherapy or do psychological counseling; reports from discussions within most professional organizations (e.g., American Cancer Society, Leukemia Society of America, Association of Pediatric Oncology Social

Workers) and most voluntary or lay groups (Candlelighters Childhood Cancer Foundation, local self-help groups) explicitly caution against such activity. Very few groups do venture onto this turf without professional assistance, but the typical group emphasis on peer support and co-counseling often creates interpersonal or group dynamics that are similar to formal counseling. In a different vein, some professionals feel that parents *should* discuss their deep feelings in a group, although still not conduct formal counseling. Groups that do not do so, that focus on having parties and raising money, or on advocating changes, may be seen by some mental health professionals as "avoiding" or "denying" real issues. What is at stake in both instances are conflicting moral judgments or values, rooted in different bases of expertise and experience, regarding what groups should do and how parents should cope.

Groups that discuss parents' feelings about the medical staff may be especially threatening to staff members. Professionals often express concern that in the midst of great parental stress and crisis, parents who talk together may inappropriately escalate one another's fears and anger, resulting in unjustifiable and uncomfortable attacks on the staff. Although this threat to professionals is understandable, and no doubt has occurred, the sharing that occurs in most groups is far more likely to dissipate or channel parental anger productively than to escalate or target it inappropriately.

Finally, groups' efforts to try to change the staff or hospital procedures also may help explain this conflict, especially when professionals feel they are already doing all that they can for their patients. For instance, when groups place direct or indirect pressure on the medical system try to change existing procedures, or when they employ some of the coercive strategies outlined above, overt and increased conflict quite naturally results. To the extent that the medical practices and protocols targeted for change are rooted in deeply held staff values or interests, conflicts over these efforts for change are likely to be intense.

A number of these underlying or structural conflicts can lead to overt clashes of culture and turf, and a need to negotiate or renegotiate established relations between providers and consumers. Since parent self-help groups are based on respect for parents' experiential wisdom, the problems of differential knowledge—technical expertise as contrasted with experiential expertise—can create difficulties in relationships between parents and staff members. After all, knowledge about the medical and psychosocial realities of childhood cancer, appropriate responses to stress, and the dynamics of small groups may be part of the expertise of many professional staff members. Groups that operate independently of the staff, and that cherish and rely upon parents' experiential knowledge, may represent a challenge or threat to staff members' sense of competence and control, as well as to their ability to support and contribute to the group. The medical staff often has its own notion of what groups "should be doing"; when their preferences are substantiated by the accumulated expertise of their profession, they may not easily renegotiate these preferences with lay persons. While staff members may be able to overcome such differences in the context of one-on-one counseling sessions, they may have to negotiate these issues much more carefully when facing a powerful collective entity such as a well-organized parent group.

It also may be difficult for professionals who care, and who feel they have relevant expertise, to sit back and not exert leadership in the parent self-help group. It may be even more difficult for them to acknowledge and encourage apparently "nonexpert" parents to exercise leadership, especially if that leadership moves in a direction not congruent with their assumptions and priorities. Moreover, when other resources such as meeting space, copying, and mailing services are readily available to staff members but difficult for parents to find, professionals may find it hard not to deliver such resources. Also, parents may find it difficult not to accept them. In these situations, professionals' commitments to provide effective help and service may clash with parents' need to exert their own form of programmatic leadership and to avoid excessive reliance and dependence on the staff.

These difficulties reflect differences between the professional culture of medicine or social service and the experiential culture of self-help. If the professional staff is composed largely of highly educated white persons of at least middle-class status, they may encounter additional cultural clashes with groups composed of families from lower-class, African American, Latino, or Asian American origins.

Staff Perceptions of the "Dangers" of Self-Help

In our study of fifty self-help groups of parents of children with cancer, we examined sixty-three professionals' (doctors, nurses, and social workers) views of potential interorganizational conflicts with the local self-help group with which they worked (Chesler, 1990b). When asked whether they "had heard the viewpoint that self-help groups could be dangerous," 90% of these professionals answered in the affirmative. When asked whether they had ever seen such dangers occur in the local group, only 24% indicated affirmatively. One nurse from a southwestern hospital first questioned even the concept of inherent danger:

Why should there be any danger? Whose goals are we trying to meet, anyway? The goal is coping and helping.

But she immediately qualified that comment by stating,

They (self-help groups) can only really be dangerous if they are used as treatment.

Such hesitant, mixed, or distrustful views of self-help groups were expressed by many professionals. Moreover, the difference between 90% of these professionals reporting that they had heard that such groups could be dangerous and only 24% responding that they had seen such dangers in their own experience is very provocative. It emphasizes the importance of considering some professionals' views of self-help groups as part of a professional or cultural ideology, and not as derived from their own empirical reality or their actual experience with group activities or processes. The low prevalence of dangers actually encountered or experienced suggests that in practice, the self-help groups that these professionals encountered were really not very dangerous, or at least not dangerous very often. These findings echo a study by Black and Drachman (1985), who reported that fully 37% of social workers in large hospitals rarely or never referred medical or psychiatric patients to self-help groups; however, the 63% who did make such referrals reported no harmful outcomes (p. 100). On the other hand, the high prevalence of "knowledge" or concern about the dangers of self-help groups suggests that professionals' perceptions of dangers are neither trivial nor haphazard; they are part of the belief system associated with a professional role and status. Whether they are learned on the job (from peer discussions) or as part of preprofessional training hardly matters, since they still may have a serious impact on professional behaviors and on local groups.[19]

The most common "dangers" mentioned by the professionals working with the fifty local groups we studied are categorized in Table 9.4.

Table 9.4. Frequency of staff reports of dangers of self-help groups

Danger cluster	Frequency ($n = 76$, $\% = 100$)
A. *Dangers to parents:*	
1. Create emotional problems for parents	20%
2. Parents learn/know too much	14
3. Spread misinformation	10
4. Parents act as professionals	5
5. Group goals and objectives	1
B. *Dangers to professionals:*	
6. Challenge the authority of professionals	23%
7. Take over professionals' job (social work)	8
8. Transfer doctors or increase medical competition	8
9. Question medical authority/judgment	8
10. Emotional attacks on professionals	3

Note: Since some informants mentioned more than one danger, the total of dangers noted (76) exceeds the number of interviews (63).

The first cluster of categories (A, representing 50% of all the responses) reflects reports of the concerns, albeit hypothetical and anecdotal, that professionals had heard regarding the negative impacts of self-help groups on members' information base or emotional health.[20] Several professionals' comments focused on parents' potential release of their emotions in the group setting, and the dangers of a lack of professional guidance or direction of this process. We suggested earlier that since some parents are overwhelmed by their own feelings, or their identification with others' situations, they may experience extraordinary pain and distress. In general, some professionals argued, parents of children with cancer experience enough emotional distress, and it is not advisable (indeed, is even dangerous) for them to be deeply involved with others' additional distress. That some parents may become confused and upset by the emotions (their own and others') rampant in a group setting has been articulated by several authors.[21] For instance, Belle-Isle and Conradt (1979) warned that

The danger of parents inappropriately sharing their concerns and unwittingly increasing each others' emotional burdens is a constant threat. With professional guidance this danger should be significantly less as staff participants are present to correct misinformation and control inappropriate exchanges. (p. 49)

In its most extreme form, this danger has been expressed in profession-als' concern that patients would "become terribly depressed, over-whelmingly anxious, even suicidal or psychotic as a result of talking together about having cancer" (Ringler et al., 1981, p. 331). Other pro-fessionals have expressed concern that over time a group may be "habit-forming," serve as a "crutch," and foster member dependency in ways that are inadvisable and inappropriate.[22] As self-help groups attempted to counter both parental dependence upon professionals and what they saw as professional orthodoxy, they were seen by some professionals as creating a potential orthodoxy of their own, placing undue pressure on people to join and urging unwilling parents to conform to group ideas and ideals about how to cope.[23] Several professionals articulated some of these views directly:

Groups also cause unnecessary depression and pain.

Parents with pathology may have that pathology supported by others who don't know how to handle it.

As facilitators, we must channel parents' emotions and needs in the right direction.

The doctors discouraged parents from talking with one another because they would intensify problems.

Even one professional who felt that the danger of a self-help group was not very great (but neither was its apparent benefit) indicated the power-ful influence of the professional ideology and culture, in the following view of self-help groups:

It is nothing more than babysitting with all their emotions. They don't really deal with the real problems most of the time.

The definition of these parents' "real problems," and the "right way" to deal with them, as seen by parents and their group or by the profes-sional staff, is at the heart of this perceived danger. Except in the most extreme cases of obviously pathological behavior, disagreement or de-bate about these issues basically involves differences over moral values and moral choices about how people "should" feel, cope, and act. It also involves different notions about who has the knowledge (technical or experiential) and competence to make such decisions.[24]

A second major concern expressed by professionals focused on the ways in which parents' discussions might manufacture misinformation and spread false ideas. Professionals expressed the fear that sharing ignorance or misunderstanding would multiply ignorance, and lead to rumors that fed false hopes, promoted confusion, or undermined trust in the medical system. In Chapter 2 we argued that one of the primary stresses of being a parent of a child with cancer involved dealing with large amounts of new information—information about the diagnosis, treatment, prognosis, and the medical staff and system itself. If meetings with other parents, and the development and sharing of experiential knowledge, were to provide misinformation as opposed to accurate information, they could well magnify these stresses.[25] Some comments from professionals concerned with this danger follow:

There is suspicion they are going to be priming the pump with pathological information.

Groups can sometimes generate misinformation.

Doctors don't want a parent giving out misinformation.

Quite a different cluster of comments involved professionals' concerns about the danger that parents might learn too much: not that they might be misinformed, but that they might become *too well-informed*. Professionals mentioning this danger suggested that when parents compared notes and information, they could attain a level of expertise that rivaled that of professionals. This concern has not been anticipated or reported in prior literature, but was reflected in the following comments:

Doctors are worried that parents will get too educated.

Professionals are afraid that parents will compare notes, compare protocols, and learn of experiments.

At first glance, a concern that parents might become too well-educated about their child's disease and treatment may not make much sense.[26] But if part of the provider-patient, parent-lay dynamic is rooted in differences between experiential knowledge and technical expertise, and if it involves differences over power and control, such concern on the part of professionals begins to make more sense. Even professionals who are strongly committed to using the power of their expertise in the best interests of children may resist its erosion—especially if they wonder about parents' abilities to serve their child's best interests. They also may not respect or approve of parents' experiential knowledge when it clashes with or goes beyond their own expertise. The perceived danger is that as parents become more educated, they may resist or ignore the staff's advice and authority. At least, they may resist professional direction that is provided without extensive and time-consuming explanations. They also may raise troublesome questions about research protocols and pursue what the staff feels are irrelevant comparisons among different children's diagnoses and treatments.

A closely related concern, that parents may "act like professionals," also may involve (mis)information, but it focused primarily on parents helping each other in ways that appeared to be therapeutic in orientation or intent. As parents conduct activities that professionals assume are beyond their lay skill and training, activities normally reserved for professionals, they may be seen as endangering themselves and others. For instance, the Leukemia Society of America's set of guidelines for family support groups, *Family Support Group Guidelines* (Leukemia Society of America, 1986, p. 8) explicitly states that "a family support group does not provide medical care, medical treatment, medical advice or psychotherapy." When peers and lay people do provide advice, as is often the case in psychosocial support sessions, Claflin (1984) noted that professionals make the "prevalent assumption that peer support groups practice group therapy (inappropriately)" (p. 125). While this is a legitimate concern for professionals and parents alike, the reality is that all such warnings are violated in practice, since they do not make sense in the informal and open atmosphere of a peer support group. People discussing their common problems do give and get medical and psychosocial advice; it is part of the development and sharing of experiential knowledge, the sharing of life experiences, and the provision of support and affirmation that people cherish about their group encounters. Although "psychotherapy" may be performed only by a formally credentialed psychologist or psychotherapist, peers who care for one another, who listen, hug, talk, and cry together undoubtedly are involved in a peer therapeutic process (sometimes called *co-counseling*), if not in peer therapy. Unfortunately, no definition of this range of therapy or psychotherapy has been offered in most published guidelines; it simply has been argued that it should not be provided by nonprofessionals. This perceived danger has raised staff fears of malpractice suits, heightened staff resistance to what are seen as unwarranted and unskillful peer interventions with their patients, and caused some local groups to defer their activities in order to pacify professional interest groups' notions of their legitimate turf. Professionals' comments relevant to these concerns included the following:

Groups may be dangerous if members do things beyond their skill and training.

Professionals feel that parents in a group are practicing medicine and psychology.

Some of the typical dynamics of all groups also have been seen as dangerous by some professionals. For instance, several writers warned of group factionalism or cliquishness, and some worried that groups' attempts to solve instrumental problems of their own management and maintenance could draw attention away from individuals' "real" psychological problems and concerns (King, 1980). Rather than seeing involvement with others in group tasks as a positive development, or as a positive way of coping with stress, some professionals may see it as an escape or diversion from the "real issues."

In addition to those dangers that professionals wanted to protect parents from experiencing, the second cluster of categories (B) in Table 9.3 (also involving 50% of all responses) notes dangers that professionals themselves were concerned about facing. Thus, not only did professionals express worry about experiencing conflict with parents regarding whether and how self-help group involvement might be beneficial or dangerous for parents, they also were concerned about experiencing more direct conflict with such groups regarding their own professional welfare.[27] The chief concern within the literature was the development by members of an anti-professional (or anti-intellectual) stance.[28] Among the dangers professionals mentioned that appeared to threaten their own status and role, challenges to their power were most common. This concern focused on the ways in which support provided in a group of parent-peers might reduce parental dependence upon the professional staff. Professionals feared that as they were less able to guide or control parent group activity, the power of their role might be compromised. In addition, the concern was raised that some parent groups might go outside normal staff channels to achieve their objectives, perhaps even mobilizing community pressure on the hospital to alter its patterns of service delivery (as reported earlier, that sometimes happened!). As some staff members noted,

Parents will become too powerful and demand things that professionals aren't prepared to meet.

Professionals are concerned with retaining control.

Doctors sometimes feel threatened by a group because parents gain momentum and power . . . through the group, parent power increases.

These comments reflected very clearly professionals' underlying concern with the dynamic of their own power and authority.

As parents provided important resources to one another, they may have been perceived as taking over professionals' roles, thereby reducing the necessity for full staff involvement. This may appear to affect the stability of personal employment or of the staff's institutional role. As Mantell (1983) noted, some professionals feared that "lay people who adopt professional activities will squeeze professionals out of their jobs" (p. 47). After all, if parent volunteers can do what a social worker or health educator can do, perhaps physicians and hospital administrators will conclude that there is no need for these paid staff members. Some professionals' comments to this effect follow:

Possibly posing competition to social workers.

Social workers are afraid someone is going to step on their space.

I feel that when I've got to refer a family to Candlelighters, I've failed at my job.

This last excerpt, from a social worker, suggesting that a referral to the local (Candlelighters) self-help group represented professional "failure," may help explain the covert and subtle basis on which much staff resistance rested. Rather than seeing the local self-help group as a complementary form of psychosocial assistance and support for parents, this social worker saw it as a last resort, as a competitive resource applicable only if her own assistance was ineffective.

A somewhat different danger was reported when parent groups were seen as encouraging the kind of information-sharing and related explorations that could escalate competition among physicians, especially competition for patients. For instance, Silverman and Smith (1984) reported that in a mutual help group for the physically disabled, a dissatisfied patient was informed that "she could choose her physician, and was not obligated to stay in the clinic. Members gave her the names of several physicians who had worked out well for people with similar problems" (p. 85). The fear that peer interaction will lead to such behavior and to a lessened need for a particular staff member's professional services, and thus to a loss of patients and personal or institutional income, was cited often as a basis of professionals' reluctance to refer people to cancer support groups (Cordoba et al., 1984; Katz, 1993).[29] It is not a trivial matter for physicians to maintain a patient load adequate to guarantee a stable income for the hospital unit, to warrant outlays for new and expensive equipment, to justify added staff roles, to provide nonreimbursable support services, or to absorb the nonreimbursable costs involved in treating patients without adequate insurance or other resources. For example, as several professionals commented,

Groups make doctors struggle to maintain their practice. Patients are money . . . they may go elsewhere for care.

Local doctors are afraid that the group will give information about other medical centers, and that parents may go comparison-shopping for doctors.

Staff fears patients will encourage others to use nonconventional treatments.

These comments reflected more than a self-interested concern about the staff's or institution's adequate patient load, or that patients who transfer to other doctors or other forms of treatment may compromise their reputation in the community; many staff members were also concerned that as a consequence children might receive a less adequate form of care.

Another threat was articulated by professionals who feared that parent groups might encourage questioning of medical authority and judgment. The concern again appeared to be with challenges to professionals' authority and omniscience, especially in a medical situation where everyone understood (perhaps silently and only in the company of other staff members) that some degree of uncertainty about treatment and treatment outcomes was the rule. Some physicians and other staff members argued that in order to prescribe and take action in an area of medical science that, despite great progress, still entailed considerable uncertainty, they must have the unquestioned compliance of patients and families. They suggested that the practice of medicine in a situation where the stakes were so high (life and death of children) was difficult enough without parents being encouraged by groups to ask what they saw as unnecessary and challenging questions. As some professionals commented,

They talked together and then went individually and confronted the doctor. That's bad. Doctors respond negatively if put on the spot.

Groups can promote too many questions.

Doctors may have to take more time to answer questions . . . they become threatened by questioning.

Groups generate questioning of doctors' judgments.

Finally, some professionals mentioned parents' emotionally inappropriate attacks on them as a potential danger of the collective sharing and action that might occur in self-help group sessions. Their primary concern was that, under great duress and distress, parental pain or anger could be inflamed by group discussion and displaced onto professionals. Some comments by professionals that reflected this concern follow:

Professionals are worried about the displacement of anger onto them.

Groups generate unwarranted criticism of professionals.

This group is typical, it is dysfunctional. They cause problems that reflect their anger, but they are aimed at staff members.

We have discussed the great stress and conflict that parents of children with cancer often experienced. No doubt this stress sometimes led to anger at inappropriate staff practices, at what they saw as medical "mistakes," or even at the hand of fate. On occasion, it also led to inappropriate displacement of their pain in the form of anger misdirected at particular staff members. But for most parents, the opportunity to share their life experiences and emotional reactions in a group of peers helped leaven that pain and direct their reactions into more appropriate channels. Indeed, buttressed by a greater experiential knowledge of their own situation, of the operations of the medical system, and of their medical and psychological options, most parents active in groups found *more rather than less* constructive ways of coping and of relating with the staff—both as individuals and as a group.

Figure 9.1 suggests how these categories of the dangers medical professionals attributed to childhood cancer self-help groups reflect some of the core themes of self-help (first elaborated in Chapter 1). Three major issues appeared to run through these professionals' views of the specific "dangers" of parent self-help groups, and they may help explain why such groups are "counternormative" or on the periphery of the U.S. system of medical treatment and psychosocial support. They are all rooted in health and medical professionals' right and power to exercise (1) control of access to the knowledge base upon which care is based (see dangers relating to parents learning too much, spreading misinformation and questioning medical authority); (2) control of practice or service in delivering medical and psychosocial care (see dangers relating to parents acting as professionals, group goals, parents taking over professionals' jobs, and transferring physicians); (3) control of the moral value frame that suggests appropriate coping behaviors and how

Figure 9.1. Core themes of self-help groups and related "dangers"

Theme	Dangers perceived by professionals
Experiential knowledge	Spread misinformation Learn too much Question authority of professionals Transfer doctors
Shared life experiences and new social identity	Create emotional problems
Support and affirmation	Create emotional problems Attacks on professionals
Improved coping skills	Learn too much Take over professionals' jobs
Collective action	Act as professionals Take over professionals' jobs Attacks on professionals Challenge authority of professionals

people should behave when in contact with illness and the health care system (see dangers relating to parents creating emotional problems, group goals, and attacking professionals). Challenge to this "triple monopoly" by assertive parent/patient organizations may be the most fundamental basis of overt conflict in health care.

Self-help groups that provide information to parents help generate an experiential knowledge base that poses implicit or explicit challenges to professionals' monopoly of expert knowledge, and thus potentially diminishes the unilateral power of the professional (Reiff, 1974). Moreover, as support groups educate parents, parents may become more active in the care of their children. As educated parents become more active (perhaps even to the point of intervening in care), they may violate the norms governing passive consumer roles and disrupt a smooth-running system.

The licensing and certification of health care professionals by state agencies establishes a monopoly of service or practice that is just as crucial to the organization of medical care as is the monopoly of expert knowledge. Concerns about challenges to the power of professionals, taking over their jobs, and promoting competition with other staffs relate to this professional monopoly. Bliwise and Lieberman (1984) note that "service delivery is rarely controlled by the client," and that "self-help organizations are unique among helping systems in that the client, rather than the professional or an external agency, has primary responsibility for care" (p. 227). As self-help groups educate parents to be more skillful in coping, they may become less dependent upon the medical staff, especially the psychosocial staff. A subtle (or not so subtle) struggle for control of the group and its activities may then ensue, since, as Claflin (1984) suggests, it is difficult for professionals to "share treatment responsibilities with patients or patient families" (p. 126). The concern about who maintains accountability and control over the delivery of services, in this case generally informational and psychosocial services, is escalated when professionals fear that group members are not only challenging or bypassing them, but that parent members may act as professionals and perhaps take over their functions. A reduction in professionals' power parallels a reduction in parent dependency upon them and upon their monopoly of informational and psychosocial services. Patients who learn to "comparison shop" present a slightly different challenge to this service monopoly. Although they do not challenge the monopoly per se, they may challenge any single professional's ability to maintain competitive control over his service sector. In a time when diminished federal funds reduce human service resources (Lavoie, 1983; Mantell, 1983), the prospect that self-help groups may encourage competition among physicians and psychosocial practitioners may be a realistic threat to some professionals' and hospitals' economic security.

The concern that groups will create emotional problems for parents is also related to professionals' values regarding the way people ought to cope and the level of stress they ought to seek or avoid (Featherstone, 1980). As self-help group members share coping strategies with one another, perhaps encouraging coping styles and life-style choices that professionals do not prefer, these choices may be experienced and labeled by professionals as inappropriate. As Katz (1984) noted, "If consumers do not conform to professional expectations, or follow the guidelines laid down by the service agency, they are thought to be resistant or refractory" (p. 233). The key to seeing a moral or value struggle here is the professional perception of "resistance" rather than "difference"; the conversion of "different" coping styles or values about services into "resistant," "wrong," or "inadequate" styles of coping obviously generates conflict.

Professionals' assumption of a monopoly in this regard may in itself create a danger for parents, if these values are used (knowingly or not) as a screen for self-interest and defense. For instance, in a startlingly forthright article, Ringler et al. (1981) discussed their own fears and perceptions, as professional staff members, about the dangers of self-help groups for cancer patients. They admitted that many of their fears were based more on their personal anxieties and defenses than on rational judgments or evidence about what went on in groups and what was good for members. As they noted, "Under the guise of 'protecting the patients', we were actually projecting our own terror at disfigurement, pain, loss of functioning, and death onto the group members. . . . [but] many of the group members were more than ready to look at those terrors (p. 339)". Ringler et al. also noted that instead of an honest exploration of these different judgments about group activities, they sought to impose their judgments on patients by controlling the group's agenda and process. Fortunately, the group resisted. Even more fortunately, Ringler et al. were attentive to their own process, learned from their errors, and were honest enough to admit it—in print!

Judgments about monopolies of moral choice regarding proper ways of coping are likely to be even more problematic when they are rooted in the demographic backgrounds and cultures common to many medical professionals: white racial groups, male-dominated medical systems, and middle-class or upper middle-class origins. Parents or parent groups who express coping styles that depart from the race, gender, and class preferences that are dominant in professional groupings are likely to encounter disrespectful and even intolerant behavior from the staff. At the very least, these parents will discover that the staff is reluctant to refer parents of newly diagnosed children to their group.[30] These social and moral, not technical and medical, choices are precisely what are at stake in parental concern or resistance to the staff's preference for or insistence upon certain types of coping behavior.

Coalitions as a Way to Deal with Conflict?

Despite inevitable interpersonal and intergroup conflict, many self-help groups and many medical institutions have experimented with new arrangements that helped mediate these conflicts. Adversarial mobilization and pressure tactics were by no means the only stances self-help groups adopted in dealing with conflicts vis-à-vis the medical system. For instance, as reported in Chapter 8, the vast majority of active members of self-help groups for parents of children with cancer felt that professionals did and should play important roles in their groups. As staff members collaborated with self-help groups, they provided some of the core resources groups needed to operate: access and referrals to new patients and families, hospital meeting rooms, contact with medical staff members, a good reputation, funds for coffee and a newsletter, links to community agencies, and so on. Some professionals also helped groups become established and consulted with them on organizational matters, teaching members how to run a meeting, educating them about the dynamics of the medical staff, helping to plan programs and educating the rest of the staff about the self-help group. When conflict escalated, some staff members even intervened between the group and other staff members to help create understanding, if not collaboration.[31] In reciprocal fashion, some self-help groups and members made important contributions to individual staff members and medical institutions. Some staff members reported earlier that they learned more about parents' needs and the ways in which they might respond helpfully to these needs from self-help group meetings and activities. And a number of medical centers changed, expanded, or improved their services as a result of parent group requests, pressure, or provision of financial resources.

Any such effort to combine informal helping systems and formal helping systems requires planning to overcome the "clash of cultures" that Froland et al. (1981) identify and that has been examined throughout this chapter. The combination of autonomy and interdependence reflected especially in the self-help groups that adopted a shared parent-professional leadership pattern suggests a coalition model of organization and organizational leadership. The basic principle underlying a coalition is the coming together of two or more parties, typically parties that have different interests or that previously have been in conflict with one another. The purpose of coalition-building is to organize at least a temporary collaborative effort that has benefits for all parties.[32] In the interest of forming coalitions of relatively equal status, all parties must wrestle with their prior experience and training, which has oriented them to traditional status, role, and power distinctions. Under stress, everyone involved is likely to retreat to traditional roles of relative dominance and subordination—reflecting their respective statuses as service providers and service consumers.[33]

The need to experiment with new interaction patterns and new forms of institutional practice speaks to another common theme in innovative discussions of professionals' roles with self-help groups. For instance, Borman (1979) predicted a less controlling conceptualization of this role, suggesting that professionals most supportive of self-help groups were changing

from a principal and solo role to a collaborative one . . . [they] were apparently a new breed, not succumbing to traditional professional models. They may be representing a paradigm shift for many human service professionals. (p. 41)

When effective, one outcome of such a shift can be a coalition that fundamentally redefines the professional-client relationship:

Both parties . . . must search for a new balance. Clients have expertise in their own experience of the problem; professionals have special supporting knowledge in the medical or welfare sphere. Relations between clients and social workers are redefined in the direction of equality in rights and status, more input by the client, and a restriction of "expert" domination. (Bakker and Karel, 1983, pp. 176, 179–180)

A coalition between professionals and self-help groups requires reconceptualizing the professional helping role as one of resource provision, as outlined in the earlier portions of this chapter. However, these resources must be negotiated with the indigenous member leadership of the group, in order to foster independence rather than dependence, and empowerment rather than powerlessness. Moreover, professionals' resources must be designed and delivered in ways that demonstrate respect for parents' contemporary crisis, experiential knowledge, courage, group skills and commitments, and the continuing role a self-help group can play in the overall psychosocial treatment of childhood cancer. The coalition solution explicitly does not require professionals to disappear, we have argued, and the evidence from the scholarly literature and from parents and professionals indicates that professionals have much to offer that parent members need and wish to receive—and vice versa.

Since a coalition involves two (or more) sets of active and committed parties, parent leaders also have critical roles to play in establishing effective and mutually empowering working arrangements with professionals. Just as it is important for groups not to be overwhelmed by and dependent upon professional authority and resources, it is important for groups to demonstrate respect and appreciation for professionals, and to utilize their resources appropriately. Group leaders must sometimes take the initiative in helping professionals learn how to interact with parent members in new ways, and must support those professionals who take risks on behalf of the group. Instead of retreating to the polarities of unilateral control or isolation/rejection, both professionals and parent group leaders must train each other to relate effectively across their different interests, backgrounds, and roles. Moreover, they must find ways of working together on programs and activities, and on issues that involve them in interorganizational as well as interpersonal relationships.

Such redefinition and coalition formation can be facilitated by parents' creation of strong and active self-help groups that advocate strongly for their own existence and for the needs of their members, and by professionals who can advocate for these groups without feeling defensive or overcommitted. Both parties can move in these directions only if the health care bureaucracies within which they interact also become more flexible. If the professional medical bureacracy cannot support active parent roles in health care, as well as active group engagement without professional control of this process, then the same system that has created the conditions and need for coalition creation will also have sabotaged its likelihood. With emphatic support from the medical establishment, the coalition between professionals and consumers may overcome the gaps in the medical care of children with cancer on three levels: (1) the *micro level* of providing compassionate and caring interpersonal support to patients and parents, through a plural set of programs and activities; (2) the *mezzo level* of providing new ideas and resources for improved service delivery and changes in the operation of medical care, through joint parent-staff fundraising, community mobilization efforts, and collaborative programs; and (3) the *macro level* of influencing the national or regional structure of health care delivery and financing, through joint lobbying, advocacy of cancer research programs, electoral campaigns, and other forms of professional-public politics.

Self-Help Groups as Social Movement Organizations?

We have explored in this chapter the possibility that some self-help groups for families of children with cancer fruitfully may be conceived as social movement organizations. First, these groups are part of a broader social movement that seeks to create greater patient/consumer awareness and activism in health care. Second, they involve people dealing with a common major conflict and threat in their daily lives; the stresses of parenting a child diagnosed with cancer, when exacerbated by the insensitive or controlling actions of medical staff members, often create a disempowered constituency. Third, they often work with their members to create a greater level of awareness of common grievances and interests, of support for and confidence in their own actions and abilities, and of the possibility of acting together for change. As with other social movement organizations, self-help groups' commitment to create environmental change is often accompanied by efforts to heal and empower individual members and to offer support to people in distress. Fourth, self-help groups often advocate for change in the medical care system: they articulate members' common concerns, target practices and practitioners that require alteration, open up lines of communication and collaboration often closed to individual consumers, and develop a power base with which to challenge resistant medical bureaucracies. Developing an articulate constituency, providing support and affirmation in the face of threat and disempowerment, targeting objectionable practices or practitioners, mobilizing constituency energy for change, and confronting power holders in an attempt to change the service delivery system are tactics practiced by many voluntary social movement organizations. They are appropriate weapons in the arsenal of groups intervening in conflicts involving parties of unequal power and resources.

While self-help groups for parents of children with cancer may be appropriately considered social movement organizations, they clearly are different from other such organizations and from much traditional thinking about social movements in general. Several theoretical stances historically have dominated thinking and research on social movement organizations (e.g., theories of absolute deprivation, relative deprivation, class conflict, resource mobilization). According to most of these approaches, self-help groups such as those discussed in this volume would not qualify as social movement organizations, nor as part of a social movement. However, more recent work has focused attention on the cultural or ideological "identity basis" of "new social movements."[34] The emphasis in this approach is more upon people's self-professed cultural identity than on their position in the class structure, on their efforts to alter information and cultural images or symbols rather than political/economic resource reallocation solely, and on efforts to transform members' lives and local institutions as well as (or sometimes rather than) the society and major institutions. Self-help groups for families of children with cancer, as discussed here, do fit this emerging broadening of views of social movement organizations in several ways: in their efforts to help parents adapt to and create a new social identity, to advance a collective sense of this identity, to create a community of concern that can support individuals under stress, to generate an experiential knowledge base and meaning system that represents an alternative to the dominant set of cultural images and messages, and to focus on changes in local institutions' practices and services. When individual involvement takes the form of self-change efforts, they respond both to the need for personal reconstruction and social action, and to the attainment of individual and group goals (Killilea, 1976). Group goals and activities, then, can be the roots of an "identity politics" approach to activism, wherein individuals identify and demand changes in the operation of social institutions in order to facilitate their own adaptation and growth.[35] For some people, such as many of the parents whose voices have been expressed in this volume, the vehicle for such personal growth, renewed or transformed identity, and collective action has been their participation in local self-help groups.[36]

However, not all self-help groups, nor all self-help groups for families of children with cancer, can appropriately be considered social movement organizations. Those that are run by professional staff members, and that focus solely on individuals' psychological needs, may be more like "rap" groups or counseling sessions. Indeed, we have indicated that some scholars would prefer not to call these variants self-help groups at all. Even some self-help groups run by parents may fail to clearly articulate conflicts and problems with the staff, may assign a low priority to external changes, and may fail to bond members together in the effort to take collective action. Nevertheless, all of these group variants have their roots in the same structural conflicts underlying patient-provider relations in the long-term care of vulnerable populations. In all such groups, there is at least an implicit challenge to the professional monopoly and ideology of service. Perhaps the professionally led groups and the internally focused parent-led groups may best be considered quasi-social movement organizations, not yet social movement organizations but with the potential to change into that form at some time in the future.

Another framework that unites many self-help groups with social movement organizations involves the process of consciousness-raising that often occurs in both settings. Most observers of social movement organizations, especially those "new social movement" organizations that include this "identity politics" orientation, see consciousness-raising and identity transformation and collectivization as early steps in the creation of an organized, committed, and active constituency that can work together for change in the surrounding community or social system.[37] The most recent literature on self-help groups reviewed in Chapter 1 and some of the empirical evidence presented in this volume suggest how consciousness-raising and identity transformation can also occur within the self-help setting. Whether or not local groups explicitly and directly undertake local change efforts, the processes of sharing life experiences and developing experiential knowledge (both of external situations and internal states of feeling) can generate a sense of personal and collective empowerment. When self-help groups do act consciously and as a collective entity for change, they are most like social movement organizations; even when they do not so act, they can be considered social movement organizations in the making—perhaps waiting for the charismatic leader or situational spark that calls for action.

The social movement perspective is important to explorations of self-help groups for several reasons. Without it, scholarship on self-help groups may be captured by powerful interests committed to maintaining current forms of psychosocial and medical service delivery. Service recipients may then be counseled to accept the help they are offered, rather than being advised to advocate for the help they need. They may be counseled to focus on only their individual concerns, to adapt passive postures, and to avoid seeking support or confirmation of their needs in the company of others. Within a social movement perspective, scholarship and practice may jointly encourage the development of (semi-)autonomous patient/family organizations, and utilize these groups to increase the active and empowered roles patients/ parents may play in advocating for themselves and others. They may even invite such groups to play a legitimate role in helping to improve the delivery of health services. Then, even in the midst of great stress, parents of children with cancer may join in the great American tradition of forming voluntary associations with people who share common interests and undertake joint action for change.

Part 5

Broader Views of Self-Help Groups: Other Bridges in Other Times and Places

In this section we extend the findings discussed in earlier chapters in several directions. In Chapter 10 we report the results of a series of revisits to the groups studied earlier, examining the ways in which the fifty groups changed over a time period of approximately ten to twelve years. This longitudinal inquiry allows us to identify both stability and change in groups' activities and operations.

In Chapter 11 we extend our findings to consider the activities and operations of other self-help groups—groups dealing with other life crises, and groups in other cultures and nations.

10

Self-Help Groups over Time
Stability and Change

Following many of the themes identified and developed previously, we explore in this chapter data gathered in 1992–1993 (referred to as Study #4 in Chapter 3 and Figure 3.1) from forty-one of the groups originally visited in the early 1980s.[1] These forty-one groups represented all of the fifty groups in the original sample that still existed in some form and were locatable in 1993. Data were gathered through revisits to each of these groups via telephone interviews with a designated local group liaison. Using these newly gathered data, we here examine the groups as they were in 1993, and in comparison to the earlier reports from field visits with group leaders and members. This provides us with a 10–12-year retrospective and longitudinal view, a comparative data base virtually absent from research with self-help groups. Updating the issues raised in Chapters 4, 5, and 7, we examine evidence of stability and change in the scope of activities and operating structures of these self-help groups. On the one hand, we might expect substantial changes to have occurred in these groups over time, as the result of the increasing privatization of portions of the public sector, the continued growth of medical and social service bureaucracies, and the expansion of psychosocial services provided by the medical system. On the other hand, inasmuch as the core dynamics of self-help touch universal and timeless human and social needs, these groups might be expected to stay the same regardless of changes in their external environments. Even though individual members may leave, and new ones enter, the groups themselves may endure.

By examining the organizational structures, priorities, and activities of these groups as they existed 10–12 years later, we may also illuminate patient-provider roles, collective action efforts by self-help groups, and problems facing parents that were not prominent when the earlier data were gathered, such as insurance barriers and special needs of long-term survivors. We raise additional questions and provide some answers to the historical relationship between self-help groups and treatment centers, exploring whether and how the two have worked more closely together or become more distinct or more similar in their agendas. In the voices of parents currently involved with these forty-one groups, we hear much about how things have changed in their groups over time, as well as stories about how they have stayed the same. Thus, we observe both stability and change in self-help and in psychosocial activities and programs for families of children with cancer. Is there an emerging complementarity between parent and professional roles in and out of treatment centers? Has the self-help basic ethos and mutual support agenda endured to the exclusion or inclusion of new group activities and agendas? We explore these questions and others as we look at the groups across the interval of the 1980s to the 1990s.

Group Continuity and Change

As indicated, forty-one of the original sample of fifty local self-help groups visited in the early 1980s were located in this restudy. Of the nine that evidently no longer existed in 1993, five had already been relatively inactive and close to extinction in the original study.[2] Moreover, six of the nine nonexistent groups were small in the original study, and seven of them were independently run groups—run by parents alone with little or no involvement on the part of professionals. Thus, a picture emerges of groups that no longer exist that much earlier were failing or had low levels of activity, and were small and independent. The independent status of the groups meant that they were not led or controlled by the professionals in the medical care system and that they may have had few effective and constructive links to the resources of this system when they began to cease operating. This interpretation is consistent with the argument in Chapter 9 about the utility of a coalition; to the extent the groups worked with professionals who could and would facilitate the process of referral and recruitment, they may have been better able to maintain stable membership levels. The independent groups' experience in this regard is in marked contrast to other groups with a shared leadership pattern that also struggled over these years, but could call upon the resources of the medical system for assistance in their most difficult periods (of recruitment, funding, changed activity, changing membership). Despite the information that over 80% of the original fifty groups did survive in one form or another over this time period, not all did, whatever the reasons. Case 5 describes some of the changes over time that were experienced by a group that no longer exists: the Share-Care group discussed in its earlier form in Chapter 5 (as Case 1).

Table 10.1 indicates that 80% (33/41) of the groups existing in 1993 considered themselves to be "the same group" that existed in the early 1980s; only 20% (8 groups) considered themselves "new groups" with few or no links to the past. This is a remarkable degree of historic continuity for local voluntary organizations. That does not mean that these "same groups" were exactly the same as their prior versions; indeed, most of these 33 "same groups" were composed almost entirely of new active members ($N = 14$), or a mix of old and new members ($N = 16$); in only 3 groups were all the same people still active and involved in leadership cadres.

Some examples of parents' descriptions of their group as a new group, and how it got (re)started, are presented below.

Table 10.1. Group history: Same group and same people, 1981–1993 ($N = 41$)

A. Is this the same group that existed in 1981?	
Same	New
80% ($n = 33$)	20% ($n = 8$)

B. Are the same (or new) people active?		
Same	New	Mixed
10% ($n = 4$)	51% ($n = 21$)	39% ($n = 16$)

Case 5. The Share-Care Group—Ten Years Later

This is an update of Case 1 in Chapter 5. It presents what we know of the Share-Care group's transitions when we gathered telephone data from them in 1993.

The Share-Care group is no longer functioning. It ceased operating six years ago. For a while after the children of two of the active—and original—parents died, those parents continued to come to the meetings, but they came less often as time went on. They didn't seem to have the energy to continue, and the other parents gradually put less and less energy into the group.

As the group's activity level fell off, one of the social workers at the hospital tried to revive it. She sent out a mailing to parents on the original list and contacted parents of newly diagnosed children, but to little avail. Without the presence of a parent who was really willing to provide co-leadership of a sustained sort, there was little response to the social worker's outreach efforts. The social worker reported that if she had wanted to establish a small, therapy-oriented group (one structured like Prof-Care; see Case 2 in Chapter 5), parents might have joined for a while, but that had not been her goal. She had wanted to stimulate a more independent parent group, and that evidently was not possible.

Since Share-Care had no official by-laws, state charter, or bank account, it simply died off after the social worker gave up her efforts six years ago. Perhaps one day in the future . . .

The old group fell apart, and I talked to Candlelighters about getting a group going again—which I have done. In the past two years we have set up a group to put the newsletter together and we got together about once a month or every other month. Also we sponsored a picnic for families of children off treatment during the summer and a boat party for the kids at cancer camp.

The old group seems to have fallen apart. A new social worker and a nurse practitioner have taken over the group. Membership fluctuates a lot.

When the big goal of building the Ronald McDonald House was gone, the group let down and fell apart. The old support group dropped off after the Ronald McDonald House. People were finding support within the House I guess. The group was rejuvenated when they built the new outpatient clinic. It was next to the inpatient service, so it provided the opportunity to meet people, and the new facility created the atmosphere for informally supporting one another.

In contrast, other parents reported that their group was not only the same group, but that nothing had changed—for better or for worse.

I think we're pretty much the same, except that some members drift away, and pretty much people come and go as they need the group.

It's no different really, and that's part of the problem. It's the same old people and there really aren't any new ideas. The group isn't as strong, needs new blood. We meet at the Ronald McDonald House; it's a good place to meet, and we don't have to pay for parking, but sometimes it's hard to come back to the memories.

Our group was not very active for a while, and then we were encouraged to get active again because the outpatient department was going to move. So in order to keep people organized around that issue I decided that a formal group was needed to keep in touch and communicate information and support.

It appears that many of the original self-help groups did endure, perhaps with a stable parent core, but that much of their membership changed over time.

Over 90% of the groups reported being "different now" (in 1993) in some ways. When asked to provide more detail about how their group had changed over time, group liaisons commented on the general level of activity; they indicated that 86% of the groups were more active now than they had been in the past.[3] Four major types of changes were reported: (1) size of membership, (2) agenda or program activities, (3) characteristics and needs of parents, and (4) group leadership. Several parents elaborated on how their group had changed in its overall size or total membership.

Membership is down. A lot more kids are off treatment, and their families have pulled away. I think they feel like they want to put it out of their minds, maybe just forget about it. The hospital does such a good job that a lot of people don't feel like they need a group, though I think they would find that we really can help them.

No fundamental difference, except I would say that the size of the group has increased significantly. The group has grown from 5–10 families (regulars) to 35–40 parents who come to meetings. There now are approximately 100 people participating in our group in one way or another.

A second kind of change, change in specific group agendas, programs, or activities, was mentioned by almost half the groups as important. These changes in particular are discussed in more detail later, but we note them here as part of a relatively common development.

Some of the issues have changed, like before a lot of kids weren't going on to school, and now we spend a lot of time working with parents on school issues.

Eight years ago, when I came to the group, they only had board meetings. Now we have parent support sessions, a bereavement subgroup, and several different camps. We do lots of special programs as the need comes up.

The need for support sessions is less, so we've shifted our focus onto education and information. We meet bimonthly, and put out a newsletter as one way of meeting the need for education. Currently we're also recognizing the need to support the children more, like we just started a treasure chest program.

A third important kind of change noted was the changing population served by the group, and by implication, the new needs that these populations presented. Reports of changes in the social characteristics of parents of children with cancer attending meetings and being actively involved in these groups suggested that some of these groups' greatest changes came about in terms of adapting or inventing programs in response to the newly identified needs of different parents.

This group is in danger of falling apart. For one thing there are a lot of bereaved parents, and among the newly diagnosed there are a lot of single parents, more single parents than before, and the group doesn't work well for them. We've had people go to meetings and not want to come back . . . part of it is they don't want to come back to meet at the hospital.

A fourth major change reported by several groups was new patterns of group leadership, perhaps reflecting broader changes in the relationship between these self-help groups and the professional staff of the medical institution.

We've had lots of changes since several years ago. When we first started, we were a parent-led group; parents took all the responsibility. Once the hospital clicked in with funding for the newsletter, they took control of the group. There is a pediatric nurse and a social worker running the group now. Also, the group is more formal now. A core of the old members are really interested in survivor issues, because it's been hard to get what we want.

There was a group in existence many years ago as a Candlelighter group, and then it wasn't very active. Then some parents reorganized that group with the help of a social worker here before me. They weren't a Candlelighter group as far as I know. The group that is active now is a Candlelighter group: it is led by parents, and we do a lot of emotional support and talking.

Figure 10.1 provides an example of a long-standing group that recently engaged in new and more assertive behavior with regard to

Figure 10.1. Excerpt from a self-help group newsletter (from the newsletter of the Seattle Candlelighters, vol. 3 [Winter 1994])

On the morning of October 11, 1994, 4 parents were invited to address the pediatric-oncology staff of CHMC. The discussion included 3 main topics: Family Support, Communication, and Pain Control. In addressing the need for family support, parents detailed what life was like at home while their child was on treatment for cancer. Specific behaviors including violent and destructive incidents during the week prior to coming into the clinic were described by parents. The home behavior was quite different from the quiet and competent child seen in the clinic. Parents also discussed the difficulty of communication with the hospital staff. Among the causes suggested: 1. parents were emotionally fragile and it was too difficult to bring things up, 2. after the long waits in the clinic families were anxious to get home and 3. the child was present and there was no place to leave the child to talk with the Dr. alone.

A questionnaire for parents was prepared by the parent panel and offered to the staff as a possible solution to help parents express their concerns. Also, a petition signed by more than 30 families requesting increased psycho-social support for pediatric-oncology families at CHMC was presented to the Dr. The issue of pain control was discussed and parents gave strong testimony to the difference in the life of their child when sedation was used for painful procedures.

Additional follow-up sessions are planned at the hospital. The parent panel felt that the discussion was well received by the staff and we each received a very gracious letter of appreciation from the Dr.

---

expressing their needs to, and collaborating with, the local medical staff.

Self-Help Group Activities—Occurrence and Frequency

A comparison of the activities common to self-help groups in 1981 and in 1993 is provided in Table 10.2.[4] The most commonly reported group activities in 1993 were still information and education, emotional sharing and support, and social activities—all predictably common activities given the earlier data. Fund-raising agendas apparently were still minimized by most groups, as were business meetings and overt public advocacy efforts. An examination of these groups at the two points in time (Table 10.2) indicates quite similar patterns of group activities, both in terms of the numbers of groups conducting various activities and the frequency of their occurrence at group meetings. There did, however, appear to be a slightly reduced focus on group efforts to raise funds and to make changes in the medical system in 1993. Quite obviously this was not true of all groups; as in the earlier data, some groups raise considerable funds, and some try to play a major role in improving local systems of medical and psychosocial care. While making change was not the most common agenda of any group, several members reported several new types of change-oriented activities in their groups, including efforts to make environmental changes or to investi-

Table 10.2. Self-help group meeting activities, 1981–1993 (*N* = 41)

Activities	Percentage of groups with these activities		Percentage of groups with high frequency of these activities (a lot or some)	
	1981	1993	1981	1993
Information and education programs	81	88	78	81
Emotional support programs	76	90	93	90
Social and recreational events	83	85	73	66
Fund-raising programs	61	49	37	27
Making changes in the medical system	42	32	32	22

gate the role of the environment in childhood cancer (five groups), and legislative changes (three groups). In most groups' reports, parents' preoccupation with their immediate experiences still meant that there was little time available for advocacy and work for change; such efforts were either slow to develop or did not make up a significant portion of many meetings.

Quests for information in the form of technical and experiential knowledge and for emotional support evidently remain as keys to why members come together. Groups across time reiterated the social and recreational aspects of a support and sharing agenda, but did not define their meetings as primarily involving social activities. Support and sharing may well be so vital to the mission of groups that it was not perceived in terms of distinct meeting activities, but as a general agenda. In addition, the specific needs of people affected by the experience of childhood cancer led to the development of some new activities. For instance, some groups increased their focus on men and fathers.

There is now a greater focus on dads and on parent-to-parent programs.

We've tried to do more things for dads, but it doesn't always work out well. Social events work the best. I've heard a lot of them say that they'll go but aren't going to talk about their feelings. But social events have turned out to be the best way to get fathers involved.

The latter report echoes a theme common in the earlier data: even if more men attended parent groups, they still seemed less interested in sessions explicitly focused on sharing feelings and generating emotional support. Social and recreational events, at which emotional and social support occurred nevertheless, seemed more attractive for men. The only exception to this pattern seemed to occur in groups that held separate sessions—or separate subgroup meetings—for fathers; there some fathers gathered together, apart from their wives and children, and shared feelings and experiences with one another. In one city, in the 1990s, when fathers of children with cancer did organize to meet separately, they confronted a particular ambivalence: on the one hand they were delighted to meet out of sight and sound of their wives, to talk about things they did not wish their wives to hear—including issues relating to their wives. On the other hand they worried that their wives would feel rejected and resentful about their desire to meet separately, and they certainly did not wish to jeopardize the larger self-help group.

As a result, these fathers attended all the regular group meetings as well as their special sessions for fathers only.

A second new programmatic emphasis appeared to be a response to issues faced by the young patients themselves, and a desire to help them get together in a group setting.

We organized a kids group that meets five times a year. The kids are the officers and make decisions, and the social worker acts as the adult leader.

We have a teen group that is activity focused. They do fun things like go to the Hard Rock Cafe, have a retreat with swimming, and we worked in some sessions on confidence-building.

We have a few teens, and we think we might have to start a group to deal with their special issues: how they look, dealing with their friends.

Closely related, a third new focus was represented by a few groups who reported that they started a group for siblings of children with cancer.

Our program is not really different, except we offer different things now like a sibling group.

In the last five years we started a bereavement group and a sib group.

A fourth major new focus of activity was on the problems faced by long-term survivors of childhood cancer.

We are in the discussion phase of a long-term survivor group.

We had a survivor day and are starting to think about a political emphasis on long-term survivors—insurance and discrimination issues, for example.

The issues have changed. Whereas before you would have issues like isolation, now its more around long-term survivors, late effects of treatment, school problems as a consequence of treatment.

Some of these new (or at least more frequent) programs, like the attention to fathers, patients, and siblings, represented extensions of the focus on psychosocial issues for all family members that have long been the concern of these self-help groups. However, the attention to long-term survivors represented a change in orientation that followed changes in medical practice itself: now that many more young people are surviving their cancer, this population is more numerous and visible. As we noted in Chapter 2, twenty—or even ten—years ago, many fewer children diagnosed with cancer lived to be long-term survivors. Thus, the needs of long-term survivors only now are emerging as a focus of concern for local self-help groups, as well as for medical and psychosocial staffs. In several locales, self-help groups and medical staffs have collaborated to hold "childhood cancer survival" events. The national Candlelighters Childhood Cancer Foundation, too, is responding to the special needs of this population. They have developed a newsletter for long-term survivors (*The Phoenix*), are organizing national and regional networks of long-term survivors, and are working actively to challenge the discrimination in equal access to schooling, insurance availability, and employment opportunities that stigmatize the social response to this population. At the national level, it has become clear that while active parents can support these survivors' activities, the long-term survivors wish to direct these programs for themselves. The extent to which local parent self-help groups can adapt to this population's quest for independence, as well as provide support for them, will help determine future operating structures and patterns of collaboration between organized groups of patients and their parents.

Group Attendance Patterns over Time

Most groups reported that their attendance was not greater than it had been a decade ago. Certainly, the evidence was clear that most mailing lists were larger in 1993, even if meeting attendance itself had not increased.[5] A report from one group about its changed attendance illuminates this general report of increased size.

The group is very much larger. I think a fair amount of the increase is due to the fact that the people who have taken leadership roles are more willing to be seen and heard. We worked to make the medical professionals more aware of the organization, and what Candlelighters are all about. We worked hard to get referrals from the staff, and through these efforts we have grown and have a higher profile now. People are more in favor of publicity now, and that's a change from eight to ten years ago. We brought the organization out of the closet, and it has become more businesslike . . . I'm not sure that's good. We have a kind of wrestling match between supporting each other, working with new families and organizational problems. But I think the medical community is more aware, and we have better lines of communication.

On the other hand, not all groups reported getting larger:

We've probably gotten smaller, and there is less participation by families.

Earlier data from the 1980s did not include direct estimates of patterns of involvement by gender and race, but reports from individual members (see Table 6.1) indicated that 90% of all of the members and nonmembers responding to our questionnaires were women. While this response rate probably was a skewed reflection of the representation of women as active members of these self-help groups, the fact remains that the majority of active group members historically have been women. In 1993, most groups (80%) reported that group meetings were still overwhelmingly attended by women, but 20% of the groups reported that attendance rates for men and women were now approximately the same. Women undoubtedly remained the most likely primary caregivers and lower-paid wage earners responding to their child's crisis, but the 1993 reports did suggest strongly that more fathers now came to meetings. About two-thirds of the groups reported in 1993 that some African Americans attended their meetings; slightly greater than half of the groups reported that some Latino parents attended meetings. In both cases, membership on mailing lists and attendance rates for people of color were greater than they appeared to be over a decade ago in almost one-third of the groups. However, even in locales with heavily African American or Spanish-speaking populations, cultural and language barriers still were perceived to exist. Although more African-American parents of children with cancer did attend these self-help group meetings, there was only slow progress being made toward truly inclusive organizations. The absolute numbers remained small, and the optimal strategies for recruiting a more diverse parent population remained to be developed, but there *was* evidence of positive change.

Diversity in Self-Help Groups: Internal Structure

Examining the indicators of groups' internal structures, Table 10.3 indicates that about half (51%) of the groups, both in 1981 and in 1993, had a relatively low level of formalization. A high degree of formalization characterized roughly one-third of the groups (34% v. 29%) at both points in time. Thus, the proportions appeared consistent over time, and the general trend toward low or moderate levels of formalization seems to have remained stable. As Table 10.2 shows, the primary focus of most groups was still information and emotional support—internally-

Table 10.3. Diversity in self-help group internal structures and operations, 1981–1993 (*N* = 41)

Internal structure/operations		Percentage in 1981	Percentage in 1993
Formalized structure	High (incorporated, differentiated)	34	29
	Intermediate (semiformal)	15	20
	Low (informal gatherings)	51	51
Size	Large (large attendance and mailing list)	17	7
	Active core (small attendance, large mailing list)	37	44
	Small (small attendance and mailing list)	46	49
Budget size	Small/none (< $1,000)	59	41
	Medium ($1–10,000)	24	28
	Large (> $10,000)	17	31
Retain parents as members after child dies	Yes	63	59
	No	37	41

oriented goals—and our earlier discussion (see Chapters 4 and 5) indicated that such activities simply did not require groups to adopt formal structures and procedures. Moreover, since groups with the lowest levels of formalization also were most likely to be led by human-service professionals, these staff members may have actively discouraged such efforts. Despite the general trend, a few groups developed an increased level of formalization.

It's not the same as it was originally. From what I understand there weren't as many families active back then. It was a smaller and more intimate group. Now it's larger, and we deal with a lot more business—more than we would like.

We are much more organized and structured now. We run like a business and do lots of programs and conferences.

Consistent with these findings about low formalization is the evidence that only 7% of the groups in Table 10.3 classified themselves in 1993 as large. Roughly 90% of the groups, at both points in time, were small or had a medium-sized membership and a small active core of parents. There is clear evidence that attendance at meetings of these groups has stayed relatively small, even if there were some reports of general attendance increasing slightly and membership lists increasing substantially. This may help explain the continuing trend toward low formalization, since smaller groups had less need of formally elected leaders, committees, and extensive charters and regulations for operating small meetings and intimate group affairs.

In terms of formal group budgets, 59% (Table 10.3) of the groups who earlier reported their budget level categorized their budget as small (less than $1,000) or nonexistent, but fewer (41%) of the groups assessed more recently identified themselves as having small or nonexistent budgets. Moreover, 17% of the groups in 1981 and 31% of the groups in 1993 reported budgets over $10,000 annually. While actual dollar figures were nominally higher in the 1993 reports, the dominant trend was still toward relatively small annual budgets, and budgetary concerns and the responsibilities they entail did not appear to be a main target for most members' or groups' limited energies.

Another indicator of groups' internal structure was their policy regarding retaining parents of deceased children as members. According to the 1993 data in Table 10.3, 59% of the groups welcomed such parents into groups with parents of living children, while 41% included only parents of living children in their groups. The earlier (1981) data from these groups showed a similar (63%/37%) split on this issue. Since there has not been any real change over time in this policy, the prevailing self-help ethos still seems to extend to helping *all* parents of children with cancer in most groups, especially in those led primarily by parents or by parent-professional coalitions. As was evident in the 1981 data, in 1993 it was also true that groups led by professionals were least likely to include parents of deceased children. These data on internal structures, as with prior data on patterns of activity, continue to suggest a remarkable degree of consistency in the nature of these self-help groups over time.

The 1993 data (not shown in tabular form) indicated that high or moderate degrees of formalization characterized groups significantly *most* likely to work for changes in the medical system, do substantial fund-raising, and conduct group business at meetings. These findings partly replicate data presented earlier (Table 5.2), which significantly linked more group fund-raising and more business meetings to greater formalization.

One group's story about its activities reflected the ways in which increased formalization was important to sustain such fund-raising:

Now that we are formally incorporated, we can tap into foundation funds. We're going to be doing extended fund-raising; we want to be able to purchase hospital meals for families, pay for parking at the hospital, and give money to families in need. Our meetings have changed also: prior to incorporation we would introduce ourselves and do updates on how families were doing, what treatments the kids had, do support and sharing, and there would be a formal program sometimes. We had a great system of phone support too.

It general, it appears that groups' higher degree of formalization is associated with more externally directed activities, and that group business, fund-raising, and working for change were not part of the agenda for groups that had less formal organizations and operations; alternatively, higher degrees of formalization permitted groups to conduct a wider variety of activities, including fund-raising and business operations. Indeed, we argued in Chapter 5 that engagement in substantial fund-raising programs explicitly (and legally) required groups to establish the highly formalized procedures that not only made internal management of funds more feasible, but that also conformed to state regulations regarding fund-raising from public sources. At least for groups with low levels of formalization, the picture was similar across time—support and sharing and other internally directed group agendas were more common than public, externally directed, or bureaucratic ones.

Diversity in Self-Help Groups: External Structure

Indicators of external group structure and operations (Table 10.4) revealed patterns that complemented the above findings on internal structures and operations of self-help groups for parents of children with cancer. Once again, there was substantial consistency in these groups' structures and processes over time. In 1993, over one-half (53%) of the groups reported getting their referrals of parents of newly diagnosed children primarily from the medical system; in the earlier data 54% of the groups identified the medical system as their main referral source. However, when parents' responses to questions about referral-system satisfaction were examined across time, some change was evident. In the 1993 data, local informants more often reported that their groups were satisfied with the referrals received from the medical

Table 10.4. Diversity in self-help group external structures and operations, 1981–1993 (*N* = 41)

External structure		Percentage in 1981	Percentage in 1993
Referral	Medical system only	54	53
source	Personal contact/outreach by parents	46	47
Meeting	Treatment center	56	69
location	Community center	34	31
	Home	10	0
Vertical links	None	22	14
	On Candlelighters Foundation list	22	43
	Use Candlelighters name	56	43
Horizontal	None	20	45
links	Few (1–2)	34	43
	Medium (3–4)	24	10
	High (5+)	22	2
Leadership	Independent	46	44
structure	Shared	25	22
	Professional	29	34

system. Overall, there appeared to be a slight change in the direction of growing positive sanctions of parent support groups by the medical system, especially by local hospitals and treatment centers. Are parents merely becoming more comfortable with their "public" voice, and the fact that the medical system is more aware of it? Or are referral sources and systems actually identifying and responding to parents' expressed needs more nowadays? Perhaps as parents have become more assured of their unique and institutionally accepted role, they have been more comfortable, more satisfied, and more able to work with the dominant referral posture of most professionals.

Groups' reports of the locations of their meetings also demonstrated that good links still existed with the medical system. Over two-thirds (69%) of the groups reported in 1993 that they met at the local treatment center; none reported meeting at members' homes. Comparison of these findings with the 1981 data revealed some change over time, since only 56% of groups in the earlier data reported meeting at treatment centers, and 12% met at individual parents' homes. Earlier anecdotal reports from parents actually put the estimate of in-home meetings and informal networking much higher, revealing frequent parental needs to get together outside of regular group meetings, especially those held in the hospital or treatment center. Practically speaking, formal or informal meetings at homes may be more work and less accessible for members. Additionally, if hospital environments were becoming more supportive of parents' psychosocial needs and of self-help group activity, it made sense for more groups to feel comfortable about holding their meetings in these clinical settings.

Case 6 describes the Living with Childhood Cancer group, first presented in Chapter 5 as Case 3, ten years later. It is an example of a group that had evolved in terms of its own structure and in terms of its coalition-building activity with the medical system.

Vertical links to the national self-help group organization—Candlelighters Childhood Cancer Foundation (CCCF)—were quite common both in 1981 and in 1993. Of the groups studied in 1981, over three-fourths (78%) either incorporated the CCCF title into their group name or appeared on the national roster with another type of group name; by 1993 this figure had risen to 86%. No formal linkage with CCCF was reported by fewer groups in 1993 than in 1981. This change may reflect the CCCF's expansion of local organizing activity, and greater recognition of their work by local medical and psychosocial treatment centers.[6] While evidence of vertical links to the national organization was abundant, horizontal community links continued to be less common, and in fact have become even rarer. In both time periods, nearly half of the groups reported only a few linkages to other local social service organizations and support groups. This pattern appeared to have increased by 1993, with almost one-half of the local groups reporting no links at all to other local community agencies.

In terms of self-help group leadership structures, the newer data revealed virtually the same proportions of groups led by professionals, by parents alone, or by shared professional-parent coalitions as did the earlier data. Certainly, self-help groups continued to rely on medical system contacts and referrals, but they were no more reliant on medical system professionals as group leaders and organizers now than in the past. However, even though the aggregate number of groups in each

Case 6. The Living with Childhood Cancer Group—Ten Years Later

This is an update of Case 3 in Chapter 5. It presents what we know about the Living with Childhood Cancer group's transition over the years, and its current status as of 1993. It is still a large group; although in the intervening years membership waxed and waned, it is now large and active. It is still led primarily by parents themselves, although two hospital staff members are now quite active in the group. It still conducts many different activities.

The Living with Childhood Cancer group has undergone several changes in leadership over the years. For two years the group was much smaller and much less active, although it retained its original committee structure and its bank account and legal status. Now the committees are all active and functioning again. There are only a few active veterans from the group described in Chapter 5, and the entire elected executive committee is new. Two parents of deceased children are on the executive committee, and a nurse and a social worker from the local hospital attend executive committee meetings, although they are not officially elected members. They help provide a close liaison with the medical team.

Meetings are held monthly, at the hospital. About twenty-five people attend these meetings, which generally include a speaker or panel presentation and time for people to talk with one another in smaller and informal groupings—typically with coffee and cookies in hand. At most meetings, sometimes before and sometimes after the presentation (depending on the topic), the five or six parents of deceased children who are attending leave to meet in a separate room. They return after a while to join in conversation with the other parents. A quarterly newsletter is mailed to about 500 families; not many of these families ever come to group meetings, but informal reports suggest they enjoy receiving the materials.

The group used its funds to hire one of its members as an official executive director about four years ago. This was at a time when the group started to get active and large again, after a two-year hiatus of relatively less activity. During the hiatus the hospital social worker tried to stay in touch with parents, and called several meetings, but very few people showed up. When two parents of newly diagnosed children said they had the interest and energy to start the group up again, the social worker was delighted to work with them, to take a "back seat," and to support them as they re-recruited members and created an active program. One of these parents has since become the executive director. She now draws a 50% salary from group funds; her salary rate is not very high, but it does provide employment for this mother and a variety of support functions for the group. Her role includes chairing the group's executive committee; planning and conducting monthly meetings; taking and distributing minutes of these meetings; writing and distributing a quarterly newsletter; maintaining inter-meeting liaison with committee chairs; meeting with the hospital staff when necessary; and chairing the group's fund-raising committee. She also has recently been elected to the national Board of the Candlelighters Childhood Cancer Foundation, and attends their yearly board meeting.

The group actively works to raise funds, with a yearly budget now of approximately $50,000. In addition to general fund-raising, the group is part of the local Community Chest campaigns, and receives a yearly allocation from that operation. They also have some good connections to leaders of corporations and labor unions in the community, and "tap" these contacts on a yearly basis for additional funding. A portion of these funds goes to pay the salary of the executive director, and for monthly meeting and newsletter expenses. In addition, the group provides about $20,000 a year to the local hospital, which is used primarily as "matching funds" for the hospital's efforts to generate grants for expanded psychosocial programs. One such program is a summer camp for families of children with cancer.

The group has just started a new committee, which is looking into the role of environmental problems in local childhood cancer statistics. There is considerable parental concern about the role of high-tension electric power lines and polluted ground water in the stimulation of childhood cancer. Several parents have been reading scientific literature, calling and talking with national experts, and meeting to talk about what they can do in this community to investigate and perhaps address their concerns. They regularly contribute a column of questions and concerns about the environment (including dietary issues) to the group's quarterly newsletter.

In the past year, Living with Childhood Cancer started a parallel support group for long-term survivors of childhood cancer. This group is comprised of about ten active young people who are (off-treatment) survivors of cancer, all between the ages of twelve and eighteen. They meet monthly, sometimes with the executive director and/or the hospital social worker in attendance. They have created a home video on what it's like to have had cancer as a child, and have arranged with the hospital staff to show this video to newly diagnosed young people with cancer. Some of them spend time on the wards and in the clinic talking with young patients in active treatment (and their parents), and some give talks at local schools about their experiences.

Living with Childhood Cancer continues to have good relations with the medical and social service staff of the local treatment center. The executive director's role and the group's ability to provide the staff with funding for some special projects seem to have created an excellent environment for cooperative work. In addition to the two staff members who regularly attend executive committee and group meetings, several physicians and other staff members are likely to show up unannounced at meetings; they are always ready to come to a meeting to give a talk, and have been very responsive to the executive director's efforts to work through problems that have arisen.

leadership category stayed approximately the same, many individual groups *did* change their leadership patterns over time. For instance, of the 12 groups (out of 41) that were led by professionals in 1981, 7 continued to be led by professionals in 1993; 2 others moved into a shared-leadership pattern, and 3 others adopted a parent-led, independent structure. Of the 19 groups that had independent, parent-led leadership patterns in 1981, only 10 continued with that pattern in 1993; 5 others adopted a shared-leadership structure, and 4 became professionally led. Of the 10 groups that had shared-leadership patterns in 1981, only 2 had retained that pattern in 1993; 5 others adopted independent leadership structures, and 3 became professionally led. As people moved in and out, and as membership or even the existence of the group waxed and waned, new people and people in new parent or professional roles rose to positions of leadership. The data indicate that the professionally led groups maintained the most stable pattern of leadership, even if they lasted for a shorter time period and were constantly being reinitiated. Indeed, professionals typically had a longer "life" in the system than did parents, and professionals had greater access to the mechanisms and resources that supported the creation and recreation of groups: office space, medical system credibility, access to parents of newly diagnosed children, and access to meeting rooms. The shared-leadership coalition evidently was the hardest pattern to sustain, and these coalitions often changed into independent or professionally led forums. These shifts are consistent with substantial theory and practical experience regarding the temporary and shifting nature of coalitions of all sorts.[7]

The 1993 data regarding the relationship of group leadership patterns to group activities and operating structure largely replicated the 1981 data reported in Table 5.3. Professionally led groups were still significantly more likely than the shared-leadership or independent groups to be small, to have lower levels of formalization, to have small budgets, and to exclude (or not include) parents of deceased children. Moreover, professionally led groups significantly less often conducted business at meetings or did substantial fund-raising. The shared-leadership groups, compared with the parent-led and the independent ones, were likely to have more highly formalized procedures and larger budgets, especially if they had forged workable and enduring coalitions with their local medical establishment. These findings provide us with continuing evidence of the degree to which parents' rely on their own expertise, of parents' and professionals' recognition of and respect for that expertise, and of the distinction that those involved in self-help groups typically make between professional support for and control of groups and group operations. These trends in parent-professional respect and collaboration also are reflected in the growth of parent-advocate or parent-representative programs. In 1993 there was evidence of paid parent roles as advocates for parent groups, and as official group liaisons to members of the medical staff, in at least eight different settings. This was a several-fold increase from the early development of such programs in Providence, Rhode Island, and Rochester, New York (Carpenter and Vattino, 1992; Pitel et al., 1985). These collaborative structures encouraged rapid communication of needs and concerns from parents to staff and staff to parents, and provided the mechanism for greater mutual accountability between medical care organizations and parent self-help groups.

Professional Roles in Self-Help Groups

Parents' reports of professionals' roles in self-help groups (not shown in tabular form) were quite similar across time. More recent data (1993) revealed that the most common professional roles continued to involve giving information about cancer and treatment (61%) and leading discussions (51%). The least common roles played by professionals in groups involved guarding parents against getting hurt (30%). Moderately common roles included running meetings, giving information about the hospital, arranging rooms, advising the group, and advocating for the group. It is interesting that over one-third (35%) of groups reported that professionals only did what parents asked, that in only 15% of the cases did professionals "make big decisions," and that in only 5% of the groups did professionals train parents in how to conduct activities or otherwise provide support. Earlier (1981) reports indicated that professionals most often referred new parents to the group, acted as referral sources for serious problems, provided information, and advocated for the group. They were least likely, according to earlier data, to have executed duties such as arranging rooms, planning group agendas, and the like. The two sets of data agree that professionals hardly ever had to guard parents against hurt.

Perhaps any observable change across time in professional involve-ment—especially where it seemed to be increasing—stemmed from the clearer visions of each other's roles that parents and professionals have developed. Professionals did not aim—now or earlier—to step into parents' shoes, and parents appear to have a keen awareness of their own potential for advocacy, collective support, and contribution to their child's care.

Aside from the roles that individual professionals played in these self-help groups, parents and groups also had to manage their in-terorganizational relationships with medical institutions' norms and practices, and with newly emerging institutional psychosocial support programs for families of children with cancer. Reports from parents in several groups illustrate the changed relationships they encountered or have created with medical institutions. For the most part, these changes have been positive.

We have better communication with the hospital. Five or six years ago most pediatricians wouldn't have known that our group exists; now they do.

Ten years ago there was a distant relationship with the staff. We've worked actively to strengthen it. We incorporated a professional on our board, and we have a good working relationship now with the staff. At first, we were a threat; they were afraid we would take money away from the hospital. Now we've become well respected, and the hospital looks good because of their association with us and our support activities.

In the past few years the comfort level of the professionals has gone up; they are not threatened by us now.

We've gone from being seen as a pain in the neck to where they're starting to see us as an asset, especially after the national Candlelighters 20th Anniver-sary Conference in Washington. That generated a lot of enthusiasm with the staff, and they've even given us some secretarial support and a grant for the newsletter.

But not all the changes have been so positive, as one parent leader noted:

The staff is less active with us now. Communication is minimal. Our group is angry about it. We wish the staff were more supportive of the group. The hospi-tal does a great job with families in the hospital, but they don't support the group, and overlook families whose children are outpatients or off treatment.

One explanation for the general report of better relationships between parent groups and local medical institutions may be the greater need some institutions had for organized parent support of their medical and psychosocial programs. As local self-help groups proved their reliability and value and as federal and state funds for psychosocial services, advanced medical procedures, and research have fallen off, parent groups may represent new sources of volunteer help and funds for the medical system.[8] Notwithstanding the serious commitment many medical and social service professionals have to parent-run self-help groups, some physicians have been quite open about their priority for groups as effective fund-raisers, or effective partners in hospital fund-raising campaigns.

Conclusions

Why might changes in these self-help groups have occurred over time? Why might few changes in these groups have occurred? Perhaps change occurred because of a changing parent core in a self-help group. However, even if the individual membership of the group, or of the parent core of the group, and some of its activities changed, the overall structure of the group seldom did. Thus, despite a new core of parents, perhaps change did not occur very often because new parents were still dealing with the same types of stresses, and searching for similar kinds of assistance in coping with these stresses. We have drawn attention to the probable effect on local programming of the needs of more recently identified subpopulations of parents and their children. As more youngsters survive their cancer, the need for programs that speak to the needs of long-term survivors have become manifest. Similarly, as more single parents seek the help of veteran members, programs must change to meet their needs as well. In an outreach effort to populations of parents who historically have experienced exclusion and oppression in the medical system, as well as in society at large, some groups have adjusted activities to respond to the needs of African-American and Latino parents. Similarly, consonant with emergent ideologies represented in governmental and corporate health plans that give parents time off to deal with childrens' health crises, many groups have instituted new programs for fathers of children with cancer.

The operations of the national self-help organization (CCCF) also have changed in the past decade, and these changes also may have affected the growth and development of local groups and their relationships with local health care systems. The CCCF staff has grown (from three to seven members), its budget has increased, it has created better liaisons with professionals and professional associations, and it has developed new publications and programs designed to assist local groups and individual parents. CCCF now has an active ombudsperson program that helps individual patients and parents deal with issues of treatment access, second opinions, educational services, and insurance and employment discrimination. The librarian in the national office fields over fifty requests a month from parents and professionals seeking information. A public relations effort, complete with Public Service Announcements, press and video releases, and a news clipping service, and a better relationship with the American Cancer Society, have improved CCCF's image with medical and social service professionals and their organizations and institutions. And the national Foundation's new newsletter (*The Phoenix*) and networking effort directed at long-term survivors of childhood cancer have helped move it to the front line of leadership in psychosocial programming and support for all those dealing with childhood cancer. Staff and board members also have reached out to visit local groups more often and greater efforts have been made to provide "hands-on" organizing and programming assistance. In several local or regional locales, self-help groups have held conferences for parents and staff featuring CCCF staff and board members as speakers. The slightly greater reported evidence of more vertical links between local groups and the national Candlelighters Foundation is sparse evidence of significant change in these relationships, but personal and anecdotal reports verify significant increases, and much greater success, in networking efforts by the national Foundation. In the 1981 data only 10% of the groups reported having been in existence for more than five years; by 1993 that figure has risen to 66% (33 of the original 50 groups reported in 1993 that they were "the same group"; 8 reported that they were "new," and 9 were not locatable). Thus, the real growth of long-lasting groups was just beginning to occur in the late 1970s and early 1980s. This was also the time when the national CCCF began to receive financial support from the American Cancer Society, to move from a house basement to an office, and to focus its efforts on outreach to local parents and groups of parents around the country.

Perhaps the attitudes and priorities of professionals and the medical system itself have changed. There is some anecdotal evidence that medical staffs are now more alert to the psychosocial issues facing families of children with cancer and are providing more psychosocial services themselves, as several group leaders stated in the 1993 interviews:

I don't think the medical system itself has changed, but social services have really competed with us in providing support to families. Maybe they've become more aware of the needs of parents by our encouraging and educating parents to speak up.

The acceptance of psychosocial support has grown over the years, and the recognition of the importance of emotional support for the whole family continues to grow.

These trends indicate that the environmental ground has shifted somewhat for families of children with cancer and for their self-help groups. If the medical system is providing a broader and greater range of psychosocial services to these families, as much recent literature suggests,[9] self-help groups can shift their focus to more specific programs that are not and cannot be provided by the treatment center and by related professionals. If the groups cannot make that shift in focus and activity, they may wither.

As the hospital relocated, and their services enlarged, in some ways the system has grown beyond us, expanded structurally, overwhelming us. We are not as important in some ways, because the hospital and the schools have become more responsive to the need to support families and children.

The expansion of psychosocial services also may reflect the impact of the role self-help groups have played over the years as pioneers and pacesetters for medical staffs in this arena.

The emphasis on experiential knowledge, on shared life experiences, on providing affirmation and support to one another, on sharing coping styles, and on taking empowered action remain the basic themes of self-help. These resources and strategies cannot be duplicated by professionals. They continue to be the core "magic" of the self-help process and the fundamental underpinnings of all of the activities and operating structures established by local groups. They continue to be the foundations for the self-help group bridge over the troubled waters faced by parents of children with cancer. When major changes in these self-help groups for families of children with cancer do not occur over time, the stability of the self-help dynamic itself and its role in responding to the crisis of childhood cancer are affirmed dramatically.

11

Other Self-Help Groups— For
Other Life Crises, in Other Cultures,
Other Nations

Generalizing about self-help groups is a risky enterprise. It appears from our explorations and the literature that some key universal elements exist in most self-help groups. In Chapter 1, we pointed to the unique nature of experiential knowledge, a community of similar others who facilitated a new social identity, a climate of shared emotions and affirming support, the availability of new resources and skills in personal coping and in helping others, and the development of new or renewed activism as universal self-help themes. Despite these common characteristics, individual groups differ from one another in many ways. Moreover, even the apparently universal characteristics of these groups mask many variations in the types of people who are members, their personal coping and interaction styles, local groups' activities and organizational structures, and their relationships with formal and professional service systems.

Three powerful factors appear to account for much of the variation in structures and processes that appear in particular self-help groups:

1. The life crisis, problem, or situation that calls people together
2. The culture and/or social background or status of people who are members
3. The national political and economic structure and ideology in which they exist

To the extent that there are unique structural and operating characteristics of self-help groups, they are determined by or derived from these three primary influences. That is, these three sets of influences, separately and in interaction, largely determine the ways in which self-help finds local expression.

While the origins of self-help may stem from the same human encounter with crisis and may result in similar social and personal processes, variation in the nature of the crisis leads to different coping strategies, support systems, and self-help group experiences. Moreover, self-help groups exist within larger social contexts that define much of a given group's scope, structural attributes, and programs or activities. Different civic and political cultures, different social and economic histories, and different health and welfare systems lead self-help groups to develop in varying ways in different nations, in different ethnic, class, or demographic groupings within nations, and around different issues. As people deal with life crises from the vantage point of their varied cultures and group interests, with varying patterns of interaction and communication, so they create a variety of coping patterns and systems of social support. Thus, while self-help groups may have universal or common characteristics, they also have important particular characteristics.

Unfortunately, systematic empirical investigation of these different forms of self-help is virtually nonexistent. Very few comparative empirical studies of several self-help groups have focused on different life crisis, even within the same culture and nation, and this is the simplest comparative design possible. There are even fewer studies of self-help groups focused on the same issue in different cultures or nations. Investigations that simultaneously cut across life crises and cultures or nations run the risk of identifying apparent universal characteristics at a very general level, while masking the realities of particular processes and activities. In part, this gap is due to the still-evolving nature of self-help as a phenomenon, as well as the state of research sophistication in this area. Problems of deciding whether and how to compare different life crises, finding common as well as differentiated themes in self-help activities, and solving problems of access bedevil such comparative efforts. In this chapter, we advance exploration of these issues by comparing data on self-help groups organized for two different crises—groups of parents of children with cancer and groups of parents of murdered children—in one national setting, the United States.

The Nature of the Life Crisis

In Chapter 2, we reviewed the stresses associated with parenting a child with cancer. We argued there, and in Chapter 1, for the need to ground self-help inquiry in the particular life crisis that calls people to membership. To do otherwise treats the group experience as abstracted from the life stresses and demands to which the group is designed to respond. As part of Study #3, we examined the life circumstances and self-help group experiences of U.S. parents facing two different life crises involving their children: childhood cancer and murdered children.[1] By bringing the experience of parents of murdered children to bear on the ongoing discussion of parents of children with cancer, we can explore the impact of the particular life crisis on self-help group phenomena.

Parents of Children with Cancer and Parents of Murdered Children

At the time of Study #3, involving 116 parents and eight self-help groups of parents of children with cancer, we also conducted investigations with 104 parents in five local self-help groups of parents of murdered children. Both are major life crises involving parenthood and children, and they stimulate many of the same stresses associated with fear, loss, coping, and social support. However, the differences in the experiences of these two populations of parents are substantial. Parental reports make it clear that the experience of being a parent of a child who has been murdered is quite different from the experience of parenting a child who has been diagnosed with cancer, or even of being the parent of a child who has died from cancer. For instance, some of the stresses faced by parents of murdered children, and indeed the chronology of stress over time, are very different. Parents of murdered children often face the shock and pain of this tragedy with anger and rage at the perpetrator of their child's demise; in the case of a murdered child, there is a human agent who created the condition.[2] In the case of childhood cancer, there is no known human agency involved in disease creation (with the exception of genetic transmission of some rare types of childhood cancer and speculations about environmental pollution in others).[3] In the case of a murdered child, the child's condition is finite and certain from the start. This is not the case in childhood cancer, where life and death are uncertain, at least for some significant time period. In the case of a murdered child, parents must relate with the police and judicial system where indeed, parents of a murdered child are the first likely suspects of police inquiry. Parents of children with cancer, in contrast, must deal with a medical system, and there is no official attempt to blame them for their child's illness, although some unthinking relatives or friends may express theories of parental etiology and blame. Even though there is often a stigma attached to having a child with cancer, it is not comparable to the depth of the stigma, rooted in societal blame and individual guilt, associated with being the parent of a child who has been murdered. Some of these important differences are summarized in Table 11.1.

Partly as a result of these inherent differences, reports from parents indicate that parents of children with cancer and parents of murdered children develop quite different coping strategies and utilize quite different sources and types of social support (Chesler, et al., 1988). For instance, parents of murdered children, more often than parents of children with cancer, reported coping in passive ways (doing nothing, not taking charge, not focusing on problems and solving them), and in private ways (trying to be alone, going off by oneself). Thus, they demonstrated a paralysis and immobility that was rooted in the objective reality that there was nothing they could do about the crisis with which they were faced. Parents of children with cancer had "work to do"; that is, they had to work with the medical staff to help heal their child physically and psychosocially. In contrast, parents of murdered children no longer had a child to heal. Moreover, as noted above, the tremendous social stigma and blame often associated with being the parent of a murdered child, and the discomfort friends felt when faced with this crisis, made it more likely that parents of murdered children would be alone, and would experience a privatization of their situation that was socially as well as individually determined.

Parents of murdered children, compared with parents of children with cancer, reported receiving less support from their spouses, children, and immediate family members. They also reported receiving less support from members of the health care staff and more from lawyers.[4] The latter result is, at face value, immediately understandable; parents of murdered children must interact with the legal system, and parents of children with cancer must interact with the medical system. However, the findings indicating a lower level of support for parents of

Table 11.1. Differences between parents of children with cancer and parents of murdered children

Life-crisis issues	Parents experiencing childhood cancer	Parents experiencing childhood murder
Chronology and temporality of stress	Uncertain, changing Irresolution Possible relapse, remission, cure	Certain, immediate resolution Finite outcome
Emotions	Hope, despite fear Uncertainty Shock	No hope Shock, pain Anger, rage
Target of feelings, emotions	Fate Physical environment	Perpetrator—human agent Fate Social environment
Interaction with social institutions	Medical system Work with staff to heal ill child	Police, legal/judicial system No possible impact on child's outcome Under suspicion
Parents' social image or stigma	Little systemic blame Sympathy and pity Some stigma of weakness	Potential initial suspects Suspicion Grave stigma of responsibility and blame
Coping	Active Often public	Passive Often private
Social support	Effective support often received from many sources	Effective support seldom received from usual sources
Family impact	Stress and tension New roles and responsibilities Potential for strengthening family bonds	Grave stress Descructive tension and suspicion Rage
Reported life changes	More positive than negative	More negative than positive

murdered children from their immediate family confirm the different personal and social meaning of their crisis experience; to the extent that immediate family members are the first suspects in a murder, this social construction of a child's murder must be at least temporarily destructive of the fabric of close family life. Parents of children of cancer also reported more often receiving help that cheered them up, and more help with practical family tasks (cooking and looking after other family members) than did parents of murdered children. Cheering up evidently did not make much sense in the instance of a child who had been murdered. Overall, parents of children with cancer reported receiving higher levels of help and support than did parents of murdered children. Data on parents' assessments of their life changes since their child's diagnosis or murder indicate that parents of children with cancer also reported more positive life change than did parents of murdered children.

Self-Help Groups for Parents of Children with Cancer and Parents of Murdered Children

On the basis of these differences in the life experience of parents of children with cancer and parents of murdered children, we would expect to discover differences in their experiences in self-help groups. Table 11.2 lists members' reports of the degree to which various activities were undertaken by the eight self-help groups of parents of children with cancer and the five self-help groups of parents of murdered children (all visited in Study #3). The Spearman rank-order correlation coefficient (rho) for these two lists was not statistically significant, indicating that the ranking of the frequencies of these activities did differ for the two types of groups. Self-help groups formed by and/or for parents of children with cancer more often engaged in fund-raising for needy families, more often held social and recreational events, and more often focused on organizational maintenance issues that kept the group going (planning group activities, discussing recruitment of new members). Groups formed by and/or for parents of murdered children more often talked about personal feelings, more often raised funds to support the parent group, and more often planned to change organizational policies and aspects of the system (police, judicial, and legislative) that affected them. The greater focus on social advocacy evident in the groups of parents of murdered children may reflect the time and energy they had available for such tasks, as well as their search for an outlet for their

Table 11.2. Members' mean reports of frequency of activities of self-help groups for parents of children with cancer and parents of murdered children

Activity	Parents of children with cancer		Parents of murdered children	
	Mean ($N = 65$)	Rank	Mean ($N = 100$)	Rank
Talk about stress on family	3.45	1	3.40	2
Learn to deal with emotions	3.32	2	3.26	4
Plan group activities	3.31	3	2.36	9
Discuss how system works	3.14	4	3.29	3
Plan to get together socially	3.09	5	2.30	10
Talk about personal feelings	3.05	6	3.51	1
Give feedback to system	2.60	7	2.57	7
Raise funds for needy families	2.57	8	1.59	12
Discuss recruiting members	2.49	9	2.06	11
Press for new social policies	2.14	10	2.79	6
Plan changes in the system	2.05	11	2.89	5
Raise money for parents	1.91	12	2.51	8

Notes: Frequency rated on a 4-point scale: 4 = a lot, 3 = sometimes, 2 = a little, 1 = never.

Spearman Rho coefficient of rank-order correlation is .42 (NS).

In the descriptions of activities, minor wording changes and one less item distinguish this list from the one in Table 6.2, so as to describe activities relevant for both sets of self-help groups.

anger—both at the crime itself and at the ways in which the police and judicial system treated them. The focus of self-help groups of parents of children with cancer was often tied to parents' immediate needs to care for and help heal their child (especially in the early stages of treatment), and to modulate whatever anger they felt with their need to maintain a collaborative relationship with the medical system caring for their child.

Table 11.3 compares the ordering of benefits reported by parents who were members of these self-help groups of parents of children with cancer and of parents of murdered children. In this case, the Spearman rank-order correlation coefficient (rho) was statistically significant, indicating that the rank-ordering of benefits reported by members of these two different types of groups did not differ—in fact they were very similar. The most discrepant mean reports of benefits occurred with

Table 11.3. Members' mean reports and rank-ordering of benefits of self-help groups for parents of children with cancer and parents of murdered children

Benefit	Parents of children with cancer Mean (N = 65)	Rank	Parents of murdered children Mean (N = 100)	Rank
Meeting others with similar problems	3.70	1	3.81	1
Talking about my child	3.66	2	3.62	3
Understanding the treatments	3.54	3	3.45	8
Being helpful to other parents	3.52	4.5	3.50	6
Learning to express compassion	3.52	4.5	3.49	7
Getting information about issue	3.49	6	3.39	11
Feeling freer to express feelings	3.46	7	3.54	4
Getting help from other parents	3.45	8.5	3.34	12.5
Feeling part of a larger group	3.45	8.5	3.53	5
Being supported/approved of	3.35	10	3.41	10
Coping with public attitudes	3.25	11	3.34	12.5
Learning to cope differently	3.23	12	3.18	15
Learning my rights as a parent	3.22	13	3.43	9
Coping with problems in my family	3.09	14	3.01	16
Learning who's on the staff	3.08	15	3.20	14
Coping with the death of my child	3.07	16	3.65	2
Developing self-confidence	3.00	17	2.95	17
Getting help from the professionals	2.92	18	2.39	22
Being an active part of the medical care system	2.83	19	2.82	18
Feeling spiritual uplift	2.74	20	2.46	21
Learning to be a leader	2.72	21	2.55	20
Changing things in the system	2.22	22	2.60	19

Notes: Benefits rated on a 4-point scale, 4 = much, 3 = some, 2 = little, 1 = none. Minor wording changes (and two fewer items) distinguish this list of benefits from the one in Table 7.1, so as to describe benefits relevant for both sets of groups. Spearman coefficient of rank-order correlation (rho) is .79 (statistically significant at $p < .01$).

respect to three items: (1) coping with the death of my child—a large difference in mean ranks; (2) getting help from professionals; and (3) changing things in the system. The benefit of the self-help group related to the death of a child was more highly ranked by parents of murdered children because for them this had already occurred, by the definition of the sample; some parents of children with cancer in the sample also had that experience, but many others had not, although all had contemplated that possibility. Parents of children with cancer rated the benefit of help from the staff more highly because, for them, the staff (medical and social service professionals) was in the business of helping to heal them and their child. The commitment of the staff dealing with parents of murdered children (in this case professional law enforcement as well as social service agencies) may not have been as clear, and mirrors our earlier discussion of these parents reporting less help and support from a variety of sources. Finally, the differential benefit from changing the "system" probably reflects the greater focus on advocacy and change-oriented activities in the support groups involving parents of murdered children. Overall, the high rank-order correlation suggests that members' benefited from both types of groups in quite similar ways, even though, as reported in Table 11.2, the groups emphasized different types of activities, and conducted them at different frequency rates. The most provocative finding illustrated in Tables 11.2 and 11.3 is the fact that the same self-help group "magic" appears to have been at work for both sets of parents who chose to get involved in these groups, even though this "magic" (the benefits) was accomplished through different programs and activity priorities/frequencies.

Professionals of various backgrounds were involved in many of these local groups. When asked to describe the most and least common roles played by professionals in their self-help groups, parents experiencing both these life crises provided similar perspectives. In both sets of groups, parents of children with cancer and parents of murdered children, members reported the following professional roles as most common:

- Refer new parents to the group
- Provide information
- Refer parents for special help
- Consult with the group on problems
- Advocate the group's existence and function

On the other hand, the following roles were reported as least commonly played by professionals:

- Train parents in how to lead the group
- Set the agenda for the group
- Plan group activities
- Supervise the group's operations

Thus, Tables 11.2 and 11.3 and this list of professional role behaviors in groups address some of the potential universalities of self-help, in terms of benefits of involvement and professional/parent relations; they also indicate some of its particular qualities in terms of how the nature of the life crisis affected different parental coping styles and therefore different self-help group activities.

Social Background as a Source of Self-Help Group Variation

In addition to the ways in which the particular crisis or issue acts as a source of potential diversity, cultural and social status differences also give rise to particular qualities of self-help groups. Different sociodemographic populations or cultural/ethnic groups within a nation may have different belief and traditions about the responsibility of person, family, community and nation in dealing with stressful life situations, different traditions about local and grass-roots mobilization of kith and kin, and differential access to state-supported services. Moreover, cultural variations in life-style values and mores may make self-help activities more or less normative in different population groups and subgroups. Thus, even if self-help activity in general is somewhat counternormative within the broader U.S. culture and social service systems, it may be more (or less) acceptable and common within certain cultural groups or demographic statuses.

Pancoast, Parker, and Froland (1983) and Richardson (1983) discuss some of the differentiating characteristics that influence the nature of the social welfare or social service apparatus and its views of self-help: economic resources, political ideology, social status, political influence, and cultural values about self-care. Several other authors studying a variety of self-help groups within given nations also report the great differences they observed across cultural or demographic groupings.[5] Weber (1982) emphasizes how group members' culturally determined beliefs about the nature of their common problem (due to fate, their own agency, identifiable actions of others, etc.) affect their views and practices of self-help. Cohen (1982) also discusses the ways in which local and cultural (or subcultural) contexts influence beliefs in self-help. He notes the importance of economic class, suggesting that inasmuch as certain beliefs may be tied to class origins and locations, they too may be considered in the same manner as cultural variables. Biegel and

Yamatani (1987) report that the membership of the ten self-help groups for families of mentally ill persons that they studied were almost exclusively made up of people who were white, female, and middle-class. Vine and Beels (1990) also examined groups for family members of mentally ill persons, and affirm the class bias in group membership. They attribute this to the group's attractiveness to highly verbal people, who have higher education and more resources, and who are intolerant of and ready to advocate resistance to the trend toward deinstitutionalization of the mentally ill. Findings regarding the largely white and middle-class (and often female) membership of a great variety of self-help groups seems to support these observations,[6] although recent studies of groups in African-American and Latina communities suggest these findings may be as much a function of researcher bias and geographic racial segregation as of truly different and racial membership patterns.

Others argue that in the United States, for instance, most organized self-help groups do not reach the potential numbers of affected persons in the barrios and ghettos.[7] Not surprisingly, in Chapter 6 we reported few persons of color in any of the 1980s samples of self-help groups for families of children with cancer, although more recent (1993) data, reported in Chapter 10, suggests groups have become somewhat more diverse. Hedrick et al. (1992) also suggest that older citizens often are not included, and that many populations underserved by the formal social service apparatus are also underrepresented in self-help groups—the very old, the very young, the very poor, people with severe disabilities, and in general those without the resources or opportunities to participate in voluntary organizations.[8] This analysis does not suggest that self-help as such does not exist in these different classes and culturally diverse settings, but that the formally organized self-help group often discussed in the literature, and emphasized throughout this volume, may not be the prevalent form. Much more evident in these communities may be informally developed networks of kith and kin involved in mutual help and support.

Involvement in formally organized groups is not the only culturally appropriate self-help framework. Self-help that is constructed in ways that are congruent with the values and life-styles of particular cultural, ethnic, or demographic groups has a better chance of being used effectively by these groups, precisely because they are *not* counter-normative for their local situation. For instance, Neighbors et al. (1990) argue that the unique cultural and material position of African-Americans in the United States leads to their special perspective on and use of informal (kith and kin) help systems. They argue that it is not possible to separate African-Americans' involvement in voluntary self-help group activities from their larger struggle for freedom, equal rights, and a meaningful role in U.S. society. In their view, African-American churches and fraternities, as well as political advocacy groups, are the historic agencies and settings within which self-help occurs for this community.[9] In a similar vein, Humphreys and Woods (1993) and Nash and Kramer (1993) document the existence of self-help groups in the African-American community, both with regard to (1) their similarity to other forms of self-help groups in their core activities and processes, and (2) their racial homogeneity, paralleling the racial homogeneity of white groups located in predominantly white geographic areas.

In another case study of self-help processes within an ethnic community in the United States, Gutierrez et al. (1990) discuss the incompatibilities between the Anglo cultural priority on functional independence and individual autonomy and the Latina orientation toward collectivism and social harmony. They assert that self-help is quite compatible with the Latina culture, but with an emphasis on neighborhood and family-oriented "mutual aid." In times of crisis Latinos do use their own indigenous and familial communal aid networks, which include the extended family, church, merchant, and social clubs.[10] The authors also suggest that Latinos are minimally inclined to join existing (mainstream and Anglo) self-help groups for various reasons: distance from their residence, language differences, awkwardness with white-led ventures, experiences of prejudice and discrimination, and a host of other practical constraints (babysitting, time, and energy) Several of these reported factors echo the reasons why some parents of children with cancer, regardless of race and ethnicity, did not join local self-help groups (see the discussion in Chapter 6).

Another example of culture's effects on self-help is the role of the professional culture, or, as Borkman calls it, the professional "frame of reference" (Borkman, 1990). The various authors in Pancoast, Parker, and Froland (1983) discuss the reactions of policy makers and profession-

als to self-help groups and processes. To the extent that professional socialization and commitment (developed through both pre-professional
training and on-the-job socialization) leads to a coherent belief system, a
professional ideology about service, service provision, and service re-
ception, it also may represent a distinctive culture (or subculture) that is
often at odds with lay cultures—and certainly with the often nonprofes-
sional (or pro-experiential) ideology of self-help group organizers and
members.[11] Moreover, to the extent that this professional culture reflects and advances values that are dominant in the Anglo and middle-
or upper-middle-class community (e.g., interpersonal distance, indi-
vidualism, and particular moral norms about proper child-rearing and
orientations to health care), it may represent a culture at considerable
variance from that of African-American, Latino, Asian-American, and
Native-American peoples and communities. In Chapter 9 we discussed
this problem as part of the "triple monopoly" associated with professional stances toward self-help; Katz (1993) also points to the power of
this professional culture when it is exercised by professionals who are
government personnel as well, given the control that governmental
agents and agencies have over funds and other programmatic resources
that self-help groups might desire and need.

Nations and National Cultures as Sources of Self-Help Group Variation

Different *nations* have different visions of the proper relationship
between individuals and the state, and organize these visions into different legal and politico-economic frameworks. They also have different
ideologies and different formal arrangements for caring for people in
stressful life situations. Specifically, they differ in ideologies regarding
the state's responsibility for people in need and thus the comprehensive-
ness and universality of public services. These frameworks, which reflect the dominant culture in a society, help both to give meaning to
human experience and to define the ways in which people should act on
their experiences. Some societies promote notions of self-sufficiency
that cause people to rely solely on their own resources in times of crisis.
Others promote a view of the general welfare that suggests citizens
should look to and rely on the state—on public and formal resource
systems—for assistance when they are in trouble. Still others promote a

view of reliance upon small groups of kith and kin in such circumstances, and emphasize the importance of families, neighborhood units, and other voluntary or informal associations that assist people in crisis.

This analysis echoes our earlier discussion of the counternormative character of self-help in the United States in general. It may help us understand the degree to which relatively small numbers of affected populations join more or less formally organized self-help groups in the United States. Moreover, it reflects both member ambivalence regarding substantial professional direction of self-help groups and professionals' ambivalence about the value of relatively autonomous self-help groups (see Chapters 8 and 9). Views on these issues may be very different in other nations. For instance, deCocq (1990) argues that in the United States, an anti–social-welfare and pro-entrepreneurial and voluntarist ideology results in a preferred image of self-help groups as relatively free of state interference and largely outside the domain of state support. When the state does support the idea of self-help in the United States, it often is done explicitly to spur voluntaristic and private alternatives to state activity and service; thus groups are likely to be independent of and even antagonistic to formal services, and in competition with them for resources.[12] Leventhal, Maton, and Madara (1988) extend this analysis, arguing that the entire self-help sector in the United States is loosely organized, partly as a function of its voluntary and nonstate nature, and partly as a result of the state's stance of nonresponsibility for self-help. Thus, the pattern of relatively independent self-help groups that constitute one end of Mellor et al.'s (1984) continuum is likely to be less common in other nations.

Some of these differences have been extended in discussions of the distinction between the Western industrialized world, where "specialized agencies of help, with professional providers who are believed to possess unique knowledge and technology" (Katz, 1984, p. 233), offer assistance, and the developing countries, where mutual assistance is offered by kith and kin in traditional and basic form (Katz, 1992). In Katz's view, self-help in the industrialized nations may be driven by dissatisfied reactions to highly formal, alienating, and bureaucratic services; in developing nations it more often may reflect traditional forms of kinship and communal responsibility. Katz (1984) suggests that in Europe there is less interest on the part of self-help groups in working harmoniously with state services, and more interest in altering the ser-

304 PART 5. BROADER VIEWS OF SELF-HELP GROUPS

vice delivery system, and indeed the social structure of the society, than in the U.S. groups.[13]

The focus on developed versus developing nations, however, may mask other important differences. For instance, deCocq (1990) argues that the welfare-state orientation of the Scandinavian and some other highly developed Western European nations fosters a national commitment to help in the formation and maintenance of self-help groups as a state responsibility. The same supportive posture appears evident in Canada (Katz, 1993). Moreover, in Israeli self-help groups the orientation to professionals' roles is markedly different from that reported by groups in the United States. Members of Israeli self-help groups for parents of children with mental illness and for parents in families of new immigrants reported the following roles of professionals in their groups as *most common* (Chesler et al., 1988):[14]

- Lead the group
- Set the group's agenda
- Plan group activities

The following roles were reported as *least commonly played* by professionals:

- Raise or provide funds
- Attend social functions and activities

This pattern was reversed in the two sets of U.S. self-help groups (parents of children with cancer and parents of murdered children)[15] where professionals more often played advisory or consultative roles, and desisted from supervisory or decision-making functions. Self-help groups in Israel appeared to be much more dependent upon professional direction and leadership than were those in the United States. This does not mean that the U.S. groups operated without or in opposition to professional assistance, but that assistance was different, and was delivered in a very different manner, than in Israeli settings. The more elaborate professional social system in Israel, backed by a state ideology and resources for the support of self-help, obviously extended into active leadership of self-help groups at the local level.

The state may be active, even to the point of organizing and enlarging the self-help sector, in other developed nations as well. For instance, van Harberden (1990; 1986) describes how the Dutch government actively supports self-help as a state responsibility, not as a substitute for formal and state-provided services. Other illustrations of the active role of the state in self-help come from nations where governments provide financial support to self-help groups or otherwise incorporate them into social welfare programs.[16] For instance, according to one report from a local Council of Voluntary Organizations,

Councils for voluntary service and other local development agencies have begun to recognize the contribution made by self-help groups by making available resources to enable and support their development. Their aim has been to smooth the path between groups and the resources they need, to enable them to make more informed choices about their goals and to improve the local climate of opinion about the value of self-help. The rationale for providing this support is clear. The task of a local development agency, expressed in its most general terms, is to enable people to participate more fully in the life of their communities by furthering the possibilities of voluntary action. Involvement in a self-help group is a type of voluntary activity which promotes the participation of some of the most vulnerable and isolated members of society. (Unell, 1987, p. 5)

Further, Trojan (1983) suggests some differences (and similarities) between the French and West German experiences with self-help. The most striking difference, he argues, is that in West Germany there were many more discussion-oriented self-help groups than in France, while in France there appeared to be more action-oriented groups and organizations of groups. He does not speculate on the nationality based reasons for such differences, except to indicate that "institutionalized rights for the participation of consumers in decision-making processes or provision of health and social services do not exist in West Germany" (Trojan, Halves, and Wetendorf, 1986, p. 22). Perhaps this gap explains the slow (or low level of) development of advocacy-oriented and well-organized self-help groups in West Germany. However, even these close links do not negate the existence of social-change-oriented and advocacy groups, some of which coexist with or even within traditional support-oriented groups.

A very different account of the structure and function of self-help is presented in Sidel's (1976) early report from the People's Republic of China. Sidel observes that the government used China's communal, family-oriented, mutual aid tradition to organize workers' cooperatives and work gangs in rural areas. Such organizations were built on the traditional affinities of people from the same geographic community;

they used grass-roots organizing methods, but had to comply with state directives and a "watchful eye" from above. This combination of the traditional communal culture and a bureaucratic national framework was also used to organize communes and residents' committees in urban areas. With particular regard to mentally ill patients in therapeutically oriented institutions, "patients . . . participate in regular study sessions, using the writings of Mao-Tse-Tung to analyze their own illnesses and points of view and to remold their attitudes" (Sidel, 1976, p. 226). Thus, the government used traditional cultures and life-styles, but added a new ideological framework and supervisory mandate. The result was an encouragement of grass-roots activity and freedom to organize on the one hand, and constraints on the issues and procedures with which self-help functioned on the other. Another example of a self-help framework introduced "from above," yet integrated into communal and workplace situations, is reported by Barath (1990). Hypertension clubs in Croatia (when it was part of Yugoslavia) were initiated by general practitioners as part of a prevention program. At the same time, these clubs were part of the "socio-political organizing structure of a local or labor community," and they worked with the "intensive cooperation of health workers" (p. 207). Once again, we see freedom to organize and design activities, but with a focus limited to reducing members' blood pressure—presumably by traditional treatment methods—and with the close supervision of professionals (and state officials).

In nations where comprehensive and universally accessible services are provided, the population may come to expect that authorities will deal with social and individual problems through formal, state-supported, professionalized mechanisms; these mechanisms are also readily available, and tend to intervene (preventively, proactively, or reactively) when required. The general relevance of the overall political and economic context within which self-help groups are formed and operate, as well as the potential for change in this context, is stressed in Gidron and Bargal's (1986) account of the Israeli experience. Gradually, what was a very centralized system dominated by a large public sector has become a more open and decentralized system, with a consequent increase in independent self-help groups and organizations. Under circumstances of expanded state services and support for self-help, Israeli professionals now are likely to generate and play potent roles in self-help activities and groups, and groups are likely to work in conjunction with public providers. Parker, Pancoast, and

Froland (1983) note that some researchers in West Germany and the United Kingdom "found a widespread acceptance of the usefulness of self-help groups among professionals" (p. 280). On the other hand, other researchers indicated an "uncertain" and "not especially enthusiastic" (p. 279) response by professionals to the role of self-help groups in the United States, France, and the United Kingdom. Contradictions such as these, within nations and within developed regions, make it impossible to conclude whether these trends in state support for self-help are due to international differences, intranational differences, or simply interresearcher differences.

Because of the diverse and often informal nature of self-help, data about its particular forms, even within a single nation, are difficult to obtain. This problem is multiplied when we attempt to examine the similarities and differences in self-help across several nations, with their own cultures, ideologies, political economies, and health and welfare systems. It does appear, however, that many more institutions and even governments now are formulating social policies vis-à-vis self-help, are building coordinating structures to link self-help groups with other support and service systems, and are establishing clearinghouses to further facilitate the use of this mode of mutual aid and community connection.[17]

Despite oft-cited desires for more effective collaboration between self-help groups and the formal sector of professionalized services, some observers caution against potential state and professional agency co-optation of self-help. In the United States, for instance, Withorn (1980) predicted that governmental rhetoric supporting self-help in the Reagan-Bush era was part of a general effort to diminish public and professional resources available to people in crisis. Similarly, McWhirter et al., (1988) express concern about the potentially pacifying role of Christian Base Communities in Latin America, especially with regard to distracting people from broader objectives of political freedom and economic democracy. Under such circumstances, what is being advanced is not a prescription for collaboration, but for co-optation and incorporation. These are especially important concerns in an age when conservative national governments are attempting to reduce the welfare state system and promote the scarcity paradigm of limited expertise, resources, and power. It may be advisable, then, for self-help groups to remain at the periphery, to emphasize their counternormative values and processes, to sustain their unique style and reliance on the resources of experiential knowledge and peer support, and to regard incorporation into the culture of professionalized services as problematic. Such incorporation is most likely to reshape self-help in the image and form of professional and formal services themselves, dramatically reducing its potential for offering alternative forms of expertise, resources, and power, and for standing as a vigorous and loving complement to established care systems.

Conclusions

The arguments made throughout this chapter for both the universal and the particular aspects of self-help dynamics and processes are crucial to the effective maintenance and further development of self-help. The specificity of particular life crises and circumstances present challenges in terms of identifying and responding to particular populations' needs. Recognizing within-crisis variation that leads self-help groups to differ in many instances, we also have argued for the commonalities that exist across life crises and, therefore, across specific groups. To the extent that these particular and universal needs are manifest in forms to which the professional service system cannot or will not respond effectively or completely, self-help efforts based upon these needs will continue to be seen as counternormative and as challenging the dominant culture's sense of what is appropriate.

To the extent that state or national ideologies and cultures truly support some of the major themes of self-help groups—for instance, the empowerment of people in crisis and the provision of support and affirmation to people facing stressful and stigmatizing life circumstances— self-help activities will not continue to be counternormative. In those situations where particular cultures accept and cherish experiential expertise and support public expressions of deeply felt emotions, self-help activities are more likely to be congruent with core norms, and even to facilitate the growth of these voluntary and democratic trends (Wuthnow, 1994). In those circumstances we also expect less tension between self-help members and professionals, and greater involvement of professionals in collaboration with self-help members, activities and groups. These are the situations where we would expect to see self-help move toward the center, rather than the periphery, of social systems' resources and individuals' legitimated options.

Part 6

Practical Guidelines and Helpful Hints: Building Your Own Bridges

Chapter 12 provides a series of "helpful hints" for parents and professionals who wish to organize and provide leadership or support to local self-help groups.

12

Practical Guidelines for
Self-Help Group
Development and Maintenance

The traditional way of concluding a monograph with a summary of theory, procedures, and findings seems to us unnecessarily repetitive and sterile. Therefore, we have elected to conclude this volume with a chapter that summarizes the main findings in a set of practical guidelines for the more successful operation of self-help groups. We hope this will prove more interesting and more useful than the standard approach.

The extraordinary worldwide growth of self-help groups has resulted in a parallel growth in efforts to help groups form and succeed in their missions. Books, articles and how-to-do-it manuals have emerged to aid in their development.[1] Across the nation, self-help clearinghouses are coordinating information and providing groups with advice, connection to others, and helpful resources.[2] In this chapter we provide a series of practical guidelines for people wishing to form self-help groups for parents of children with cancer, using as a basis the issues and findings presented in this volume. We have argued throughout that there appear to be some *relatively universal characteristics and themes in all self-help groups*, regardless of their demographic appeal, sociocultural setting, and the specific issue or life condition that is their focus. At the same time, we have also argued that *groups in different nations and cultures, or groups focusing on different life conditions, often develop relatively distinctive characteristics*. Thus, while some of the universal "magic" of self-help may be relevant to all initiators and organizers, there are specific organizing principles and activities that are most appealing to parents of children with cancer.

In order to be effective, local self-help groups of parents of children with cancer need a variety of resources: ideas about program and purpose, the wherewithal to implement programs and activities effectively, parents who join and become active members, parents who are willing and able to undertake leadership roles, collaborative links with medical and social service professionals, and access to the materials, advice and staff of the CCCF. We direct this chapter to the above issues and build suggestions from the central questions guiding the inquiries reported in prior chapters—questions such as the following:

• What are these groups all about?
• What do they do, and how do they operate?
• Why do people join them, and how do members benefit from involvement?
• How do these groups relate with formal care systems—to professional medical and social service staffs and institutions?
• Do (or how do) these groups change over time?

Here we focus on some additional and more practical questions such as,

• How can interested parents start a local self-help group?
• How can members be recruited?
• What kinds of programs and activities are most important for a local group?
• How can interested parents find out what other parents in other groups are doing?
• How can a group prepare for changes in its leadership or membership over time?
• What roles should professionals play in parent groups?

Basic Assumptions and Themes

The most important practical principle to recognize in facilitating self-help groups and activities for parents of children with cancer is that they are *grass-roots phenomena, that they grow out of the needs of relatively normal people experiencing a particular stressful life circumstance.* Parents of children with cancer are not a psychopathological population, in need of psychotherapy or deep psychological counseling. They are, however, in need of psychological and social support, especially the unique kind of support that comes from others "who have been there." Thus, while outsiders—professionals, and friends and neighbors of people directly afflicted—have important and helpful roles to play, they may not be as central to the self-help process as are other people who are in the same situation. For the most part, these self-help groups are not organizable and sustainable from outside the community of fellow sufferers, and they rely upon the resources of other parents of children with cancer to survive and grow.

We have argued elsewhere (Chesler and Barbarin, 1987) that *parents of children with cancer need a great deal of psychosocial and social support* in order to deal with this frightening and stressful life situation. Some of the support they require is tangible and material, as in physical transportation, childcare, and perhaps financial aid; other helpful support is social and emotional in nature, as in formal counseling, informal friendship, and love and affirmation. These various forms of support may come from various sources: professionals, kith and kin, and community agencies. But in self-help groups, parents of children with cancer come into contact with a very different source of support—other parents who have traveled the same path, who have navigated the same "troubled waters" of childhood cancer. Our focus on the support available in these self-help group settings does not obviate or trivialize these other sources and forms, for they are all important. But it also is important to focus on this unique setting and its possibilities, for there are resources and support promised and available *in self-help groups that are not available anywhere else!*

Self-help groups and their members have a special kind of assistance they can offer, an "experiential expertise", that is quite unique. This special expertise is rooted in *experiential knowledge*, the sharing of which is one of the central dynamics of most self-help groups. Through such sharing, people in stressful life situations gain information about the disease and its treatment, about the hospital and staff, about the typical strains and stresses of parenting a child with cancer, about coping techniques and tricks, and the like. In the context of intimate group conversations, people *share experiences with one another and often form a new sense of self-in-situation, a new social identity.* This process of identifying with the new role of a parent of a child with cancer is based upon parents' personal experience with childhood cancer and on comparing experiences and knowledge shared by other parents. As people share experiences in these groups, they find *support and affirmation from others* and a social setting in which they can counter the stigma so often associated with serious childhood illness. Many people find others who know the bridges they are crossing, and who may even become life-long friends and companions. As experienced parents *share coping skills and tactics* with others, they help others new to the situation learn how to handle the many practical problems they face. They also may find new ways to heal themselves as they offer healing balm to others. The "benefits" of self-help often lead to a sense of *(re)empowerment of oneself as an individual and of the group as a collectivity*, as difficult situations are coped with and perhaps action taken to improve the quality of medical and psychosocial care.

These five themes or underlying processes appear to be central to most self-help groups, and they are particularly useful responses to the stresses of parenting a child with cancer. Parents of children with cancer often experience several categories of psychosocial stress (outlined in Table 2.1): intellectual or informational, practical or instrumental, inter-personal or social, emotional, and existential. The unique nature of these particular stresses distinguishes the experience of childhood cancer from other stressful life conditions, and defines the parameters of self-help group activity that may respond successfully to these stresses. *People interested in forming self-help groups for parents of children with cancer need to attend to these particular stresses, and to their prevalence in the particular parent populations with which they wish to work.* Then they can develop some of the group activities or programs that respond to these stresses, which we summarize below.

How Do Parents or Professionals Go About Starting a Group?

The first important task is to create or initiate a group where none exists or to re-initiate an old group that has gone out of existence. *In order to initiate a group, one must have several different resources:* an energetic and (ideally) charismatic parent of a child with cancer, (usu-ally) a helpful member of the professional staff, a list of names of parents of children diagnosed with cancer at the local treatment center or in the community, a way of calling, or mailing to, or otherwise contacting these parents, a meeting place, and an agenda for the first meeting that is likely to attract people and interest them in future meetings. Luke, Roberts, and Rappaport (1993) suggest that first meetings of self-help groups are crucial for future member participation and retention. At these first meetings parent organizers need not only to make the group's mission and purpose clear, but also to listen to new members' needs and desires, in order to create the best possible "person-group match at the outset" (p. 235). Although there is "magic" in parents meeting other parents, just meeting others is not sufficient to start a group; *a clear mission, agenda, and plans for meeting again and having certain activities is crucial.*

Among the important ongoing maintenance activities are those that involve *recruiting new members.* This usually involves establishing a good relationship with the medical staff, so that the staff will refer parents of newly diagnosed children to the group, and in general will legitimize the group in the eyes of parents. In some cases, groups can recruit parents directly, without intervention or assistance from the medical staff, through their own visits to clinics and the hospital's wards. In almost all cases, recruitment involves personal contacts (face-to-face greetings, telephone conversations, rides to meetings) between parent group organizers and potential new members. Sometimes members are overcautious in reaching out to parents of newly diagnosed children, not wishing to intrude into their already stressed lives. At the same time, many parents of newly diagnosed children are justifiably cautious or confused about whether they want to meet other parents of children with cancer, let alone go to an organized group meeting. The transition from the shock of having heard that one's child has cancer to being part of a group of parents who are actively identifying with and dealing with this situation is neither easy nor rapid. But veteran parents can reach out and introduce themselves to others, can say the magic words, "My child has cancer too, and I know something about what you are going through," and can model the reality that despite this diagnosis they are standing, talking, working, caring, and offering a gift of comradeship and love amidst the struggle.

What Should Groups Do?

Self-help groups can and do undertake a wide variety of activities. The most useful activities are those that speak to the special needs of people affected by the life condition or situation that is the focus of the group. Group activities that address these needs are most likely to be sustained and, in turn, to sustain active members and a working group (see Table 4.1). Some groups undertake a local needs-assessment effort to discover the specific needs of their particular populations. A *formal* needs assessment usually involves systematic surveys of the local catchment population identified through group or hospital records, and the subsequent analysis of the results. More *informal* assessments of parent populations can be accomplished by using group mailing lists or telephone networks to ask parents questions such as the following:

- What do you want to know about the treatment and prognosis of different kinds of childhood cancer?
- What questions do you have about schooling issues? About nutritional supplements?
- Do you want to talk with other parents whose child has the same diagnosis as your child? What would you ask them?
- Do you need help in working with your insurance company? In getting time off from work? In meeting your bills?
- Are you feeling stressed out? Overwhelmed? In need of a break? Do you want to know how others handle stress?
- Do you know where to go to get help in enabling your child with cancer to live a (relatively) normal life? In dealing with siblings' reactions? In dealing with marital stress?

Such assessments help groups identify the existing and potential needs of parents, and thus help them to plan the activities that will best suit their members' needs. Among the most common activities of self-help groups for parents of children with cancer are the following:

- Lectures, materials, and *information sessions* that illuminate the nature of childhood cancer, its prognoses, and treatments.
- Lectures and *discussions of different ways of coping* with the practical and emotional stresses associated with childhood cancer.
- *Social and recreational events* for all family members.
- *Peer counseling or "rap" sessions*, in which members share their feelings or concerns and help each other solve their coping problems.
- Opportunities to *form new friendships.*
- Opportunities to express parents' needs and *seek improvements in the system of medical care* (including lobbying efforts to generate external community support for the medical system and its programs).
- *Fund-raising events* to benefit individual families, the group's program, or the medical system's service and research agenda.

- *Visits to other parents and children* who are hospitalized.
- *Telephone networks* or personal visits to families.

Effectively implemented activities benefit all members, but it is the fit between group activities and the unique needs of individual members that is critical to the success of a local group. Not all local groups can or should undertake all of these activities, and certainly not at the early stages of their initiation or development. *Different local groups, with somewhat different relationships with the treatment center, and perhaps somewhat different membership, need to shape these common activities for their own purposes, populations, and resources.*

A diversity of activities can better accommodate the variety of needs and stresses that different parents face, or the relative strength of each of those stresses. *Groups characterized by a diverse set of activities, offering numerous options for members, seem to attract and retain parents more effectively than do groups with a more limited activity focus.* Thus, if some parents would like to listen to medical experts, and others would like to talk with one another, and others would like to go bowling together, only a group providing such a variety of activities can be expected to appeal to all these parents. Or, if some parents have been coming to group meetings for quite a while and now have children out of treatment, while others are newcomers fresh from their child's initial diagnosis, only a broadly organized set of activities can accommodate such disparate needs.

The ability of local self-help groups to meet these parents' needs, to provide useful and satisfying activities and programs that support parents in times of difficulty and that improve their own and their children's coping capacities, is the true test of their utility. We *should not assess group success by size*—the number of people who come to meetings—*or by longevity, or by fund-raising capacity.* Good and important things can happen in small meetings of two to three people as well as in large meetings of thirty to forty people. Several sessions of high-quality sharing and caring may be more important than a several-year history of dull and boring meetings. Sharing life experiences and developing intimate bonds may be more vital for people's health and outlook than creating a large bank account. Different self-help groups will develop different standards for success, but our hope is that they will stay focused on the fundamental human dynamics of self-help: sharing life experiences, developing experiential expertise, supporting and affirming one another, sharing coping skills and tactics, and empowering one another to take appropriate personal and collective action.

How Should Groups Operate?

Aside from program-focused activities, there are a number of other tasks a group must accomplish in order to survive over time. These "maintenance activities" maintain or ensure the life of the group, and differ from the services or programs that groups provide for members.[3]

Decisions about where and when to meet can differ greatly among groups. These are important choices; some parents hesitate to return to the treatment center more often than they have to, and so will shun meetings held there. Popular alternatives include Ronald McDonald houses, churches and community centers, or members' homes. On the other hand, the treatment center often is a central and well-known location, and it provides easy access to medical professionals, wards, and libraries. With regard to the timing of meetings, groups that create activities wherein members share their personal experiences and stories probably will elect to meet more often (perhaps once a month or more) than will groups meeting primarily for social purposes.

Groups also may differ in the *degree to which they formalize their operations.* Some, but not all, successful groups create a charter and by-laws, gain tax-exempt status, have regular elections of officers, and use committee structures for getting work done. Generally speaking, a more formal organization is necessary when substantial funds are being raised from the general public and when the group gets quite large. Another aspect of formalization often involves the *choice of whether to meet always as a single group or to create subgroups for specific purposes or subpopulations.* One common pattern is for an entire group to meet together for a while, and then to separate so that parents who are struggling with children in particular situations (e.g., undergoing a bone marrow transplant, going off treatment, dealing with brain tumors) or with specific concerns (about schooling, about toilet training in infancy, about adolescent dating) can talk together and then reconvene as a whole group before closing a meeting. It also is common for groups to subdivide into discussions that allow mothers and fathers to talk separately about their own concerns, such as differences in child-rearing responsibilities, work roles, marital problems, and the like. Subgroups or even separate self-help groups specifically for teenagers, siblings, or parents of deceased children also have emerged out of regular group structures and meeting times.

Groups that do not manage their internal affairs well often lose members and eventually cease to exist. *Good management of internal operations generally requires good leadership that avoids factionalism and cliquishness.* When a lack of leadership skill or energy, or conflicts over leadership, prevents groups from delivering needed and useful activities, everyone suffers. It appears especially important to guard against those leadership issues that often plague small voluntary organizations: "ego-tripping," control by original founders who are unable to let go or take a back seat, factionalism and cliquishness by a small group of close friends, excessive resistance to working with the staff and the adoption of a beleagured "bunker mentality" with regard to the medical staff, or excessive "buttering up" of the staff and a willingness to be coopted. Some of these leadership issues become especially potent at times of transition, when one set of leaders drops out of the group and others move in, or when the group undergoes any sort of major change in its activity focus or level. *New leaders must be developed and trained* in order to prepare for these changes and to ensure smooth transitions.

In addition to the successful operation of these internal group activities and procedures, all groups must attend to their relationships with their external environments. The most important external operational link for self-help groups operating within the medical system is *good working relationships with the medical staff.* Different groups, and different medical staffs, handle this linkage in different ways.[4] Some groups develop close ties with the staff, involving them in many aspects of group life, while others maintain a somewhat distant relationship. In some unusual cases, staff members have become leaders and members of local self-help groups, and in some unusual instances, parent representatives have become regular members of the medical staff.

Other important external links that groups, group leaders, or initiators need to consider are *connections to resources in their local communities,* such as self-help groups for other forms of childhood illness, community service agencies, and the like. *Most groups also benefit by linking their operations with the national organization of self-help groups for families of children with cancer. The Candlelighters Child-*

hood Cancer Foundation. The Candlelighters Foundation makes available to local groups information hotlines and booklets or manuals, an ombudsperson program, consultation on group problems, leadership training programs, regional and national meetings, and their extensive files on group activities and sources of professional and lay assistance; they also link to professional associations, the cancer research and treatment establishment, and health care policymakers. We think it very important for local groups to link to this national networking organization. In addition, *local chapters, officers, and affiliates of the American Cancer Society (ACS) and the Leukemia Society of America (LSA) may have valuable help to offer.* However, the staffs of ACS, LSA, and other relevant *organizations often must be educated about the value of self-help groups* for families of children with cancer; then they may be predisposed more often to respond proactively to local self-help groups.[5] Over and above the help that ACS, LSA and similar agencies provide to individual families in need, they can also be very helpful to organized groups—with regard to medical referrals and recruitment, public relations, community legitimacy, and funding for group programs such as conference attendance and newsletter distribution.

How Can Groups Attract Members and "Sell" Themselves?

Most groups try to appeal to a wide variety of parents, to parents of children with different diagnoses, to parents of children being treated at different local clinics or hospitals, to parents with different coping styles, and to parents of varying class and ethnic backgrounds. Most self-help groups recruit and retain parents whose children have died from cancer as well as parents whose children are living with the disease. *Parents of deceased children can be especially helpful to parents of living children, and vice versa.* Indeed, we have argued that many different kinds of parents join and stay active in self-help groups, depending upon how groups are operated and the activities they provide.

Despite the value of heterogeneity in a group, it is not easy to create and sustain. For instance, in most self-help groups, *mothers predominate.* It also appears that *white people (anglos), and people from relatively middle-class backgrounds seem to predominate,* especially in groups that meet in suburban areas. It may even happen that parents who are "active copers," or who are more comfortable talking about normally private matters in public, predominate, at least in group meetings and discussion. Overall, and despite their positive value, most self-help groups are reaching only a small proportion of the local families and parents affected by childhood cancer. *Special recruitment efforts must be made to reach other people.*

Some key strategies for recruitment, based on reported information about why some parents do not join or stay active in local self-help groups include the following:

- Realize that few parents join in the first three months after diagnosis; give families time to respond to the initial shock, but try to reach out and help them through this period.
- Remember that parents are often overwhelmed by physical and emotional stress.
- Time and energy are at a minimum; give parents a reason to get involved and provide assistance in terms of transportation and childcare.
- Minimize travel time and distance from parents' homes to the group meeting place.
- Remember that some parents are afraid that group discussion will increase anxiety and anger.
- Remember that everyone has their own coping strategies (and ways of dealing with or denying stress); not every parent will (or should) choose to come to the group regularly, or at all.
- Keep the group open, reduce factions and cliquishness, and keep time spent on group "business" to a minimum (let those who love to do business do it at separate meetings).
- Perception of the group as all white, or all middle-class, or all women, or all anything, will turn some people away.
- Have the medical staff talk in positive terms about the group to parents of newly diagnosed children.
- Make some group activities visible with posters and announcements in clinics and on hospital wards.
- Provide a wide range of activities, at different times, so that parents with different needs can all find assistance within the group.

Group *newsletters and telephone networks can keep members in touch* with parents who may temporarily be unable to attend group meetings. Social work staff who follow up with parents of deceased children and children off treatment can facilitate access to these families. Parents of both living and deceased children who have never participated in a self-help group while their child was in treatment may be willing to get involved later, when they have more time and energy or distance from the stress of the illness, especially if they continue to see and hear about the group in the clinic, in the media and in the community.

Since *"meeting other people in a similar situation" stood out as the most commonly reported and highly ranked benefit* of group involvement, meeting times should focus on building communication among parents, encouraging the sharing of experiences and problems, and developing the strong emotional bonds of friendship that sustain many parents and their groups. Providing information about medical treatments and common ways of coping with stress also should be a high priority. Both parents and professional staff members can share such information.

Members of self-help groups report greater positive changes in their own mental health, in their sense of being able to influence the medical environment, and in their overall satisfaction with friends and family members than do parents of children with cancer who are not self-help group members. Although we do not believe that all parents will benefit from self-help group involvement, *the ability of such groups to make a positive difference in many people's lives* is undeniable. Positive outcomes of participation should be *identified, publicized, and utilized in recruitment tactics* as a way of appealing to new members, as well as a way of gaining cooperation from the medical staff and community agencies.

Working with Professional Staffs

Along with other self-help group members, we continually state and believe that professional *members of the medical staff have many valuable resources to offer to self-help groups and their members.* There are, however, many versions of the good, better, and/or best ways for professionals to provide those resources. Most of the differences among these versions center around the *degree of control professionals should or should not exercise in the life of the group, and the balance of leadership among professionals and parent members.* Some mutual support groups are led and directed by professional staff members, while others are led primarily by parents. These *different kinds of support groups all have value*, whether they are led by professionals, by parents, or by some mix. But since our primary interest is not in the delivery of professional therapy or counseling, not even professional counseling conducted in a group environment, we have emphasized throughout the particular operations and activities of parent-led self-help groups. To the extent that these groups are and should be examples of grass-roots voluntary organizations, primary leadership should be in parents' hands, with effective collaboration and coalitions with staff members.

Since physicians are the heads of clinics and hospital departments serving children with cancer, their support for and legitimation of the group in the medical system is crucial. However, in practical terms, *the most important member of the medical staff for the self-help group usually is the social worker.* These staff members have been trained to understand and deal with the psychosocial stresses and situations of parents of children with cancer, and many of them also have skills in group dynamics and organization building. Thus, they can be useful and helpful in a variety of ways. Some of the most important roles that professional social workers (and other medical staff members) can play vis-à-vis the local self-help group include the following:

- Publicizing and advocating the group to parents of newly-diagnosed children
- Referring new members
- Gaining the cooperation of the senior medical staff
- Providing the group with access to hospital facilities and resources (rooms, printing facilities, etc.)
- Attending the group when invited and providing information on childhood cancer, coping strategies, etc.
- Consulting with the group on the problems it is having.

Parent self-help groups also can be very helpful to the medical staff. Some groups, for instance, raise considerable funds that they provide to the staff for research purposes or for adding staff, equipment, facilities, and services. For treatment centers operating on tight budgets, this is an extra source of needed funds. In addition, parent groups that develop special expertise in meeting the psychosocial needs of parents of children with cancer can assist the medical staff in responding to those needs, thus perhaps decreasing the burden on the staff and increasing the total psychosocial resource base available to patients and their families. In some treatment centers, parent group leaders are invited to meet with and even join the staff, to provide a parental perspective in staffing sessions. In this way, and also through group meetings with the staff, parents can inform and educate the staff about their needs and how the staff may better meet them.

While social workers and other medical professionals can be very helpful to local self-help groups, and vice versa, it is also possible that *groups and staffs may come into conflict with one another. This is natural and normal* in situations where people and organizations with similar purposes (service to children and families of children with cancer), yet some very different backgrounds, experiences, and ways of working on these issues, must interact with one another. For instance, some parent group leaders are very concerned about staff intrusion into parents' personal lives and into a group's program and activities. Some professional staff members object to self-help groups, feel they do more potential damage than good for parents, worry about groups harming parents if they operate without professional supervision and guidance, and are concerned that groups will make their own work more difficult and encourage challenges to medical authority. Some of the particular problems staff members often face in working closely with a local self-help group are illustrated in Figure 8.1. Professionals experiencing these problems may impede recruitment efforts, fail to refer parents of newly diagnosed children to the group, and otherwise make the group's operations difficult. Thus, there are certain things that professionals working with self-help groups should *not* do: be threatened by the existence of parent initiative and activism, attempt to overcontrol the parent group's direction or activities, act like a parent of a child with cancer, fail to recognize parents' unique expertise, do for parents what they can do for themselves and for each other, or treat parents as if they are not part of the treatment team.

Parent group *leaders and members must anticipate these problems*, recognize the likely conflicts, and try to work with professionals to overcome them. The most promising model for creating collaboration between a self-help group and the staff is a *coalition*. In this type of relationship both parties (group and staff) have their separate agendas and spheres of activity and influence, but they work together and help each other.

The Long Haul

The findings from our studies both support and challenge the common proposition that self-help groups' activities and operations "are determined primarily by the shared problems and experiences of the members" (Katz, 1981, p. 141). Members' social backgrounds and life situations clearly play a major role in shaping self-help group activities. In addition, the five elements of "magic" that we have argued are evident in almost all self-help groups determine what does and does not occur. However, groups' relationships with external organizations, including the health care system, the local community, as well as the national culture and political economy, are also powerful factors. Certainly, small associations, such as self-help groups, can expect neither to substitute for individual parents' efforts to solve their unique problems, nor to solve all social problems. However, they can mediate between the individual and institutions, such as medical systems, and can help buffer individuals' major stresses. Since most research on self-help groups, and the energy of most members and practitioners, have focused on groups' internal processes and dynamics, it is important that more attention be paid to these external forces.

Self-help groups are an increasingly popular response to people's needs and to problems in our nation's current health care practices. They generate programs and activities that respond to the major stresses experienced by parents of children with cancer. The studies of self-help groups for parents of children with cancer reported in this volume indicate that *the most effective and satisfying activities are* (1) emotional support sessions; (2) practical assistance such as providing transportation, meals, child care, and funds; (3) information on the disease and treatment, staff and facilities; (4) sharing successful coping strategies and techniques; (5) one-to-one networking and peer co-counseling; and (6) efforts to improve the character and quality of medical and psychosocial care.

The major problems that groups appear to encounter include (1) finding and maintaining consistent and effective parent leadership; (2)

recruiting parents of newly diagnosed children; and (3) creating positive yet noncontrolling relations with the medical and social service staff.

Many self-help groups for parents of children with cancer have been in existence for ten or twenty years. Although it is obvious that permanence is not necessarily a good criterion for assessing the utility of these groups, their sheer survival does suggest that good things have been happening. Good things can continue to happen as more parents reach out to others and start groups, imagine and create new activities, and develop innovative ways of getting and staying organized.

Appendices

Notes

Bibliography

Index

Appendix A:
Methods of Inquiry

The information provided in the text of this volume contains detail on some, but not all, of the variables, measures, and analytic procedures utilized in the various studies. In this appendix we illustrate how we assessed and analyzed variables not otherwise specified in detail in the text. We include information on both quantitative and qualitative data, gathered and analyzed at either the group level or the individual level.

Key Organization-Level Variables

Organizational or group-level variables were the primary research focus of Studies #2 and #4.

Formalization

Indicators of formalization included the existence of a group's charter and by-laws, legal incorporation and/or not-for-profit and tax-exempt status, formal committees, other forms of structural differentiation such as separate sub-groups for different activities, and formal budget processes. An index was created out of these items, such that groups were characterized with high, moderate, or low levels of formalization.

Leadership Patterns: Parent, Professional, Shared

The fifty groups in Studies #2 and #4 were divided into three categories: (1) those in which parents were the sole leaders, (2) those in which professionals provided primary leadership, and (3) those in which members and professionals worked closely together, while parents exerted primary leadership. Information for assigning groups to these categories came from responses in on-site interviews and follow-up "group information sheets" (Study #2), or from telephone inquiries (Study #4), to several questions regarding group participation and leadership: "Who attends meetings? Who runs meetings? Who sets the agenda and plans meetings? What roles do professionals play? Do professionals set agendas and plan meetings? Do they attend meetings?" Some definitions of self-help groups would omit professionally led support groups from this sample. However, we included them for two reasons. First, they comprise one empirical and logical endpoint on the continuum of institutionally controlled to independent parent groups, and as such can elucidate some of the dynamics of all groups. Second, the professionally led groups provide a useful contrast group in comparative analyses with the independent and shared-leadership categories.

External Links to Other Organizations and Resources

The concept of linkage was used to help understand groups' relationships with their external environment. Horizontal links involved groups' connections with like organizations in their communities serving families of ill children generally, or children facing problems in school. The number of horizontal links for a given self-help group in Studies #2 and #4 was determined from responses in the on-site interview to the following question: "Does this group link to other groups doing similar things?" Probes asked informants to report on self-help groups serving other populations, local cancer-related agencies, social service resources, and civic organizations. The information was then coded into a count of the number and type of organizational links thus identified, and reduced to categories.

Vertical links involved groups' connections with the national network of groups organized by/for families of children with cancer, The Candlelighters Childhood Cancer Foundation. Three categories of vertical linkage emerged from the data in Studies #2 and #4: (1) Low-linkage groups had no known connections to or knowledge of regional or national organizations or networks of parents of children with cancer, (2) moderate-linkage groups were on the national CCCF mailing list but considered themselves locally autonomous; these groups may have had names identifying themselves locally (often specifying a medical institution or a community), but their presence on the national list established them as part of a network of groups with a similar purpose, and created the potential for intergroup contact; (3) high-linkage groups used the name "Candlelighters" and were on the official Candlelighters mailing list. The official Candlelighters affiliation is not a highly restrictive one; there are no strict rules regarding structure, membership, or activities for Candlelighters groups. However, the name is copyrighted, and its use must be approved by the national office.

Key Individual-Level Variables

Most assessments of individual parent (member and nonmember) orientations and perspectives were generated by Study #3, although some individual-level data from Study #2 are presented throughout this volume.

Outcomes

Two different ways of measuring the outcomes of one's experience with childhood cancer, or the adequacy of coping with this crisis, were used in Study #3. The first asked parents to respond to the following question: "In general, how well have you handled your child's illness?" Three response categories were provided: (1) "very well," (2) "fairly well," and (3) "not well at all." In addition, parents were asked to indicate which issues or situations they felt they had handled "well," and which they felt they had handled "less well."

As a second way of measuring coping outcomes, four scales were designed to tap different dimensions of perceived change in parents' lives since their child's illness: (1) mental health, (2) activism, (3) physical health, and (4) life satisfaction. These four scales (presented in Table A.1) were developed from a set of items documenting parents' reports of life changes over the course of their child's illness. Responses to these items were coded as "worse," "same," or "better," and scaled as -1, 0, or $+1$, in order to clarify the direction of reported change.

Coping Styles

In study #3, five scales of coping strategies were constructed from a set of items coded on frequency of reported usage: "a lot" (4), "sometimes" (3), "seldom" (2), and "not at all" (1). The scales were designed to assess help-seeking, coping alone, passive coping, active coping, and sharing feelings and emotions (see Table A.1).

Support and Help

Also in Study #3, separate items designed to assess the helpfulness of various sources of support were rated by parents and coded on a 1–4 basis, ranging from "very helpful" (4) to "not helpful" (1). These items, documenting individual sources of perceived support, were combined into five scales. In addition, four scales were constructed from items designed to assess different types of support. Parents indicated for each item whether they received each type of support "a lot" (4), "some" (3), "a little" (2), or "none at all" (1). Items and scales for both assessments of social support are included in Table A-1.

Civic Attitudes and Involvement

Parents involved in Study #3 were asked about their views of the importance of being involved in voluntary organizations and about their actual involvement in a range of civic activities.

Data-Analysis Procedures

Since some of the data from these studies were gathered via qualitative methods and some via quantitative measures, we used both qualitative and quantitative techniques in their analysis and presentation.

Table A.1. Components of scales used for self-help group individual-level analyses (Study #3)

Scales	Item components
Reported life-change scales	
Mental health (alpha = .64)	Your own mental health
	Your sense of personal control over your life
	Your sense of loss
	Your sense of who you are
Activism (alpha = .80)	Your sense of what you as an individual can do
	Your willingness to join up with others to change things
Physical health (alpha = .63)	Your own physical health
	Your physical health compared to other men/women your age
Satisfaction (alpha = .51)	Your satisfaction with life in general
	Your satisfaction with family life
Coping-style scales	
Help-seeking (alpha = .57)	Get help in solving problems
	Seek professional help
	Seek help from friends
	Seek help from the medical staff
	Seek help from relatives
Coping alone (alpha = .46)	Try to be alone
	Keep feelings to myself
	Go off by myself
Passive coping (alpha = .49)	Accept things as they come
	Avoid thinking about problems
	Do nothing
Active coping (alpha = .38)	Keep family life normal
	Change family plans
	Reassign work around house
	Take charge of things
	Focus on problems and solve them
Sharing feelings and emotions (alpha = .56)	Share inner feelings with spouse
	Share feelings with others
	Talk it out as a family
	Talk about things to someone

Sources-of-support scales

Medical professionals (alpha = .47)
Social workers
Physicians
Nurses

Community (alpha = .26)
Lawyers
Church leaders
School people
Funeral directors
Social service agents

Family (alpha = .56)
Spouse
My parents
My child with cancer
My other children
My in-laws

Friends (alpha = .59)
Close friends
Other friends in general
Neighbors
Co-workers

Similar others (alpha = .63)
Other parents with ill children
The parent support group

Types-of-support scales

Emotional (alpha = .63)
Comfort or emotional support
Listening to you talk about your private feelings
Cheering you up
Hearing what others did in a situation that was similar to yours

Action (alpha = .69)
Someone to go with you to take some action
Suggestion for some action that you should take

Family (alpha = .56)
Care of ill child
Cooking meals and doing chores
Looking after other family members

Practical (alpha = .46)
Giving you information
Money
Providing you with transportation
Referrals for assistance
Health insurance

Qualitative Data Analyses

Three different forms of qualitative analysis were presented in this volume. One form used the principles of narrative analysis (discussed in Chapter 3) to let parents tell their own stories about their experiences with their children's cancer and about their group experiences. A second form involved selecting and presenting excerpts from individual or group interviews that best exemplified a point made by the quantitative data or otherwise expounded in the text. A third form of qualitative analysis utilized the principles of inductively grounded theory development. As an illustration of this analytic process, we elaborate here the qualitative analysis leading to the results presented in Chapter 9 on professionals' views of the dangers of self-help groups. Forty-eight professional members of different medical staffs (doctors, nurses, social workers) responded to the question, "What do professionals mean when they talk about the dangers of self-help groups?" This was one question asked in the context of a longer open-ended interview.

Once the interviews were transcribed verbatim, the raw text in response to this item was read carefully, and all mentions of a danger were underlined. Here we departed from some approaches to grounded theory development, because we approached the total data set with the specific question of "dangers" in mind, and limited our analysis of the interviews to this issue. *In vivo* coding, coding that utilizes informants' own language and imagery, done directly on the text, line by line, was the first step in preparing a coding and analysis scheme (Charmaz, 1983; Corbin, 1986). Following are several examples of professionals' responses and our *in-vivo* underlining process:

Social worker, Group 3: The professionals are afraid people will be *repeating misinformation*, that *people will compare one diagnosis to another* and come back and say, "Why aren't we getting XXXXX." There is a fear that they will *get people who are obsessed with the disease*, and *not coping well*, and totally *fixated on getting the secondary gains* from the disease. Frankly, I've seen that happen in a few individual cases.

Nurse, Group 6: Groups perhaps generate *unwarranted criticism of professionals*.

Social worker, Group 7: Professionals are afraid that a group could *get out of hand, take power*, or just *be harmful* in some way.

The next step involved reducing the wording of the key phrases and organizing them into clusters. This step was done several times, as different clustering patterns were tried, altered as phrases were moved to another cluster, and tried again. This iterative procedure is a core element in the "method of constant comparison" (Glaser and Strauss, 1967). Since the articulation of one cluster of phrases as distinct from another cluster involved making comparisons, only an ongoing and progressive process of comparisons enabled us to feel secure not only about the creation of a conceptually distinct set of categories, but also about our careful avoidance of data overreduction. This process involved "fracturing the data, then conceptually grouping it into codes (Glaser, 1978, p. 55)."

Three examples of the resultant clusters of phrases, with cluster labels, are presented below. Some of the items in these clusters come from the interview excerpts above and some from other interviews.

- Control will be taken away
    proprietary control
    concerned with retaining control
    fear of loss of control
    compare diagnoses

- Parent power will increase
    take power
    gain power
    get out of hand

- Create misunderstanding/misinformation
    generate misinformation
    repeat misinformation
    misinformation circulating
    giving out misinformation
    misinformation can be exchanged
    won't understand what's happening

The completion of this step resulted in forty apparently distinct clusters, some with only one entry and one with eleven entries. We felt that forty clusters were unnecessarily differentiated from one another and probably too great a number for feasible analysis. The next step involved the use of constant comparisons once again, in a process of pattern coding or metacoding (Charmaz, 1983; Miles and Huberman, 1984). These expanded code categories entailed a greater level of abstraction, moving away from the prior level of concreteness. The final result was the creation of the ten metaclusters of professionals' meanings of the dangers of self-help groups presented in Table 9-4 and discussed in the surrounding text.

The next steps required generalizing about the phrases in each cluster and generating mini-theories that provided an explanatory framework for the coded entries. They are typical steps in any scientific analysis, except that we undertook them here on an inductive rather than deductive basis; that is, we did not test or try to apply an a priori theory or generalization (no more than we developed and used an a priori coding scheme) from prior research, but to discover or generate themes that underlay the clusters and intercluster connections in this particular data set. In Chapter 9 we discussed the general meanings of each cluster and explained why professionals may have seen these kinds of dangers in self-help groups.

Quantitative Analyses: Group-Level Data

The transformation of the organizational-level information collected in Study #2's field interviews into variables suitable for analysis involved a multi-step process. (1) Tapes from each interview were first reviewed by trained coders on the research team to transfer more complete information to the interview schedule that had been used for informal note-taking in the field. In several cases, contradictions between the field investigator's notes on this form and the material on the tape led to more detailed conversations with the field interviewer, which resulted in capturing details of events that had occurred in private and untaped conversations, for example, on the way to the airport or at dinner. (2) Information from all interviews about a single group was then assembled onto a single summary form. This was first done using written notes, then completed in more detail by re-reviewing the tapes. (3) The third step involved transforming the information into variables and then into variable clusters and indices by consolidating interview and follow-up information into a single format. (4) The next step involved formal coding of variables for categorical analysis. In Study #4, similar coding procedures were used, although several of the earlier steps were omitted because there was only one source of data—the 1992–93 follow-up telephone interviews with group leaders and liaisons.

To clarify this process of the transformation of information from multiple sources into analytic variables, and in some cases typologies, a step-by-step example is provided from the data. (1) In response to one of our first questions, "When was this group formed?" answers from different informants about the same group might be "two or three years ago," "a couple of years ago," and "July 1979." (2) These answers would be lifted from their various interview schedules and placed side-by-side on the group summary form. (3) In the following step, coders would transform this information into a response to the item "age of group at time of interview," so that if the interviews were conducted in July 1982, the age of the group would be listed as "3 years." If there was serious conflict between the answers provided by different informants, we used one of two procedures: (a) a review of the balance of evidence from various forms or informants, or (b) a call-back to local informants posing the contradictions to them for clarification and resolution. (4) After entering information for each group on the coding sheet, the data were organized in a histogram. Groups clustered in age under 3 years, then a smaller number of age 3–5 years, and a few others in existence for more than 5 years. This clustering, and the predominance of younger groups, seemed consistent with our independent observation that most groups had encountered a "succession crisis" about 4–5 years after they were founded. This succession pattern is discussed in Chapters 5 and 10.

For the most part, Chi-square statistics were utilized in analyses of bi-variate distributions to systematically compare organizations (or types of organizations) with one another, and to examine the relationships among different organizational variables (see especially the tables in Chapters 4 and 5). The advantage of analyzing types or categories of organizations, rather than only individual units, is especially clear in investigating a complex problem such as the relationships of organizations to their environments. By looking at the relative strength of the relationships between group environments and group type, as well as individual characteristics of groups, it is easier to distinguish between systematic and idiosyncratic effects. This also facilitates the task of generalizing to self-help groups outside this sample, and perhaps to local voluntary organizations more broadly. The dangers and potential disadvantages of comparative analyses via a typology (such as the one involving parent-professional leadership structures) also are clear. Should we err in developing the categories and assigning groups to them, or should those classifications fail to reflect the concrete reality of the organizations, such an analysis could be grossly misleading. Overdependence on a categorization scheme also could fail to do justice to the rich and detailed character of the data, and to the variety of unique and interesting groups within the sample. Thus, we have used both individual and categorical forms of organizational analysis as well as composite case studies, throughout this volume. The varieties of data are verified in several ways across the various studies. Group interviews, group summary form information, and group-level follow-up interviews allow for the triangulation of organizational-level findings.

Quantitative Analyses: Individual-Level Data

In the analysis of individual-level variables, analysis of variance and regression techniques were used throughout the tables presented in Chapters 6, 7, and 8. The multiple-item scales described earlier were used to measure life change outcomes, coping strategies, sources and types of support, and perceived self-help group benefits. Reliability coefficients, presented earlier, confirm that these scales are statistically reliable, bringing together items that are empirically related. This speaks to the validity of measures that attempt to organize concepts into theoretically driven clusters for analysis.

One-way, single-factor analyses of variance procedures examined, for example, the significance of the major scales by self-help group membership. Multiple regression analyses examined the relationship of each block of independent predictor variables to the dependent variables via investigator-defined iterative models (nonautomatic stepwise procedures). The regression analyses used the "full model" approach to understand how self-help group membership, in combination with other independent variable measures, helped explain variation in parents' reported life changes.

Participatory Action Research

The material presented in this appendix focuses on the measures used to gather, format, and analyze data. However, the measures alone do not tell the full story of how these individual studies were conducted, and how our agenda for action and agenda for inquiry fit together. They do illustrate how we worked with members of these informant groups and the national CCF to create an integrated action research enterprise. We hope they do not obscure the fact that we also used ourselves as major sources of insight—as experiential as well as scholarly experts for the theoretical analyses and interpretations presented in this volume. We refer readers to a fuller discussion of the action research model and of our particular ways of working with that epistemological, methodological, and political framework in Chapter 3. Unless we and others pursue the potential utility of these alternative models of social scientific research, we risk replicating, with informants and ourselves, the typical patterns of power and privilege that currently dominate both traditional positivist paradigms of research and traditional patterns of medical/social service delivery.

Appendix B
A Note for Parents Seeking a Group

Individuals wishing more information about self-help groups for parents and families of children with cancer, who wish to initiate or make contact with a group in their local area, or who wish to know more about psychosocial services and programming for children with cancer and their families should call or write to:

The Candlelighters Childhood Cancer Foundation
7910 Woodmont Ave. (Suite 460)
Bethesda, Maryland 20814
Tel: 301-657-8401 or 1-800-366-2223
Fax: 301-718-2686

Notes

Chapter 1. Introduction to Self-Help and Self-Help Groups

1. See, for example, the writings of Katz and Bender (1990a). Katz and Bender (1976), Killilea (1976), Madara and Meese (1990), Neighbors et al. (1990), Powell (1987), and Trojan et al. (1986).

2. Discussions of informal help contained in exchange theories are found in Homans (1961) and specified as part of a helping process by Clark (1983).

3. Moreover, the boundaries between self-help groups and other types of groups and associations are often blurry. For instance, Wuthnow (1994) examines a wide variety of associational settings, including Bible study groups, Sunday school classes, political action groups, sports and hobby clubs, as well as self-help groups, in his extensive and insightful study of the small-group movement in the United States. Sometimes his treatment makes the distinction between self-help groups (estimated participation: 5% of the population) and the other forms of small groups (estimated participation: 40% of the population) clear and sometimes not.

4. Biegel and Yamatani (1987), Borman (1992), Katz and Bender (1990c), Levy (1976), Lieberman (1979), Romeder (1990).

5. Gaventa (1993), Hall, Gillette, and Tandon (1982).

6. We see parallel epistemological challenges to traditional knowledge forms and concentrations in efforts to develop alternative pedagogies of instruction (student-centered or discovery-oriented rather than teacher-centered), psychological treatment (client-centered), and social science research methods (participatory research, critical thinking). Wuthnow (1994) argues that these challenges became popular in the United States during the cultural reformation of the 1960s and 1970s.

7. Similar themes arise in discussions of movement between "the personal" and "the political" that occur in consciousness-raising groups (Culbert, 1976), especially feminist consciousness-raising groups (Freeman, 1979;

Kravetz, 1980; Lieberman and Bond, 1976). Freeman (1979) notes that in early feminist consciousness-raising groups, "women who met to discuss women's oppression and to develop strategies for changing it found themselves talking more and more about their own personal experiences" (p. 180).

8. In addition, this phenomenon is discussed in some detail by Hedrick et al. (1992) and Richardson (1983).

9. The concept of an experiential learning community as developed by Borkman (1976) refers to the creation of an environment within which each person and the entire group learn about their problem or situation. Such experiential knowledge cannot be bestowed on, imposed on, or transmitted to people; they must learn it themselves in a trusting community of others like themselves.

10. The concept of a *reference group* has a long history in social psychology (Merton and Kitt, 1950; Newcomb, 1950; Sherif, 1953; Turner, 1956). Although there has been substantial debate about its specific meanings, it usually identifies the group an individual sees herself as part of, or wishes to be part of. As a result of this identification, the person takes on behaviors and attitudes that are consistent with those of the group that is the *referent*.

11. See, especially, Borman (1992), Katz and Bender (1976), Klass (1992), Mullan (1992), and Richardson (1983).

12. Brickman and his colleagues (1982) have developed four models of the helping process, based on the interplay of the two factors noted: (1) a medical model, based on situations that the individual is not responsible for having created and from which he is not responsible to recover, (2) a moral model, based on situations that the individual is responsible for having created and from which she is responsible to recover; (3) a compensatory model, based on situations that the individual is not responsible for having created but from which he is responsible to recover; (4) an enlightenment model, based on situations the individual is responsible for having created but from which he is not responsible to recover.

13. With regard to evidence of health benefits, see Baider and De-Nour (1989), Cohen, Adler, and Mintz (1983), Spiegel et al. (1989), Spiegel (1993), Telch and Telch (1986), and Vugia (1991). With regard to improvements in problem-solving capacities, see Bakker and Karel (1983), and Kurtz (1990b).

14. Chesler and Chesney (1988), Gidron et al. (1990), Gutierrez, et al. (1990), Haber (1992), Hedrick et al. (1992), Mullan (1992), Neighbors et al. (1990).

15. With regard to evidence on increased self-reliance, see Marieskind (1984); with regard to evidence on increased ability to cope and take responsibility for solving personal problems, see Chesler and Chesney (1988), Borkman (1990), and van Harberden (1990); with regard to evidence on making changes in one's life, see Hamilton (1990), and Katz and Bender (1976); and with regard to a more informed consumerism, see Mullan (1992).

16. Borman (1992), Gartner (1990), Hedrick et al. (1992), Klass (1992), Riessman (1965), Theirs (1987), van Harberden (1990).

17. Gartner (1990), LeVeck (1982), Levy (1976), Mellor et al. (1984), Steinman and Traunstein (1976), Videka-Sherman (1990).

18. Katz (1981), Katz and Bender (1976), Mellor et al. (1984), Steinman and Traunstein (1976), Videka-Sherman (1990).

19. Chesler (1991), Gamson et al. (1982), McCarthy and Zald (1973; 1977).

20. They come to this conclusion on the basis of two forms of evidence: (1) analysis of the common activities and processes of ten self-help groups for families of people with mental illness that they studied; and (2) comparison of the ordering of activities and benefits of these ten groups with similar data from Levy's (1982) study of a large number of behavioral control and stress-coping groups.

21. Hinrichsen, Revenson, and Shinn (1985, p. 67); see also Chesler (1991), Gottlieb (1982), Kagey, Vivace, and Lutz (1981), Knight et al. (1980).

22. See especially Katz and Bender (1976), Neighbors et al. (1990), Trojan et al. (1986), and Powell (1987).

23. Powell points first to groups designed for member-motivated elimination of "narrowly defined habits," which would include the "addiction organization" in the Katz and Bender typology. A second mission category includes groups focused on "improving general coping patterns," such as the "stress reduction" groups in Figure 1.3. Groups organized for or by victims of discrimination and social stigma constitute a third type, ones with the mission of mutual support and efforts "to change the offending practices" (Powell, 1987, p. 149). This category is quite similar to the "social advocacy/action" and "alternative life-style" groups in Katz and Bender's scheme. A fourth type of mission Powell discusses is characterized by groups for significant others of people experiencing trauma or illness; Katz and Bender include these groups within their "therapeutic" category. The fifth category of group Powell identifies includes most of Katz and Bender's "therapeutic" group category, disease-specific groups that have the mission of serving persons with a given chronic condition or persons who have undergone a significant physical change.

24. This is part of a much larger critique and analysis of contemporary society. The prescriptions that Bellah and his colleagues (1985) offer are a new series of "habits of the heart," and are remarkably consistent with the major themes of self-help.

25. Bellah et al. (1985) update DeTocqueville's (1957) classic faith that "associational life" would be the bulwark against anomie and mass society in American life.

26. The key differences between Wuthnow's (1994) notion of small groups at the core of U. S. society and our argument that they are at the periphery stems from the different conception of groups involved. Wuthnow applies a very broad definition of "small groups," including political clubs, neighborhood associations, Bible study groups, and so on. Our discussion of self-help groups focuses on a particular form of small group or association, one that by its nature implicitly challenges currently bureaucratized forms of professional service delivery in favor of lay expertise and support, and of alienated community life in favor of intimate and affirming relationships. Thus, while self-help groups are

an increasingly common form of small group or voluntary association in the United States, and do reflect some of our culture's historic values, they also challenge and stand at the periphery of public politics and mainstream organizational forms.

Chapter 2. The Challenge of Childhood Cancer

1. See Chesler and Barbarin (1987), especially Chapters 2 and 3, for an extended discussion of these stresses.

2. Unless otherwise specified, these and other comments by parents in this chapter are taken from our individual and group interviews, conducted as part of Study #3. See Chapter 3 for an explanation.

3. Useful discussions of these different coping strategies can be found in Lazarus (1981), Menaghan (1983), Silver and Wortman (1980).

4. While there is some controversy over the extent to which coping processes are staged (Lazarus and Folkman, 1984), there is little disagreement that individuals' perceptions of and responses to their environment, especially those portions of it that present threats and potential mental or physical harm, may change over time.

5. See, for instance, Mattlin, Wethington, and Kessler (1990), Pearlin and Schooler (1978). This complexity helps to explain why, despite individual preferences, there is so little consensus in the scientific literature about "good," "better," and "worse" coping strategies for people dealing with stress. Actually, research and theory suggest that having and being able to use a large repertoire of coping behaviors may be more important than the use of any one coping strategy (Aldwin and Revenson, 1987; Folkman and Lazarus, 1980; Pearlin and Schooler, 1978).

6. Recent research has begun to counter the negative findings and images of parental and family disaster reported in early research on the psychosocial aspects of childhood cancer in families. See Chesler and Barbarin (1987), Chesney and Chesler (1993), Daiter et al. (1988), Kalnins (1983), Kupst et al. (1982), and Lansky et al. (1978).

7. Billings and Moos (1981), Pearlin and Schooler (1978).

8. See, for example, DiMatteo & Hays (1981), Gottlieb (1983), House (1981), and Kahn and Antonucci (1980).

9. This emphasis on the subjective view is detailed in House (1981), Israel and Rounds (1987), and Wethington and Kessler (1986).

10. See Chapter 1 for a discussion of how norms of self-reliance and autonomy may make it hard to seek help. Empirical research and commentary that document the negative effects of help-seeking in these circumstances is contained in Brickman et al. (1983), Merton et al. (1983), and Pilisuk and Parks (1980).

11. This notion replays one of the four models of helping discussed by Brickman et al. (1983) and referred to in Chapter 1.

12. See, for example, Chesler and Barbarin (1984a), Dunkel-Schetter (1984), Fisher et al. (1983), Froland et al. (1981), and Pearlin (1985). This con-

cern also echoes the discussion of "exchange theories" of helping discussed in Chapter 1.

13. Dunkel-Schetter (1984) and Rowland (1989) discuss the positive impact of social support for families dealing with cancer in general; Broadhead et al. (1983) focus on its positive effects for families of chronically ill children; and the positive value of support for families of children with cancer, in particular, is reported in Barbarin (1987), Chesler and Barbarin (1987), Krulik and Florian (1986), and Morrow et al. (1984).

14. See research reported in Chesler, Barbarin, and Lebo-Stein (1984), Stein (1986), and Morrow et al. (1982).

15. Israel et al. (1988), Schulz et al. (1993), Swift and Levin (1987), Withorn (1980), Zimmerman (1990).

16. After all, a parent cannot prevent a child from getting cancer, and there is not much a parent can do to facilitate physical recovery from this illness. Although there is some argument that various psychosocial coping techniques (e.g., visualization, laughter, engaging the will to fight) may not only improve one's mental health, but the physical condition itself, there is scant reliable empirical evidence to support this stance. As far as we know, the power to heal and cure physically, to the extent that it exists, lies in the hands of highly trained medical professionals.

17. Examples of such (re-)empowerment are discussed in Frank (1988), Kieffer (1983–84), Rappaport (1987), Rosenberg (1979), and Scotch (1988).

18. Gamson (1975), Gutiérrez (1988), McCarthy and Zald (1977), Schensul and Schensul (1982).

19. Dunst et al. (1988), Morrow, Carpenter, and Hoagland (1984), Spinetta and Deasy-Spinetta (1981).

20. Discussion of the "cognitive antidote" is contained in Antze (1976), Lieberman (1988), and Videka-Sherman 1982); new social networks are discussed in Belle-Isle and Conradt (1979), and Martinson (1976); new identities are discussed by Levine (1988); additional coping resources are examined by Klass (1984–85), and Thoits (1986); and change efforts are reported in Chesler (1991), and Chesney and Chesler (1993).

21. Borkman (1984; 1976), Lynam (1987), Monaco (1988).

22. Vugia (1991), Weiss (1976), Wechsler (1976).

23. Abrahams (1976), Chesler and Barbarin (1987), Weiss (1976), Dunkel-Schetter, 1979).

24. Chesler & Barbarin (1987), Kartha & Ertel (1976), Lynam (1987).

25. Chesler and Chesney (1988), Chesney (1989), Stewart (1990), Vugia (1991).

Chapter 3. Action Research with Self-Help Groups

1. The study was funded in part by the University of Michigan Committee on the International Year of the Child and the Spencer Foundation (Chesler and Barbarin, 1987).

2. This work was funded in part by the Candlelighters Childhood Cancer Foundation and in part by a grant from the University of Michigan's Rackham Fund.

3. This investigation was part of a larger international comparison study of self-help groups focused on families experiencing a variety of life crises in Israel and the United States, funded by the U.S. Department of Health and Human Services (Chesler, et al. 1988; Chesler, Chesney, and Gidron, 1990; Gidron, Chesler, and Chesney, 1991). The University of Michigan's Program on Conflict Management Alternatives also provided pilot and start-up funds for this effort.

4. The study was funded in part by the Candlelighters Childhood Cancer Foundation.

5. We did not use the "purest" model of P-A-R, since final control over most decisions and their implementation stayed with our research staff. However, the senior investigator's personal identification and involvement as a parent of a child with cancer, a self-help group member and organizer, and a leader of the national organization of self-help groups for families of children with cancer always kept these studies rooted in a participatory as well as investigatory mode. Almost all other investigators and assistants in these studies also had direct experience with cancer, either as young adult survivors of childhood cancer or as family members of a person with cancer. In addition, several of the key studies in this series were funded, and decisions about them approved, by the Foundation's officers (themselves members and/or representatives of the informant population).

6. See, for example, Cancian and Armistead (1990), Lincoln and Guba (1985), and Whyte (1986).

7. First elaborated by Lewin, discussions of action research date back to the immediate post–WWII period; seminal works or commentary include Chein et al. (1948), Elden (1981), Lewin (1946), Sanford (1970), and Tichy and Friedman (1983).

8. Brown and Tandon (1983), Carr and Kemmis (1983), Fals-Borda (1984), Gaventa (1988).

9. Brown and Kaplan (1981), Susman and Evered (1978).

10. Freire (1973), Israel, Schurman, and House (1989).

11. The procedures of editing and presenting selected portions of parents' stories involved us as co-creators of their narratives. As noted by Weigers (1994), investigators' roles and interactions with informants in the interviewing process and in analysis or selection of materials to present inevitably reflect the mutuality of narrativity as a form of inquiry. Increasingly in the social sciences there are varying definitions of and approaches to the design and use of narratives as a technique for data gathering and data analysis, and for the construction of social theory (Hart, 1992; Ortner, 1991; Polkinghorne, 1988; Somers, 1992).

12. This point is emphasized in Tiebes and Kraemer's (1991) observation

that researchers (or their sponsors) and self-help group members probably will view and evaluate a group's impact from different perspectives.

13. See, for example, Cancian and Armistead (1990), Gaventa (1988), and Hall et al. (1982).

14. As Tiebes and Kraemer (1991) argue, there are clear logistical limits to the control that researchers can have over the activities, intervention processes, and outcomes of self-help groups. These groups' antibureaucratic, democratic, and voluntaristic nature mitigates against standardization and control from external sources—administrative or research sources.

15. The relevance of P-A-R to the study of self-help groups has been illustrated or discussed by Borkman and Schubert (in press), Chesler (1991), Lavoie (1984), Rappaport et al. (1985), and Wollert et al. (1984). The relevance of narrative analysis to the study of self-help groups has been discussed by Rappaport (1993) and Wuthnow (1994).

16. This is undoubtedly one explanation for the resistance to research reported by such sensitive self-help scholars as Lieberman and Borman (1979), Powell (1987), and Rappaport et al. (1985).

17. In addition, group leaders and liaisons often invited the research staff to stay at their homes, eat with their families rather than in local motels and hotels, and celebrate family birthdays and anniversaries with them. The meal most often served to us was lasagna (except in Texas and Florida, where barbecue was the standard fare). This is an important detail: lasagna is not the kind of meal served to "important" and high status external visitors; steak or fish would be more appropriate in those circumstances. Lasagna is a family meal, an informal dish that implies one's welcome as a friend or family member.

Chapter 4. What Self-Help Groups Do

1. Adams (1979), Belle-Isle and Conradt (1979), Chesler and Chesney (1988), Gilder et al. (1976), Heffron (1975), Kartha and Ertel (1976), Martinson (1976), Yoak and Chesler (1985).

2. Indeed, sometimes it has been labeled as such in the formal psychosocial and social service literature (Gilder et al., 1976; Kartha and Ertel, 1976).

3. Elaboration of these issues and problems in professional vs. lay leadership occurs in Chapters 5, 8 and 9.

4. Adams (1978), Belle-Isle and Conradt (1979), Chesler and Chesney (1988), Gilder et al. (1976), Heffron (1975), Kartha and Ertel (1976), Martinson (1976), Yoak and Chesler (1985).

5. See, for example, *Oncology Handbook for Parents* (1977; 1978), *Parent/Child Handbook* (1980), and Schweers, Farnes, and Foreman (1977).

6. We return to this theme in Chapters 8 and 9, in a fuller discussion of the relationships between local groups and the caregiving system.

7. Substantial research has indicated some of the difficulties that children with cancer face in trying to maintain a normal schooling experience—absenteeism due to extended hospitalization, teasing by peers, ignorance or

insensitivity on the part of teachers, and physical or cognitive disabilities requiring special resources (Barbarin and Chesler, 1983; Deasy-Spinetta and Irvin, 1993; Lansky et al., 1975). Barbarin and Chesler (1983) provide descriptions of several other educational workshops addressing these issues, including detailed evaluations of one such example.

8. We discuss these details of self-help organization and structure, and their impact on group members and activities, in Chapter 5.

9. Despite the growth and power such identity and role transitions may have provided, the creation and adoption of a new social identity was not a simple or comfortable process (Goffman, 1968; Lieberman and Borman, 1979; Powell, 1975; Voysey, 1972; Wortman and Dunkel-Schetter, 1979). The self-help group setting evidently provided parents with the support and affirmation necessary to test and to help each other "try out" new ways of conceiving of and presenting themselves.

10. The acts of contributing to others at a time when they needed help themselves often operated as a form of "helper-therapy" (Dory and Riessman, 1982; Gartner and Riessman, 1977; Riessman, 1965; Silverman, 1974).

11. This distinction has been made several times, and it may help us understand the report in Table 4.2 that even groups that did not report regular emotional support programs felt that emotional sharing and support happened often and was a priority for them.

Chapter 5. How Groups Are Organized and Operated

1. These case studies are composites; they represent no single group but are our construction of illustrative types of groups, based on data about several similar groups.

2. Staff members concerned with the medical ethics of preserving patient privacy were justifiably cautious about sharing patient information or patient caseload lists with self-help groups without the patient's or family's permission. Self-help group members understood these concerns, but their priority on reaching out to and caring for other parents of children with cancer led them to disagree with, or to try to get around, this policy in practice.

3. This option, described by Carpenter and Vattino (1992) and Pitel et al. (1985), is discussed in more detail in Chapter 8.

4. Chapin and Tsouderos' research on voluntary associations resulted in the following generalizations concerning size: "Associations with large memberships were found, in general, to tend toward impersonal criteria and an elaboration of a code of behavior, i.e., ritual, rules for membership recruitment, etc., while associations with small memberships tended toward personal discretion. In general, . . . it seems that associations with large memberships (with a declining frequency of general meetings, . . . increased frequency of formal reporting to membership . . .) tend to have more formalized codes than do associations with a small membership" (Chapin and Tsouderos, 1956, pp. 343–44).

5. Indicators that have been used in research on voluntary organizations propose that formalization can be identified by the presence of rules, codification of operating procedures and structures, and specification of roles or committees (Hage and Aiken, 1970; Hall, Haas, and Johnson, 1967; Scott, 1981).

6. As we report in Chapter 6, the great majority of active members in most self-help groups for parents of children with cancer, as in most self-help groups of all types, are women.

7. This was the case in Providence, Rhode Island, and Rochester, New York.

8. Chapter 10 presents 1992–1993 data gathered through telephone revisits to all of the original fifty groups still in existence. These groups were reassessed ten to twelve years later, and more detail is provided on key issues, such as leadership succession and transition.

9. Nash & Kramer (1993) used a similar typology in their study of the leadership roles of professionals in 104 groups for people with sickle-cell disease. At the time of their interviews, members were running 29.8% of the groups, and 38.8% had a shared leadership pattern, while 27.3% were led primarily by professionals.

10. These findings about professionally led groups appear at first glance to confirm Stolberg and Cunningham's (1980) report that *all* childhood cancer parent support groups were generally small and short-lived. However, their data were gathered from medical professionals at twenty-five major children's cancer clinics throughout the nation, and undoubtedly reflected the limited perceptions of these medical professionals and the limited reality of professionally led support groups. Most of the literature on childhood cancer groups, written by and for professionals, has concentrated solely on groups with this type of professional leadership pattern.

11. These findings are consistent with other data regarding the organizational prerequisites for effective fund-raising campaigns and activities (e.g., a more formal organization, a longer-lasting organization), and make sense in terms of the active community connections that are required to do effective local fund-raising.

12. Whether the initiative came solely from local parents, from knowledgeable intermediaries, or from the national office of the Candlelighters Foundation, most groups eventually established relationships (formal or informal) with CCCF. However, local parents' and groups' knowledge about the Foundation often was spotty. One attempt to increase local parents' and groups' knowledge about CCCF and its resources that they could call upon was undertaken by Nathanson (1987), in a handbook developed especially to aid local leaders' efforts to develop and sustain their groups.

13. Original founders included Grace Ann Monaco, Julie Sullivan, Minna Nathanson, and several other parents of children who had died from childhood cancer in the Washington, D.C., metropolitan area. Since that time it has grown enormously, has employed a national staff, and has evolved into the

premier educational, peer support, and advocacy organization concerned with childhood cancer.

14. As noted above, the Foundation has been supported by a yearly grant from the American Cancer Society, by a variety of grants for research and services, and by contributions from parents, professionals, local groups, and interested individuals. The Foundation also acts as a self-help group itself; eighteen of the twenty National Board members of the Foundation are themselves either parents of children with cancer (some living, some deceased) or long-term survivors of childhood cancer themselves. Further information is available in Appendix B.

Chapter 6. Self-Help Group Participation

1. Battaglino (1987), Gottlieb (1982), Medvene and Krauss (1989), Potasznik and Nelson (1984), Videka-Sherman (1982).

2. See, for example, Gutiérrez et al. (1990), Humphreys, Mavis, and Stoffelmayr (1992), Neighbors et al. (1990), and discussions of the role of kith and kin in communities of lower-class people and people of color.

3. Humphreys and Woods (1993) and Nash and Kramer (1993) argue not only that traditional forms of self-help do exist in the African-American community, but that different cultural and geographic settings may generate variations on common self-help themes. These authors also argue that, as a result of social patterns of racial separation and discrimination, African-Americans tend to join self-help groups in major urban areas, where they are likely to be in the majority (and therefore accepted and comfortable), while whites tend to join groups in suburban areas and small cities, where they are likely to be in the majority (and therefore accepted and comfortable). Humphreys and Woods caution researchers not to overlook the influence of these structural realities and to not assume a "universal quality" of white middle-class self-help groups based on their own (predominantly white and middle-class) vantage point.

4. This range of coping strategies has been studied and illustrated by several scholars. The use of passive strategies has been detailed by Chesney (1989) and Silver and Wortman (1980); active or problem-solving strategies have been analyzed by Menaghan (1983), Lazarus (1981), and Pearlin and Schooler (1978); Barbarin (1987) has discussed, especially with regard to parents of children with cancer, information-seeking coping strategies.

5. Indeed, the distinction between the use of generic coping strategies (assessed via questionnaire) and the search for childhood cancer-specific coping skills and information (reported in parents' own words) may help explain the lack of significant difference between members' and nonmembers' generic coping strategies.

6. This sense of gain from efforts to help others is another illustration of the theme of "helper therapy" that is so prevalent in self-help groups of various kinds (see the discussion in Chapter 1, and Riessman, 1965).

7. As indicated in Chapter 3, we have available in one of our studies (re-

ferred to as Study #3) samples of nonmembers. Our study design and the reality of access to individual families experiencing childhood cancer did not permit the creation of "a completely comparable" or ideally random or representative nonmember sample. Thus, analyses and inferences of nonmembers' responses have limited generalizability. These nonmember samples cannot provide definitive answers to the issues at hand, but they are valid enough to shed some light on the question of why some parents of children with cancer did not join local self-help groups. Moreover, in this inquiry into nonparticipation we also may illuminate further the issue of why others did become members of groups.

8. See note 5 above.

9. See the citations in note 1, above.

10. Chesler and Barbarin (1987, pp. 32–37) report similar stress timelines in their study of parents of children with cancer.

11. In his study of the "small group movement," Wuthnow (1994) also concludes that active group members are more likely to be involved in more political and volunteer organizations than are group nonmembers or members who are not very active. In addition Gottlieb and Peters (1991) report that self-help group members are from the same population base as members of other types of voluntary associations. These patterns of differential involvement may reflect the higher level of education typical of members (see Table 6.1), and an association between higher education and generalized civic activism. They emphasize, once again, the powerful phenomenon of voluntary civic activism in our nation.

12. One approach to this problem of understanding parents' decisions to participate in self-help groups could have been, or might still be, to try to "predict" which parents would participate based upon their background characteristics and the explanations developed in this chapter. Alternatively, one could, as we did, try to understand their "narratives," their own attempts at explaining their decisions and the decisions of others. While statistical prediction certainly was and always is possible, real prediction would have required gathering data from all parents of children newly diagnosed with cancer in a common pool, and then collecting data from them over time, as they made their decisions about self-help group participation. This was logistically impossible for us, and will be very difficult for other observers as well. Retrospective analysis—whether statistically manipulated or narrative in format—may once again be the most feasible option.

Chapter 7. How People Benefit from Self-Help Groups

1. These themes are elaborated in Chapter 1. Also relevant to this discussion is the analysis of the reasons why many members decided to join a group in Chapter 6, and the major stresses reported by parents of children with cancer reviewed in Chapter 2 and Table 2.1

2. Prior studies emphasizing this feature of self-help groups include Bloch and Seitz (1985), Chesler and Chesney (1988), and Levy (1976). It is

an example of Wuthnow's (1994) report that the "feeling that (one) is not alone" was the most common type of support experienced by small group members (p. 169).

3. Discussion of the process of adopting this new social identity can be found in Chesler and Chesney (1988), Wechsler (1976), and Weiss (1976).

4. This phenomenon is another example of the process of "helper-therapy" (Riessman, 1965).

5. See the discussion in Chapter 1 of the communal basis of help in self-help groups, contrasted with the exchange basis of reciprocal obligations so characteristic of everyday relationships.

6. The common concern about such responses, about whether one is re-acting to this stress in a "normal" or "bizarre" manner, has been discussed in Chesler and Barbarin (1987), Lynam (1987), Stein (1986), and Wortman and Dunkel-Schetter (1979).

7. Wuthnow (1994) reports that 88–90% of members mentioned the importance of the emotional support they received in their small group.

8. For example, Chesler and Barbarin (1987), Cohen (1994), Kalnins (1983), Kupst et al. (1982), and Lansky et al. (1978).

9. In a prior study (Chesler and Barbarin, 1987), 81% of parents of children with cancer indicated that they coped "extremely well" or "good," and 18% indicated "fair" coping. Thus, there is consistency in responses to these questions across two samples of parents of children with cancer.

10. The specific items in the four life-change scales of *mental health, activism, physical health,* and *life satisfaction* are included in Table A-1 in Appendix A.

11. None of the typical measures of parents' demographic or social status—income, education, age, gender, marital status—were significantly correlated with these coping outcomes. Only one measure of coping strategy was related significantly to coping adequacy: parents who more often reported coping alone less often reported coping very well. With regard to coping outcomes assessed via the life-change scales, none of the coping strategies were positively associated with either mental health or life satisfaction. However, parents who reported more often coping actively, seeking help, and sharing feelings reported significantly higher changes for the better in terms of activism, and parents who more often reported coping alone or passively reported significantly lower positive changes in activism. Thus, coping alone stood out as a strategy that was related repeatedly to less positive outcomes.

12. Both these outcome measures, and others used throughout our studies, are based on self-report information, and need to be viewed within the inferential limits and advantages of such data. In order to assess the outcomes of parents' efforts to deal with childhood cancer, and thus of the potential role of self-help groups in this experience, we solicited and listened to parents themselves as the most valid source of information. Obviously different parents responded to these measures and to the request for open-ended responses from varying

perspectives, thus opening the door to varying interpretations of their voices. We acknowledge that other investigators may prefer to reduce this source of variation by using more standardized and reliable measures of parental self-reported outcomes or external assessments (by social service professionals) of parental coping and life change. Clearly, this option also has its limitations.

13. Some of these "strategies of self-presentation" are discussed by Goffman (1968) and Wortman and Dunkel-Schetter (1979). In addition, Katz's (1993) concept of "cognitive restructuring," whereby in the context of collective sharing and discussion one reformulates her problem and behavior, is relevant here.

14. There is beginning to be a trend in the empirical research on stress in general to argue against the traditional emphasis on people's vulnerability, and to look instead for demonstrations of strength in the face of stress and crises (Thoits, 1994).

15. Clearly, the idea methodological scenario for such studies would be a longitudinal panel study that visited and revisited parents prior to (logistically impossible, given the inability to know ahead of time which parents will have a child diagnosed with cancer) or early in their childhood cancer experience (possible, but difficult given the level of emotional stress and myriad practical tasks early in the process) and repeatedly throughout treatment, remission, and death or long-term survival. Despite the difficulties, the opportunity to verify perceived and actual life changes and coping adequacy, and their relationship to involvement in self-help groups, with multiple inquiries of the same population of parents is the ideal model for future explorations.

16. See, for example, Back (1981), Kiefer (1983–84), Rappaport (1985), Stewart (1990), and Zimmerman (1986). Spiegel (1993) argues further that self-help groups for cancer patients can improve their physical health, but this intriguing stance is not yet supported by sufficient data, and is in fact contradicted by our data.

17. Roughly 5% (physical health) to 16% (activism) of the variance in reported life changes is explained by self-help group membership alone. In the set of "full model" analyses that explored the impact of the wider set of variables on each of the four life-change outcome measures, the full predictor set explained 43% of the variance in reported changes in mental health, 51% of the variance in reported changes in activism, 39% of the variance in reported changes in physical health, and 53% of the variance in reported changes in life satisfaction. In all four analytic models, each investigating a different life-change measure, membership in the self-help group was the most enduringly significant contributor to explained variation in reported life changes.

18. Specific aspects and benefits of group leadership roles are discussed in Rappaport (1987) and Yoak, Chesney, and Schwartz (1985).

19. As a final exploration of parents' reports of the outcomes of self-help group involvement, we considered examining the issue of intergroup variation. Restricting such analyses to reports from members only, and stratifying parents' responses by the eight self-help groups in this sample, resulted in relatively

small numbers of members in each group. Partly as a result, there was little variation among the eight local self-help groups with regard to levels of specific benefits members reported, and little difference among groups in members' reported life changes. This issue cannot be put to rest on the basis of these data and analyses. Groups that operate differently, that provide different activities and programs, and that are led differently by parents or by professionals may well facilitate different outcomes for parents. However, a full test of these hypothesized relationships must await larger and more tightly controlled samples and studies.

20. It is clear that the data reported in this chapter, as provocative as they are, do not fully solve the relationship between self-help group participation and personal outcomes. We need to know more about this relationship, and especially about its causal nature. We have noted the flaws inherent in our approach to answering this question fully, and have taken our data as far as we can. Fuller answers will require different (although very difficult) research designs, ones that go beyond sole reliance on retrospective data.

Chapter 8. Roles of Professionals in Self-Help Groups

1. The formal and technical knowledge of the professional is not the same as the informal and personal knowledge of the parent. While both may be necessary inputs into effective treatment (e.g., knowing how a particular child may respond to removal from the home, extended hospitalization, or being held in mother's arms during an intravenous insertion), they are not the same. In Chapter 1 we discussed these different bases of knowledge—"expertise" and "experience"—as analyzed by Borkman (1990) and Powell (1990).

2. This general characteristic of professionals' roles is described in detail by Friedson (1970) and Parsons (1951), among others.

3. For example, some chief physicians have tried to convince parent groups to help raise funds for their local hospital or pediatric oncology clinic. While some groups have been quite interested in such activities, others have preferred to focus their time and energy on emotional rap sessions or social events. Under these circumstances in particular, and in a broad range of like circumstances, there was little support from the medical establishment for a social worker's active role with a "deviant" or "uncooperative" parent self-help group. As one of the lowest-status persons on the medical team, social workers were in difficult and low power positions on such matters.

4. Bakker and Karel (1983), Bryant (1990), Chutis (1983), Dory and Riessman (1982), Gottlieb (1982), Katz and Bender (1990b), Klass and Shinners (1982–3), Levy et al. (1984), Lurie and Shulman (1983), Newton (1984), Powell (1987), Silverman (1992), Videka-Sherman (1990).

5. Bakker and Karel (1983), Chutis (1983), Gottlieb (1982), Katz and Bender (1990b), Medvene (1990), Lurie and Shulman (1983), Remine et al., (n.d.), Scott and Doyle (1984), Toseland and Hacker (1982), Wempner (1984).

6. Black and Drachman (1985), Browning et al. (1984), Coplon and Strull

(1983), Dory and Riessman (1982), Gottlieb (1982), Katz and Bender (1990b), Klass and Shinners (1982–83), Knight et al. (1980), Lurie and Shulman (1983), Newton (1984), Powell (1987), Remine et al. (n.d.), Scott and Doyle (1984), Toseland and Hacker (1982), Wempner (1984).

7. Bryant (1990), Chutis (1983), Klass and Shinners (1982–83), Katz and Bender (1990b), Lurie and Shulman (1983), Pheifer (1992), Remine et al. (n.d.), Toseland and Hacker (1982), Videka-Sherman (1990), Wempner (1984).

8. Browning et al. (1984), Klass and Shinners (1982–83), Lurie and Shulman (1983), Remine et al. (n.d.), Videka-Sherman (1990), Wempner (1981).

9. Bryant (1990), Haber (1992), Katz and Bender (1990b), Remine et al. (n.d.), Toseland and Hacker (1982).

10. Bryant (1990), Chutis (1983), Klass and Shinners (1982–83), Lurie and Shulman (1983), Powell (1987), Remine et al. (n.d.), Silverman and Smith (1984), Toseland and Hacker (1982), Videka-Sherman (1990).

11. Browning et al. (1984), Klass and Shinners (1982–83), Remine et al. (n.d.), Toseland and Hacker (1982).

12. Bakker and Karel (1983), Borman (1982), Bryant (1990b), Haber (1992), Katz and Bender (1990b), Knight, et al. (1980), Masiak et al. (1981), Toseland and Hacker (1982), Videka-Sherman (1990).

13. Foster and Mandel (1979), Klass and Shinners (1982–83), McCollum and Schwartz (1972), Pitel et al. (1985), Ross (1980), Stuetzer (1980).

14. Bakker and Karel (1983), Black and Drachman (1985), Chutis (1983), Coplon and Strull (1983), Gottlieb (1982), Knight et al. (1980), Newton (1984), Remine et al. (n.d.), Toseland and Hacker (1982).

15. Bakker and Karel (1983), Borman (1982), Chutis (1983), Dory and Riessman (1982), Jertson (1975), Masiak et al. (1981), Newton (1984), Toseland and Hacker (1982), Yoak and Chesler (1985).

16. Tulsky and Cella (1992).

17. Chutis (1983), Dory and Riessman (1982), Gottlieb (1982), Klass and Shinners (1982–83), Wempner (1984).

18. Bakker and Karel (1983), Black and Drachman (1985), Borman (1976; 1982), Bryant (1990), Dory and Riessman (1982), Gottlieb (1982), Gutiérrez et al. (1990), Haber (1992), Katz (1992), Masiak et al. (1981), Pheifer (1992), Scott and Doyle (1984), Silverman (1992), Toseland and Hacker (1982), Videka-Sherman (1990).

19. See Chapter 1 and Figure 1.1 from Mellor et al. (1984), and Chapter 5's findings, for fuller discussion regarding "independent," "shared-leadership," and "professionally led" groups.

Chapter 9. Consumer-Provider Conflict and the Mobilization of Consumer Activism

1. See especially Chesler (1991), Katz (1981), and Toch (1965).

2. Antonovsky (1980), Friedson (1970), Mechanic (1978), Parsons (1951), Starr (1982), Waitzkin (1983).

3. Ehrenreich (1978), Sidel and Sidel (1983), Starr (1982).

4. Ehrenreich (1978), Friedman & DiMatteo (1979).

5. Note the extended discussion of some of these stresses in Chapter 2, and the exploration of self-help groups' roles in responding to them in Chapters 4 and 7.

6. Cassileth and Hamilton (1979), Friedson (1970), Meadow (1968), Mechanic (1964), Parsons (1951).

7. Abbott (1983), Fox (1989), Friedson (1970), Parsons (1951).

8. Antonovsky (1980), Featherstone (1980), Lorber (1975), Taylor (1979).

9. See Chapter 2 for a discussion of this problem as a key element of the informational stresses associated with childhood cancer.

10. DiMatteo (1979), Haug (1975).

11. See related discussions of structural violence in Galtung (1969), and Wehr (1979). This type of conflict can be distinguished from "behavioral conflict," which is created by and evident in individuals' overt actions and reactions.

12. Becker and Maiman (1980), DiMatteo and Hays (1980), Ware, Davies-Avery, and Stewart (1978).

13. At one extreme, Levine (1975) discusses the "hero" element present in some staff members' self-concepts, and the conflict created when such conceptions of oneself cannot be realized in practice. Many medical staff members care deeply and personally about their young patients, and when these youngsters die, or when tense interpersonal relations are experienced with these patients and family members, staff members may experience frustration and "burn-out." Interestingly, several researchers suggest that it is often the most talented and compassionate professionals who experience burn-out; in part their expectations and commitments, and consequent disappointments, may be the highest (Cherniss, 1980; Freudenberger, 1974; Maslach, 1976; Stone, 1983; Vachon, Lyall & Freeman, 1978).

14. "Conflict that was hard to resolve" was reported by 52% of the 74 parents in the Chesler and Barbarin (1984b) sample. Other commonly reported problems with the medical staff (reported by over 25% of the sample) included "poor interpersonal contact," "nonacceptance of parental efficacy," "staff's lack of competence," "lack of empathy with the child," "poor communication," and "inadequate transmission of information."

15. Whether it was intervention that caused conflict and tension leading to dissatisfaction, and thus to bonding with other parents, or whether self-help group membership led to dissatisfaction and the trend toward intervention cannot be determined from these associational data.

16. This last point has been made, in broader contexts of social protest and change, by Coser (1966), Dodson (1960), and Himes (1966).

17. The argument that disparate interests and roles make overt conflict more or less inevitable, and therefore that influence, pressure, and coercion are most likely to occur, is made by Katz (1981) and Kleiman, Mantell, and Alexander (1976).

18. The argument that mutual interest can be fashioned amidst structural

conflict is presumed by Lenrow and Burch (1981), Levy (1978), and Lieberman and Borman (1979).

19. The difference between dangers "heard about" (90%) and dangers "experienced" (24%) in our sample of professionals from fifty groups, or in Black and Drachman's (1985) report about the difference between successful referral experiences of some professionals and no referrals by others, is quite striking. In a related study, Meissen, Mason, and Gleason (1991) argue that their findings of positive attitudes toward self-help groups among Kansas graduate students were somewhat mitigated by the students' lack of understanding of the real nature of self-help. Thus, more negative attitudes and perceptions of "dangers" may come primarily from information and "understanding" gained on the job, as students are oriented by veteran professionals into what Rappaport (1993) has called "professional centrism." One hopes that more positive views will be forthcoming from more recent graduates, and that they can be sustained by professionals' actual experience, even in the face of older professionals' ideology.

20. This view is mirrored in some of the professional and scholarly literature: Belle-Isle and Conradt (1979), Deneke (1983), Mantell et al. (1976), Ringler et al. (1981), and Rosenberg (1984).

21. See, for instance, Belle-Isle and Conradt (1979), Binger et al. (1969), Heffron (1975), Johnson and Stark (1980), Kartha and Ertel (1976), and Ringler et al. (1981).

22. Mantell et al. (1976), Toseland and Hacker (1982).

23. Henry (1978), King (1980), Rosenberg (1984).

24. In a similar vein, some authors considering these dangers have worried about even the positive things that have occurred as a function of relatively autonomous group activity. For example, Knapp and Hansen (1973) reported some of the positive actions members performed in a preventive therapy group they conducted for parents of ill children (collecting blood for accident victims, sending cookies to American soldiers in Vietnam, participating in church functions). As they noted, however, "Underlying all these efforts was a need to help others, and do good, perhaps in the hope that it might save their child" (p. 73). The authors provided no evidence for the attribution of this parental motive of a self-interest "bargain" with the fates of God ("save their child"). Was the hope of saving their child really the basis of involvement in good works? This sort of attribution may have led some observers and professionals to unwittingly convert positive outcomes and processes of self-help groups into negative outcomes or dangers. More positive interpretations of the motivational base of people in crisis have been offered by Riessman and his colleagues' (Riessman, 1965; Dory and Riessman, 1982) discussion of the "helper-therapy" principle.

25. That this might occur, and thereby give rise to false fears and unrealistic hopes and plans, has also been cautioned against by Belle-Isle and Conradt (1979), Deneke (1983), and Mantell et al. (1976).

26. Katz (1993) also notes that one set of fears professionals have regarding self-help groups is that of members becoming so well informed that they will

"discourage group members from consulting with qualified professionals in situations of need" (p. 76).

27. Mantell (1983), Ringler et al. (1981), Silverman & Smith (1984), Wollert et al. (1984).

28. See Henry (1978), Mantell et al. (1976), Rodolfa and Hungerford (1982), Rosenberg (1984), and Toseland and Hacker (1982). This stance was seen as working to the clients' disadvantage, as they might not avail themselves of necessary or appropriate services (Deneke, 1983), but also to the disadvantage of professionals, as they might encounter resistance to the use of their services.

29. As an antidote to these fears, the Leukemia Society of America's guidelines for facilitators of cancer support groups took pains to point out that it is a "neutral organization and does not support one institution in the community over another" (*Family Support Group Guidelines*, 1986, p. 10).

30. This dynamic once again highlights the special value of self-help groups articulated by Katz (1984) as he noted that self-help groups often have the "corollary (social) benefit of reducing monopolistic *social* controls by professionals" (p. 234).

31. Other sources that discuss the staff's role in providing access to resources include Remine et al. (n.d.), and Toseland and Hacker (1982). Sources that explore the staff's role in consulting with the group include Chutis (1983), Dory and Riessman (1982), and Wollert and Barron (1983). Sources that articulate the role of a staff member as an educator of the rest of the staff include Bakker and Karel (1983), Masiak et al. (1981), and Toseland and Hacker (1982). Finally, sources that discuss the staff member as an intervenor in group/system conflict include Chesler and Barbarin (1984b), Foster and Mandel (1979), and Klass and Shinners (1982–83).

32. Studies of coalitions have a long history in the social sciences; some general principles have been articulated by Chesler (1981) and Hinckley (1979).

33. Much of the coalition literature addresses the dangers of nonequal status coalitions; dominant groups (professionals) may continue to co-opt or covertly dominate previously subordinate groups (parents), only with a newly formed veneer of collaboration. This theme is addressed with specific regard to coalitions between self-help groups and professionals by Kleiman et al. (1976).

34. See, for instance, Cohen (1985), Hyde (1992; 1991), Melucci (1989), Snow and Benford (1988), and Touraine (1985).

35. Anspach (1979), Culbert (1976), Gamson (1975), McCarthy and Wolfson (1992), McCarthy and Zald (1977), Schensul and Schensul (1982).

36. See the "outcome" data presented in Chapter 8, along with Chesney (1989) and Rappaport (1987).

37. See above, notes 34 and 35.

Chapter 10. Self-Help Groups over Time

1. The original study began in 1981 and concluded in 1983; for the sake of simplicity we refer to it here as the 1981 or the 1980s study.

2. Interestingly, Wuthnow's (1994) study of "the small group movement" notes that four out of every five groups had been in existence for more than five years. He argues, "They may be fluid and diverse, but they are not one-night stands" (p. 343).

3. "The past" in this context did not necessarily mean the early 1980s; it could have meant the early 1980s or any time after that when there had been a lull in group activity of which the informant was aware. Thus, while we make comparisons between the early 1980 data and the 1993 data, it should not be assumed that this is a straight-line relationship; groups' activity levels could have risen and fallen several times during the intervening years.

4. Note that the figures in the column for the 1981 data do not exactly conform to the data for these groups reported in Table 4.2, because in Chapters 4 and 5 we reported data for the total original sample of fifty groups, while in this chapter we focus the comparison only on information from those forty-one groups that were assessable in both time periods.

5. However, the increased size of mailing lists may have represented simply the addition of several years' worth of names, not necessarily that more people were involved actively.

6. It also may be explained in part by the fact that we reported names and addresses of all groups visited in the early 1980s to the national CCCF Foundation, and they were then placed on the Foundation's mailing lists. Since our studies were conceived as action-research efforts to improve as well as study local groups' and CCCFs operations, this was a deliberate "intervention."

7. See the discussion of coalitions as temporary systems in Chapter 9, as well as the earlier discussion of self-help groups as temporary systems in Chapter 5.

8. Some scholars and physicians have suggested that as treatment for the "common" and "uncomplicated" forms of childhood cancer have become standardized, much of this care has been taken over by local community hospitals. The very standardization of such care has also standardized insurance payments. Advanced and complicated or unusual cases are still sent to the major childhood cancer treatment centers; these cases are not only hard to treat, but also require vast expenditures of funds and experimental procedures that often are not fully reimbursed by health insurers or dwindling federal research programs. As a result, many major treatment centers find themselves in serious financial straits.

9. See, for example, Chesler (1993), Chesler et al. (1993), and American Cancer Society (1993).

Chapter 11. Other Self-Help Groups

1. We acknowledge the collaboration of our friend and colleague, Dr. Steven Sunderland, an activist and scholar working with Parents of Murdered Children. Sunderland is the originator of many of the comparative ideas about

parents of murdered children and parents of children with cancer discussed in these pages and in Table 11.1.

2. See the discussions in Gaylin (1982), McGee (1983), and Sunderland (1984).

3. In the case of some environmental disasters (e.g., Chernobyl, Love Canal), there is evidence of increased birth disorders and escalated rates of childhood cancer. There is also speculation about the involvement of high-tension radio transmission towers, toxic dump sites, radon, asbestos, and the like in causing childhood leukemia. By and large, however, there is little sound epidemiological evidence regarding the etiology of childhood cancer, and thus seldom is there an individual or corporate agent to "target" as the hereditary or environmental cause.

4. See the extended discussion of these findings, and their interpretation, in Chesler, et al. (1988).

5. See for example, reports from Trojan in West Germany (1989), Levy in England (1982), Gidron and Bargal in Israel (1986), Neighbors and Jackson in the African-American community in the United States (1984), and Pilisuk and Minkler in the elderly community in the United States (1980). At the same time, Nash and Kramer's (1993) studies of self-help groups for African-American sickle-cell disease patients in the United States show great similarity in group activities to our reports from groups of parents of children with cancer.

6. See the discussion in Chapter 6, and Battaglino (1987), Borman (1982), Edwards (1966), Humphreys and Woods (1993), Lieberman and Borman (1976), Medvene and Krauss (1989), and Videka-Sherman (1982).

7. For instance, see Hamilton (1990) and Hedrick et al. (1992).

8. Evidence supporting this argument is provided by Bartalos (1992) and Gottlieb and Peters (1991).

9. Maton and Rappaport's (1984) observations of a male prayer group in an African-American church affirms Neighbors and Jackson's (1984) argument. In addition, Rodgers and Tartaglia (1990) discuss the growth of the United Black Fund as a culturally unique form of self-help activity aimed at community self-improvement and self-empowerment, especially in the face of elite white control of social services and charitable resources.

10. See also Barrera (1981).

11. Some of the literature on self-help, and some of the attitudes of professionals, appear to confuse this pro-experiential orientation with an aprofessional or even antiprofessional stance (Borkman, personal note). As the discussion in Chapters 8 and 9 indicates, self-help members' and groups' valuation of and commitment to generating and using the experiential wisdom and resources of fellow sufferers does not necessarily lead to rejection or antagonism regarding professional's technical expertise, helpful resources, or involvement in group activities.

12. See further argument along this line in Asch (1986) and Withorn (1980).

13. Early research into self-help groups in the United States seemed to

support Katz' view of a priority on a personal change versus social change agenda; however, more recent work, including that reported in this volume, suggests that self-help groups in the United States do undertake local (and even national) change agendas.

14. Not discussed elsewhere in this volume, Study #3 gathered data from members of two types of self-help groups in Israel: groups of parents of children (or young adults) with mental illness and groups of parents in families of new immigrants. Other comparisons involving U.S. and Israeli parents and groups are found in Chesler et al. (1988), Chesler et al. (1990), and Gidron et al. (1991). In this international portion of our investigations, we encountered some of the typical problems in conducting cross-cultural research, including finding common themes active in various cultures, developing instruments with common wording, working across spatial barriers, finding funding, and so on. While some of the findings of the international aspect of this study are, therefore, not as directly comparable and not reported in this volume, the material on professionals' roles and self-help group members' preferences for professional involvement appears to be quite reliable and in line with other literature reported herein.

15. See reports from parents of children with cancer in Chapter 8. Data regarding how parents of murdered children viewed the roles of professionals in their self-help groups are not reported extensively in this volume, but are referred to earlier in this chapter and are available in Chesler et al. (1988).

16. This issue is discussed in general, with examples, in Gidron (1991) and Katz (1984). Further detail about specific arrangements in England, West Germany, and the Netherlands is found in Humble and Unell (1989) and van Harberden (1990).

17. Self-help clearinghouses are agencies specifically designed to offer technical expertise, consultation, publicity, and other forms of support to a wide range of (generally local) self-help groups. An example of the groups identified by a New Jersey self-help clearinghouse is provided in Figure 1.2, and discussion of these agencies is contained in Leventhal, Maton and Madara (1988), Madara (1985), Pancoast et al. (1983), and Reynolds (1982).

Chapter 12. Practical Guidelines for Self-Help Group Development and Maintenance

1. See, for example, Madara and Meese (1990) and Silverman (1992), and for the particular case of groups for parents of children with cancer, Nathanson (1987).

2. The useful roles of self-help clearinghouses were noted briefly in Chapter 11, and have been discussed and/or evaluated by Borck and Aronowitz (1982), Madara (1985), and Madara, Kalafat, and Miller (1988).

3. Listings of how the groups in this study organized themselves to manage some of these tasks are provided in Tables 5.1 and 5.4.

4. Some of the ways in which the groups we studied managed their rela-

tions with the medical staff and the influence of these decisions on groups' activities (or vice versa) are illustrated in Table 5.5 and Chapters 8 and 9.

5. Too often these agencies, and sometimes hospital staffs as well, are concerned about control and "ownership" of the childhood cancer population, and the effect that self-help group success might have on their own agenda, fund-raising capacities, and standing in the community. Then they cannot truly be helpful to local parents and groups.

Bibliography

Abbott, A. 1983. Professional ethics. *American Journal of Sociology* 88(5): 855–85.

Abrahams, R. 1976. Mutual helping: Styles of caregiving in a mutual aid program—The Widowed Service Line. In G. Caplan and M. Killilea, eds., *Support Systems and Mutual Help: Multidisciplinary Explorations.* New York: Grune & Stratton.

Adams, D. 1979. *Childhood malignancy: The psychosocial care of the child and his family.* Springfield, IL: C. C. Thomas.

Adams, M. 1978. Helping the parents of children with malignancy. *Journal of Pediatrics* 93 (5):734–38.

Aldwin, C., and Revenson, T. 1987. Does coping help? A reexamination of the relation between coping and mental health. *Journal of Personality and Social Psychology* 53: 337–48.

American Cancer Society. 1990. *Cancer Facts & Figures.* New York.

American Cancer Society. 1993. *Cancer Facts & Figures.* New York.

American Hospital Association. 1980. *American Hospital Association Guide to Health Resources.* Chicago.

Anderson, B. 1988. Considering whether to participate in research. Boston: Federation for Children with Special Needs (mimeo).

Anspach, R. 1979. From stigma to identity politics: Political activism among the physically disabled and former mental patients. *Social Science and Medicine* 13A: 765–73.

Antonovsky, A. 1980. *Health, Stress, and Coping.* San Francisco: Jossey-Bass.

Antze, P. 1976. The role of ideologies in peer psychotherapy organizations: Some theoretical considerations and three case studies. *Journal of Applied Behavioral Science* 12(3): 323–46.

362

Asch, A. 1986. Will populism empower the disabled? *Social Policy* 16(3): 12–18.

Ayers, T., and Chesler, M. 1987. Leading self-help groups: Report on workshop for leaders of childhood cancer support groups. Working paper #351. Ann Arbor: University of Michigan, Center for Research on Social Organization (December).

Back, K. 1981. Small groups. In M. Rosenberg and R. Turner, (eds.), *Social Psychology: Sociological Perspectives.* New York: Basic Books.

Baider, L., and De-Nour, A. 1989. Group therapy with adolescent cancer patients. *Journal of Adolescent Health Care* 10(1): 35–38.

Bakker, B., and Karel, M. 1983. Self-help: Wolf or Lamb? In D. Pancoast, P. Parker, and C. Froland, eds., *Rediscovering Self-Help.* Beverly Hills: Sage.

Barath, A. 1990. Hypertension clubs in Croatia, Yugoslavia. In A. Katz and E. Bender, eds., *Helping One Another.* Oakland, Calif.: Third Party Publishing.

Barbarin, O. 1987. Psychosocial risks and invulnerability: A review of the theoretical and empirical bases of preventive family-focused services for survivors of childhood cancer. *Journal of Psychosocial Oncology* 5, 25–41.

Barbarin, O., and Chesler, M. 1983. *Children with Cancer: School Experiences and Views of Parents, Educators, Adolescents, and Physicians.* Maywood, Ill.: Eterna Press.

Barbarin, O.; Hughes, D.; and Chesler, M. 1985. Stress, coping, and marital functioning among parents of children with cancer. *Journal of Marriage & The Family* 47(2): 473–80.

Barrera, M. 1981. Social Support in the Adjustment of Pregnant Adolescents. In B. Gottlieb, ed., *Social Networks and Social Support.* Beverly Hills: Sage.

Bartalos, M. 1992. Illness, professional caregivers and self-helpers. In A. Katz, H. Hedrick, D. Isenberg, L. Thompson, T. Goodrich, and A. Kutscher, eds., *Self-Help: Concepts and Applications*, Philadelphia: The Charles Press.

Battaglino, L. 1987. Family empowerment through self-help groups. In A. Hatfield, ed., *Families of the Mentally Ill: Meeting the Challenges.* New Directions for Mental Health Services, No. 34, San Francisco: Jossey-Bass.

Bauman, L.; Garvey, R.; and Siegel, K. 1992. Factors associated with cancer patients' participation in support groups. *Journal of Psychosocial Oncology* 10(3): 1–20.

Becker, M., and Maiman, L. 1980. Strategies for enhancing patient compliance. *Journal of Community Health* 6: 113–35.

Bellah, R.; Madsen, R.; Sullivan, R.; Swidler, A.; and Tipton, S. 1985. *Habits of the Heart.* Berkeley and Los Angeles: University of California Press.

Belle-Isle, J., and Conradt, B. 1979. Report of a discussion group for parents of children with leukemia. *Maternal Child Nursing Journal* 8(1): 49–58.

Biegel, D., and Yamatani, H. 1987. Help-giving in self-help groups. *Hospital and Community Psychiatry* 38(11): 1195–97.

Billings, A., and Moos, R. 1981. The role of coping responses and social resources in attenuating the stress of life events. *Journal of Behavioral Medicine* 4: 139–57.

Binger, C.; Albin, A.; Feuerstein, R.; Kushner, J.; Zoger, S.; and Mikelsen, C. 1969. Childhood leukemia: Emotional impact on patient and family. *New England Journal of Medicine* 280: 414–18.

Black, R., and Drachman, D. 1985. Hospital social workers and self-help groups. *Health and Social Work* 10: 95–103.

Black, R., and Weiss, J. 1990. Genetic support groups and social workers as partners. *Health and Social Work* 15 (May): 91–99.

Bliwise, N., and Lieberman, M. 1984. From professional help to self-help: An evaluation of therapeutic groups for the elderly. In A. Gartner and F. Riessman, eds., *The Self-Help Revolution.* New York, Human Sciences Press.

Bloch, J., and Seitz, M. 1985. *Empowering Parents of Disabled Children.* Syosset, N.Y.: Variety Pre-schooler's Workshop.

Bogue, E., and Chesney, B. 1987. *Making Contact: A Parent-to-Parent Visitation Manual.* Washington, D.C.: The Candlelighters Childhood Cancer Foundation.

Borck, L., and Aronowitz, E. 1982. The role of a self-help clearinghouse. In *Helping People to Help Themselves.* Valhalla, N.Y.: Westchester Self-help Clearinghouse.

Borkman, T. 1976. Experiential knowledge: A new concept for the analysis of self-help groups. *Social Service Review* 50: 445–56.

Borkman, T. 1984. Mutual self-help groups: Strengthening the selectively unsupporting personal and community networks of their members. In A. Gartner and F. Riessman, eds., *The Self-Help Revolution.* New York: Human Sciences Press.

Borkman, T. 1990. Experiential, professional and lay frames of reference. In T. Powell, ed., *Working with Self-Help.* Washington, D.C.: NASW Press.

Borkman, T. 1993. Personal communication with the authors (September).

Borkman, T., and Schubert, M. In press. The participatory action research paradigm for studying self-help groups internationally. *Prevention in Human Services.*

Borman, L. 1976. Self-help and the professional. *Social Policy* 7(2): 47–48.

Borman, L. 1979. Characteristics of growth and development. In M.

Lieberman and L. Borman, eds., *Self-Help Groups for Coping with Crisis.* San Francisco: Jossey-Bass.

Borman, L. 1982. Kalmuk Resettlement in America. In G. Weber and L. Cohen, eds., *Beliefs and Self-Help: Cross-cultural Perspectives and Approaches,* New York: Human Services Press.

Borman, L. 1992. Introduction: Self-Help/Mutual Aid Groups in Strategies for Health. In A. Katz, H. Hedrick, D. Isenberg, L. Thompson, T. Goodrich, and A. Kutscher, eds., *Self-Help: Concepts and Applications.* Philadelphia: The Charles Press.

Brickman, P.; Kidder, L.; Coates, D.; Rabinowitz, V.; Cohn, E.; and Karuza, J. 1983. The dilemmas of helping: Making aid fair and effective. In J. Fisher, A. Nadler, and B. DePaulo, eds., *New Directions in Helping.* Vol. 1. New York: Academic Press.

Broadhead, W.; Kaplan, B.; James, S.; Wagner, E.; Schoenbach, V.; Grimson, R.; Heyden, S.; Tibblin, G.; and Gehlbach, S. 1983. The epidemiologic evidence for a relationship between social support and health. *American Journal of Epidemiology* 117: 521–37.

Brown, D., and Kaplan, R. 1981. Participative research in a factory. In H. Reason and J. Rowan, eds., *Human Inquiry.* London: Wiley.

Brown, D., and Tandon, R. 1983. Ideology and political economy in inquiry: Action research and participatory research. *Journal of Applied Behavioral Science* 19(3): 277–94.

Browning, P.; Thorin, E.; and Rhoades, C. 1984. A national profile of self-help/self-advocacy groups of people with mental retardation. *Mental Retardation* 22(5): 226–30.

Bryant, N. 1990. Self-help groups and professionals: Cooperation or conflict. In A. Katz and E. Bender, eds., *Helping One Another: Self-Help Groups in a Changing World.* Oakland, Calif.: Third Party Publishing.

Cancian, F., and Armistead, C. 1990. Participatory research: An introduction. Irvine, Calif.: Department of Sociology, Univ. of California, Irvine. Mimeo.

Caplan, R. 1979. Patient, provider, and organization: Hypothesized determinants of adherence. In S. Cohen, ed., *New Directions in Patient Compliance.* Lexington, Mass.: Heath.

Caplan, G., and Killilea, M., eds. 1976. *Support Systems and Mutual Help: Multidisciplinary Exploration.* New York: Grune & Stratton.

Carpenter, P., and Vattino, C. 1992. Development of a parent advocate program as part of a Pediatric Hematology/Oncology Service. *Journal of Psychosocal Oncology* 10(2): 27–38.

Carr, W., and Kemmis, S. 1983. *Becoming Critical: Knowledge Through Action Research.* Victoria, Australia: Deakin University Press.

Cassileth, B., and Hamilton, J. 1979. The family with cancer. In B. Cassileth, ed., *The Cancer Patient: Social and Medical Aspects of Care.* Philadelphia: Lea and Febiger.

Chapin, F., and Tsouderos, J. 1956. The formalization process in voluntary associations. *Social Forces* 34: 342–44.

Charmaz, K. 1983. The grounded theory method: An explication and interpretation. In R. Emerson, ed., *Contemporary Field Research.* Boston: Little, Brown.

Checkoway, B.; Chesler, M.; and Blum, S. 1990. Self-care, self-help and community care for health. In T. Powell, ed., *Working With Self-Help.* Washington, D.C.: NASW Press.

Chein, I.; Cook, S.; and Harding, J. 1948. The Field of Action Research. *American Psychologist* 3: 43–50.

Cherniss, G. 1980. *Staff Burnout: Job Stress in the Human Services.* Beverly Hills: Sage.

Chesler, M. 1981. The creation and maintenance of interracial coalitions. In B. Bowser and R. Hunt, eds., *The Impact of Racism on White Americans.* Beverly Hills: Sage.

Chesler, M. 1988. Community support systems. In T. Dowell, D. Copeland, and J. Van Eys, eds., *The Child with Cancer in the Community.* St. Louis: C. C. Thomas.

Chesler, M. 1990a. Action research in the voluntary sector: A case study of scholar-activist roles in self-help groups. In S. Wheelan, E. Pepitone, and V. Abt, eds., *Advances in Field Theory.* Beverly Hills: Sage.

Chesler, M. 1990b. Professionals' views of the 'dangers' of self-help groups, In T. Powell, ed., *Working with Self-Help.* Washington, D.C.: NASW Press.

Chesler, M. 1991. Mobilizing consumer activism in health care: The role of self-help groups. *Research in Social Movements, Conflict and Change* 13: 275–305.

Chesler, M. 1993. Introduction to psychosocial issues. *Cancer* 71(10): 3245–50.

Chesler, M., and Barbarin, O. 1984a. Difficulties of providing help in a crisis: Relationships between parents of children with cancer and their friends. *Journal of Social Issues* 40(4): 113–34.

Chesler, M., and Barbarin, O. 1984b. Relating to the medical staff: How parents of children with cancer see the issues. *Health and Social Work* 9(1): 49–65.

Chesler, M., and Barbarin, O. 1987. *Childhood Cancer and the Family.* New York: Brunner-Mazel.

Chesler, M., Barbarin, O.; and Lebo-Stein, J. 1984. Patterns of participation in a self-help group for parents of children with cancer. *Journal of Psychosocial Oncology* 2 (2/3): 41–64.

Chesler, M.; and Chesney, B. 1988. Self-help groups: Empowerment attitudes and behaviors of disabled or chronically ill persons. In H. Yuker, ed., *Attitudes Toward Persons with Disabilities*. New York: Springer Publications.

Chesler, M.; Chesney, B.; and Gidron, B. 1990. Israeli and U.S. orientations toward self-help groups for families in crisis. *Nonprofit and Voluntary Sector Quarterly* 19(3): 251–62.

Chesler, M.; Chesney, B.; Gidron, B.; Hartman, H.; and Sunderland, S. 1988. Self-help groups: A comparative international study of social support and social action. Final report to DHHS on contract #90-PD-0119. Ann Arbor: University of Michigan (September).

Chesler, M.; Hainey, S.; Perrin, G.; Monaco, G.; Kupst, M.; Cincotta, N.; Katz, E.; Deasy-Spinetta, P.; Whittam, M.; and Foley, G. 1993. Principles of psychosocial programming for children and cancer. *Cancer* 71(10): 3210–12.

Chesler, M., and Yoak, M. 1984. Self-help groups for parents of children with cancer. In H. Roback, ed., *Helping Patients and Their Families Cope with Medical Problems*. San Franciso: Jossey-Bass.

Chesney, B. 1989. Empowering parents of children with cancer: The role of self-help groups. Unpublished doctoral dissertation. Ann Arbor: University of Michigan.

Chesney, B., and Chesler, M. 1993. The activism potential of self-help group membership: Reported life changes of parents of children with cancer. *Journal of Small Group Research* 24 (2): 258–73.

Chutis, L. 1983. Special roles of mental health professionals in self-help group development, *Prevention in Human Services* 2(3): 65–73.

Claflin, B. 1984. Mutual support in a suburban setting. In A. Gartner and F. Riessman, eds., *The Self-Help Revolution*. New York: Human Sciences Press.

Clark, M. 1983. Reactions to aid in communical and exchange relationships. In J. Fisher, A. Nadler, and B. DePaulo, eds., *New Directions in Helping*. Vol. 1. New York: Academic Press.

Coe, R. 1978. *Sociology of Medicine*. 2d ed. New York: McGraw-Hill.

Cohen, C.; Adler, A.; and Mintz, J. 1983. Network interventions on the margin: A service experiment in a welfare hotel. In D. Pancoast, P. Parker, and C. Froland, eds., *Rediscovering Self-Help*. Beverly Hills: Sage.

Cohen, J. 1985. Strategy or identity: New theoretical paradigms and contemporary social movements. *Social Research* 52: 663–716.

Cohen, L. 1982. Cross-ethnic comparisons. In G. Weber and L. Cohen, eds., *Beliefs and Self-Help: Cross-cultural Perspectives and Approaches*. New York: Human Services Press.

Cohen, P. 1994. Survivors of childhood cancer: Patterns of perception and adap-

tive response among mothers and young adults. Unpublished doctoral dissertation. Ann Arbor: University of Michigan.

Collins, A., and Pancoast, D. 1976. *Natural Helping Networks*. Washington,
D.C.: National Association of Social Workers Press.

Coplon, J., and Strull, J. 1983. Roles of the professional in mutual aid groups.
Journal of Contemporary Social Work (May): 259–66.

Corbin, J. 1986. Coding, writing memos and diagramming. In C. Chenitz and
J. Swanson, eds., *From Practice to Grounded Theory*. Reading, Mass.:
Addison-Wesley.

Cordoba, C.; Shear, M.; Fobair, P.; and Hall, J. 1984. *Cancer Support Groups*.
San Francisco: American Cancer Society.

Coser, L. 1966. *The Functions of Social Conflict*. Glencoe, Ill.: The Free Press.

Cousins, N. 1979. *Anatomy of an Illness as Perceived by the Patient: Reflections
on Healing and Regeneration*. New York: Norton.

Cronbach, L., and Meehl, P. 1955. Construct validity in psychological tests.
Psychological Bulletin 82: 281–302.

Culbert, S. 1976. Consciousness-raising: A five-stage model for social and organizational change. In W. Bennis, K. Benne, R. Chin, and K. Corey, eds.,
The Planning of Change. 3d ed. New York: Holt, Rinehart & Winston.

Daiter, S.; Larson, R.; Weddington, W.; and Ultmann, J. 1988. Psychosocial
symptomatology, personal growth, and development among young adult
patients following the diagnosis of leukemia or lymphoma. *Journal of Clinical Oncology* 6(4): 613–17.

Darling, R. 1988. Parental entrepreneurship: A consumerist response to professional dominance. *Journal of Social Issues* 44: 141–58.

Davis, S.; Chesler, M.; and Chesney, B. 1990. Coping with cancer: Life
changes reported by patients and significant others dealing with Leukemia
and Lymphoma. Working Paper #427. Center for Research on Social Organization Ann Arbor: University of Michigan (August).

de Cocq, G. 1990. European and North American self-help movements:
Some contrasts. In A. Katz and E. Bender, eds., *Helping One Another:
Self-Help Groups in a Changing World*. Oakland: Third Party Publishing
Company.

De Tocqueville, A. 1957. *Democracy in America*. New York: Vintage.

Deasy-Spinetta, P., and Irvin, E., eds. 1993. *Educating the Child With Cancer*.
Washington, D.C.: Candlelighters Childhood Cancer Foundation.

Deneke, C. 1983. How professionals view self-help. In D. Pancoast, P. Parker,
and C. Froland, eds., *Rediscovering Self-Help*. Beverly Hills: Sage.

Denzin, N. 1977. *The Research Act: A Theoretical Introduction to Sociological
Methods*. New York: McGraw-Hill.

DiMatteo, M. 1979. A social psychological analysis of physician-patient rapport: Toward a science of the art of medicine. *Journal of Social Issues* 35(1): 12–33.

DiMatteo, R., and Hays, R. 1980. The significance of patients' perceptions of physician conduct: A study of patient satisfaction in a Family Practice Center. *Journal of Community Health* 6 (Fall): 18–34.

DiMatteo, M., and Hays, R. 1981. Social support and serious illness. In B. Gottlieb, ed., *Social Networks and Social Support*. Beverly Hills: Sage.

Dodson, D. 1960. The creative role of conflict reexamined. *Journal of Intergroup Relations* 1: 5–12.

Dory, F., and Riessman, F. 1982. Training professionals in organizing self-help groups. *Citizen Participation* 3(3): 27–28.

Dunkel-Schetter, C. 1984. Social support and cancer: Findings based on patient interviews and their implications. *Journal of Social Issues* 40 (4): 77–98.

Dunst, C.; Trivette, C.; Davis, M.; and Cornwell, J. 1988. Enabling and empowering families of children with health impairments. *Children's Health Care* 17: 71–81.

Edwards, G. 1966. Who goes to Alcoholics Anonymous? *Lancet* 2: 382.

Ehrenreich, J., ed. 1978 *The Cultural Crisis of Modern Medicine*, New York: Monthly Review Press.

Elden, M. 1981. Sharing the research work: Participative research and its role demands. In H. Reason and J. Rowan, eds., *Human Inquiry*. New York: Wiley.

Emerick, R. 1990. Self-help groups for former patients: Relations with mental health professionals. *Hospital and Community Psychiatry* 41(4): 401–7.

Fals-Borda, O. 1984. Participatory action research. *Development: Seeds of Change* 2: 18–20.

Family Support Group Guidelines. 1986. New York: Leukemia Society of America.

Featherstone, H. 1980. *A Difference in the Family*. New York: Basic Books.

Fine, M., and Asch, A. 1988. Disability beyond stigma: Social interaction, discrimination, and activism. *Journal of Social Issues* 44: 3–21.

Fisher, J.; Nadler, A.; and Whitcher-Alagna, S. 1983. Four theoretical approaches for conceptualizing reactions to aid. In J. Fisher, A. Nadler, and B. DePaulo, eds., *New Directions in Helping*. Vol. 1. New York: Academic Press.

Folkman, S., and Lazarus, R. 1980. An analysis of coping in a middle-aged community sample. *Journal of Health and Social Behavior* 21: 219–39.

Foster, Z., and Mandel, S. 1979. Mutual help group for patients: Taking steps toward change. *Health and Social Work* 4(3): 82–98.

Fox, R. 1989. *The Sociology of Medicine*. Englewood Cliffs, N.J.: Prentice Hall.

Frank, G. 1988. Stigma: Visibility and self-empowerment of persons with congenital limb deficiencies. *Journal of Social Issues* 44: 94–115.

Freeman, J. 1979. Resource mobilization and strategy: A model for analyzing social movement organization actions. In M. Zald and J. McCarthy, eds., *The Dynamics of Social Movements*. Cambridge, Mass.: Winthrop.

Friedman, H., and DiMatteo, R. 1979. Health care as an interpersonal process. *Journal of Social Issues* 35(1): 1–11.

Freidson, E. 1970. *Profession of Medicine*. New York: Dodd & Mead.

Freire, P. 1973. *Education for Critical Consciousness*. New York: Seabury.

Freudenberger, H. 1974. Staff burn-out. *Journal of Social Issues* 30: 159–65.

Froland, C.; Pancoast, D.; Chapman, N.; and Kimboto, P. 1981. *Helping Networks and Human Services*. Beverly Hills: Sage.

Froland, C.; Pancoast, D.; and Parker, P., eds. 1983. Introduction. In D. Pancoast, P. Parker, and C. Froland, eds., *Rediscovering Self-Help*. Beverly Hills: Sage.

Galtung, J. 1969. Violence, peace and peace research. *Journal of Peace Research* 3: 167–92.

Gamson, W. 1975. *The Strategy of Social Protest*. Homewood, Ill.: Dorsey Press.

Gamson, W.; Fireman, B.; and Rytina, S. 1982. *Encounters with Unjust Authorities*. Homewood, Ill.: Dorsey Press.

Gartner, A. 1990. A typology of women's self-help groups. In A. Katz and E. Bender, eds., *Helping One Another: Self-Help Groups in a Changing World*. Oakland, Calif.: Third Party Publishing.

Gartner, A., and F. Riessman. 1977. *Self-Help in the Human Services*. San Francisco: Jossey-Bass.

Gartner A., and Riessman, F., eds. 1984. *The Self-Help Revolution*. New York: Human Sciences Press.

Gaventa, J. 1993. The powerful, the powerless and the experts: Knowledge struggles in an information age. In P. Park, B. Hall, and H. Jackson, eds., *Voices of Change: Participatory Research in the United States & Canada*. Westport, Conn.: Bergin & Garvey.

Gaventa, J. 1988. Participatory research in North America. *Convergence* 21 (2/3): 41–46.

Gaylin, W. 1983. *The Killing of Bonnie Garland*. New York: Penguin.

Gidron, B. 1991. Stress and coping patterns of parents of the mentally ill in Israel. *International Social Work* 34: 159–70.

Gidron, B., and Bargal, D. 1986. Self-help awareness in Israel: An expression of structural changes and expanding citizen participation. *Journal of Voluntary Action Research* 15(2): 47–56.

Gidron, B.; Chesler, M.; and Chesney, B. 1991. Cross-cultural perspectives on self-help groups: Comparison between participants and nonparticipants in Israel and the United States. *American Journal of Community Psychology* 19(5): 667–81.

Gidron, B.; Guterman, N.; and Hartman, H. 1990. Participation in self-help groups and empowerment among parents of the mentally ill in Israel. In T. Powell, ed., *Working With Self-Help*, Washington, D.C.: NASW Press.

Gilder, R.; Buschman, P.; Sitarz, A.; and Wolff, J. 1976. Group therapy for parents of children with leukemia. *American Journal of Psychotherapy* 30: 276–87.

Glaser, B. 1978. *Theoretical Sensitivity: Advances in the Methodology of Grounded Theory.* Mill Valley, Calif.: Sociology Press.

Glaser, B., and Strauss, A. 1967. *The Discovery of Grounded Theory.* Chicago: Aldine.

Goffman, E. 1968. *Stigma: Notes on the Management of Spoiled Identity.* London: Penguin Books.

Gottlieb, B. 1982. Mutual help groups: Members' views of their benefits and of roles for professionals. *Prevention in Human Services* 1(3): 55–67.

Gottlieb, B. 1983. *Social Support Strategies.* Beverly Hills: Sage.

Gottlieb, B., ed. 1981. *Social Networks and Social Support.* Beverly Hills: Sage.

Gottlieb, B., and Peters, L. 1991. A national demographic portrait of mutual aid group participants in Canada. *American Journal of Community Psychology* 19 (5): 651–66.

Green, D., ed. 1989. *Long-Term Complications of Therapy for Cancer in Childhood and Adolescence.* Baltimore: Johns Hopkins University Press.

Gutiérrez, L. 1987. Empowerment and social work theory. Mimeo. Ann Arbor: University of Michigan.

Gutiérrez, L. 1988. Coping with stressful life events: An empowerment perspective. Working Paper. School of Social Work. Ann Arbor: University of Michigan.

Gutiérrez, L.; Ortega, R.; and Suarez, Z. 1990. Self-help and the Latino community. In T. Powell, ed., *Working with Self-Help*, Washington, D.C.: NASW Press.

Haber, D. 1992. Self-help groups and aging. In A. Katz, H. Hedrick, D. Isenberg, L. Thompson, T. Goodrich, and A. Kutscher, eds., *Self-Help: Concepts and Applications.* Philadelphia: The Charles Press.

Hage, J., and Aiken, M. 1970. *Social Change in Complex Organizations.* New York: Random House.

Hall, B.; Gillette, A.; and Tandon, R. 1982. *Creating Knowledge: A Monopoly.* New Delhi and Toronto: Society for Participatory Research and International Council for Adult Education.

Hall, R.; Haas, E.; and Johnson, N. 1967. Organizational size, complexity and formalization. *American Sociological Review* 32: 903–12.

Hamilton, A. 1990. Self-help and mutual aid in ethnic minority communities. In A. Katz and E. Bender, eds., *Helping One Another: Self-Help Groups In a Changing World.* Oakland, Calif.: Third Party Publishing.

Hart, J. 1992. Cracking the code: Narratives and Political Mobilization in the Greek resistance. *Social Science History* 16(2): 26–47.

Hasenfeld, Y. 1987. Power in social work practice. *Social Science Review* 61: 469–83.

Haug, M., and Sussman, M. 1969. Professional autonomy and the revolt of the client. *Social Problems* 17: 153–61.

Haug, M. 1975. The deprofessionalization of everyone. *Sociological Focus* 8(3): 197–213.

Hedrick, H.; Isenberg, D.; and Martini, C. 1992. Self-help groups: Empowerment through policy and partnerships. In A. Katz, H. Hedrick, D. Isenberg, L. Thompson, T. Goodrich, and A. Kutscher, eds., *Self-Help: Concepts and Applications.* Philadelphia: The Charles Press.

Heffron, W. 1975. Group therapy sessions as part of treatment of children with cancer. In C. Pochedly, ed., *Clinical Management of Cancer in Children.* Acton, Mass.: Science Group.

Henry, S. 1978. The dangers of self-help groups. *New Society* 22: 654–56.

Himes, J. 1966. The function of racial conflict. *Social Forces* 45 (1): 1–10.

Hinckley, B. 1979. Twenty-one variables beyond the size of winning coalitions. *Journal of Politics* 41 (1): 192–212.

Hinrichsen, G.; Revenson, T.; and Shinn, M. 1985. Does self-help help? An empirical investigation of scoliosis peer support groups. *Journal of Social Issues* 41(1): 65–87.

Homans, G. 1961. *Social Behavior: Its Elementary Forms.* New York: Harcourt Brace.

House, J. 1981. *Work, Stress and Social Support.* Reading, Mass.: Addison-Wesley.

Humble, S., and Unell, J. 1989. *Self-Help in Health and Social Welfare: England and West Germany.* London: Routledge.

Humm, A. 1984. The changing nature of lesbian and gay self-help groups. In A. Gartner and F. Riessman, eds., *The Self-Help Revolution.* New York: Human Sciences Press.

Humphreys, K.; Mavis, B.; and Stoffelmayr, B. 1992. Involvement in mutual help groups one year after substance abuse treatment: Are 12-step programs appropriate for disenfranchised groups? Presented at International Conference on Self-Help and Mutual Aid. Ottawa, Canada.

Humphreys, K., and Woods, M. 1993. Researching mutual help group participation in a segregated society. *Journal of Applied Behavioral Science* 29(2): 166–81.

Hyde, C. 1991. Did the New Right radicalize the women's movement? A study of change in feminist social movement organizations, 1977–1987. Unpublished doctoral dissertation. Ann Arbor: University of Michigan.

Hyde, C. 1992. The ideational system of social movement agencies. In Y. Hasenfeld, ed., *Human Services as Complex Organization*. Beverly Hills: Sage.

Israel, B., and Rounds, K. 1987. Social networks and social support: A synthesis for health educators. *Advances in Health Education and Promotion* 2: 311–51.

Israel, B.; House, J.; Schurman, S.; Heaney, C.; and Mero, R. 1988. The relation of personal resources, participation, influence, interpersonal relationships and coping strategies to occupational stress, job strains and health: A multivariate analysis. Mimeo, School of Public Health. Ann Arbor: University of Michigan.

Israel, B.; Schurman, S.; and House, J. 1989. Action research on occupational stress: Involving workers as researchers. *International Journal of Health Services* 19: 135–55.

Jacobs, J., and Dopkeen, L. 1990. Risking the qualitative study of risk. *Qualitative Sociology* 13(2): 169–81.

Jacobs, M., and Goodman, G. 1989. Psychology and self-help groups. *American Psychologist* 44(1): 536–45.

Jertson, J. 1975. Self-help groups. *Social Work* 20 (March): 144–50.

Johnson, E., and Stark, D. 1980. A group program for cancer patients and their family members in an acute care teaching hospital. *Social Work in Health Care* 5 (4): 335–49.

Kagey, J.; Vivace, J.; and Lutz, W. 1981. Mental health primary prevention: The role of parent mutual support groups. *American Journal of Public Health* 71(2): 166–67.

Kahn, R., and Antonucci, T. 1980. Convoys over the life course: Attachment, roles and social support. In P. Baltes and O. Brim, eds., *Life Span Development and Behavior*. Vol. 3. New York: Academic Press.

Kalnins, I. 1983. Cross-illness comparison of separation and divorce among parents having a child with a life-threatening illness. *Child Health Care* 12(2): 72–77.

Kartha, M., and Ertel, I. 1976. Short-term group therapy for mothers of leukemic children. *Clinical Pediatrics* 15: 803–6.

Katz, A. 1981. Self-help and mutual aid: An emerging social movement. *Annual Review of Sociology* 7: 129–55.

Katz, A. 1984. Self-help groups: An international perspective. In A. Gartner and F. Riessman, eds., *The Self-Help Revolution*, New York: Human Science Press.

Katz, A. 1992. Professional/self-help group relationships: General issues. In A. Katz, H. Hedrick, D. Isenberg, L. Thompson, D. Goodrich, and A. Kutscher, eds., *Self-Help: Concepts and Applications*, Philadelphia: The Charles Press.

Katz, A. 1993. *Self-Help in America.* New York: Twayne Publications.

Katz, A., and Bender, E., eds. 1976. *The strength in us: Self-help groups in the modern world.* New York: New Viewpoints/Vision Books.

Katz, A., and Bender, E., eds. 1990a. *Helping One Another.* Oakland, Calif.: Third Party Publishing.

Katz, A., and Bender, E. 1990b. Professional self-help group relationships. In A. Katz and E. Bender, eds., *Helping One Another.* Oakland, Calif.: Third Party Publishing.

Katz, A., and Bender, E. 1990c. Social learning and group dynamics in self-help. In A. Katz and E. Bender, eds., *Helping One Another.* Oakland, Calif.: Third Party Publishing.

Katz, A., and Bender, E. 1990d. Toward definitions and clarifications of self-help groups. In A. Katz and E. Bender, eds., *Helping One Another.* Oakland, Calif.: Third Party Publishing.

Kaufman, C. 1993. Roles for mental health consumers in self-help group research. *Journal of Applied Behavioral Science* 29(2): 257–71.

Kaufman, C.; Freund, P.; and Wilson, J. 1989. Self-help in the mental health system: A model for consumer-provider collaboration. *Psychosocial Rehabilitation Journal* 13(1): 5–21.

Keller, E. 1985. *Reflections on Gender and Science.* New Haven: Yale University Press.

Kieffer, C. 1983–84. Citizen empowerment: A developmental perspective. *Prevention in Human Services* 3(2–3): 9–36.

Killilea, M. 1976. Mutual help organizations: Interpretations in the literature. In G. Caplan and M. Killilea, eds., *Support Systems and Mutual Help.* New York: Grune & Stratton.

King, C. 1980. The self-help/self-care concept. *Nurse Practitioner* (May/June): 34–39.

Klass, D. 1984–85. Bereaved parents and the compassionate friends: Affiliation and healing. *OMEGA; Journal of Death and Dying* 15: 353–73.

Klass, D. 1992. The dynamics of self-help in healing parental grief: The role of The Compassionate Friends. In A. Katz, H. Hedrick, D. Isenberg, L.

Thompson, T. Goodrich, and A. Kutscher, eds., *Self-Help: Concepts and Applications*. Philadelphia: The Charles Press.

Klass, D., and Shinners, B. 1982–83. Professional roles in a self-help group for the bereaved. *OMEGA: Journal of Death and Dying* 13(4): 361–75.

Kleiman, M.; Mantel, J.; and Alexander, E. 1976. Collaboration and its discontents: The perils of partnership. *Journal of Applied Behavioral Science* 12(3): 403–09.

Knapp, V., and Hansen, H. 1973. Helping the parents of children with leukemia. *Social Work* 18(4): 70–75.

Knight, B.; Wollert, R.; Levy, L.; Frame, C.; and Padgett, V. 1980. Self-help groups: The members' perspectives. *American Journal of Community Psychology* 8(1): 53–65.

Kravetz, D. 1980. Consciousness-raising and self-help. In A. Brodsby and R. Hare-Mustin, eds., *Women and Psychotherapy*. New York: Guilford Press.

Kropotkin, P. 1972. *Mutual Aid: A Factor in Evolution*. New York: New York University Press.

Krulik, T., and Florian, V. 1986. Support groups for parents of children with cancer. An alternative source for social support. Paper presented at the Fourth International Conference on Cancer Nursing. New York (September).

Kupst, M.; Schulman, J.; Honig, G.; Maurer, H.; Morgan, E.; and Fochtman, D. 1982. Family coping with childhood leukemia: One year after diagnosis. *Journal of Pediatric Psychology* 7 (2): 157–74.

Kurtz, L. 1990a. The self-help movement: Review of the past decade of research. *Social Work with Groups* 13(3): 101–15.

Kurtz, L. 1990b. Twelve-step programs. In T. Powell, ed., *Working with Self-Help*. Washington, D.C.: NASW Press.

Lansky, S.; Cairns, N.; Clark, G.; Lowman, J.; Miller, L.; and Trueworthy, R. 1979. Childhood cancer: Non-medical costs of illness. *Cancer* 43: 403–08.

Lansky, S.; Cairns, N.; Hassamien, R.; Wehr, J.; and Lowman, J. 1978. Childhood cancer: Parental discord and divorce. *Pediatrics* 62: 184–88.

Lansky, S.; Lowman, J.; Vats, T.; and Gyulay, J. 1975. School phobia in children with malignant neoplasms. *American Journal of Disabled Children* 129: 42–47.

Lavoie, F. 1983. Citizen participation. In D. Pancoast, P. Parker, and C. Froland, eds., *Rediscovering Self-Help*. Beverly Hills: Sage.

Lavoie, F. 1984. Action research: A new model of interaction between the professional and self-help groups. In A. Gartner and F. Riessman, eds., *The Self-Help Revolution*. New York: Human Sciences Press.

Lavoie, F. 1990. Evaluating self-help groups. In J. Romeder, ed., *The Self-*

Help Way: Mutual Aid and Health. Ottawa: Canadian Council on Social Development.

Lazarus, R. 1981. The costs and benefits of denial. In J. Spinetta and P. Deasy-Spinetta, eds., *Living with Childhood Cancer.* St. Louis: Mosby.

Lazarus, R., and Folkman, S. 1984. *Stress, Appraisal and Coping.* New York: Springer.

LeVeck, P. 1982. Self-help in a Manic Depressive Association. In G. Weber and L. Cohen, eds., *Beliefs and Self-Help: Cross-cultural Perspectives and Approaches,* New York: Human Services Press.

Lenrow, P., and Burch, R. 1981. Mutual aid or professional services: Opposing or complementary. In B. Gottlieb, ed., *Social Networks and Social Support.* Beverly Hills: Sage.

Leventhal, G.; Maton, K.; and Madara, E. 1988. Systemic organizational support for self-help groups. *American Journal of Orthopsychiatry* 58 (4): 592–603.

Levine, A. 1975. Support systems for the patient with cancer. *Cancer* 36: 813–20.

Levine, M. 1988. How self-help works. *Social Policy* 19:39–43.

Levy, L. 1976. Self-help groups: Types and psychological processes. *Journal of Applied Behavioral Science* 12(3): 310–22.

Levy, L. 1978. Self-help groups viewed by mental health professionals: A survey and comments. *American Journal of Community Psychology* 5: 305–13.

Levy, L. 1982. Mutual support groups in Great Britain: A survey: *Social Science in Medicine* 16: 1267–75.

Levy, L. 1984. Issues in research and evaluation. In A. Gartner and F. Riessman, eds., *The Self-Help Revolution.* New York: Human Sciences Press.

Levy, L.; Knight, B.; and Wollert, R. 1984. Make today count: A collaborative model for professionals and self-help groups. In A. Gartner and F. Riessman, eds., *The Self-Help Revolution.* New York: Human Sciences Press.

Lewin, K. 1946. Action research and minority problems. *Journal of Social Issues* 2(4): 34–46.

Lieberman, M. 1979. Analyzing change mechanisms in groups. In M. Lieberman and L. Borman, eds., *Self-help Groups for Coping with Crises.* San Francisco: Jossey-Bass.

Lieberman, M. 1988. The role of self-help groups in helping patients and families cope with cancer. *CA-A Cancer Journal for Clinicians* 38: 162–75.

Lieberman, M., and Bond, G. 1976. The problems of being a woman: A survey of 1,700 women in consciousness-raising groups. *Journal of Applied Behavioral Science* 12: 363–79.

Lieberman, M., and Borman, L. 1976. Epilogue: Self-help and social research. *Journal of Applied Behavioral Science* 12(3): 455–63.

Lieberman, M., and Borman, L., eds. 1979. *Self-Help Groups for Coping with Crisis.* San Francisco: Jossey-Bass.

Lincoln, Y., and Guba, E. 1985. *Naturalistic Inquiry.* Beverly Hills: Sage.

Lipsky, M. 1980. *Street-Level Bureaucracy: Dilemmas of the Individual in Public Services.* New York: Russell-Sage.

Lorber, J. 1975. Good patients and problem patients: Conformity and deviance in a general hospital. *Journal of Health and Social Behavior* 16(2): 213–25.

Luke, D.; Roberts, L.; and Rappaport, J. 1993. Individual group context and individual-group fit: Predictors of self-help group attendance. *Journal of Applied Behavioral Science* 29(2): 216–39.

Lurie, A., and Shulman, L. 1983. The professional connection with self-help groups in health care settings. *Social Work in Health Care* 8(4): 69–77.

Lynam, M. 1987. The parent network in pediatric oncology: Supportive or not? *Cancer Nursing* 10: 207–16.

Mack, S., and Berman, L. 1988. A group for parents of children with fatal genetic illnesses. *American Journal of Orthopsychiatry* 58(3): 397–404.

Madara, E. 1985. The Self-Help Clearinghouse operation: Tapping the resource development potential of I & R Services. *Information and Referral* 7(1): 42–58.

Madara, E. 1992. The primary value of a self-help clearing house. In A. Katz, H. Hedrick, D. Isenberg, L. Thompson, T. Goodrich, and A. Kutscher, eds., *Self-Help: Concepts and Applications.* Philadelphia: The Charles Press.

Madara, E.; Kalafat, J.; and Miller, B. 1988. The computerized self-help clearinghouse: Using 'high tech' to promote 'high touch' support networks. *Computers in Human Services* 3(3/4): 39–54.

Madara, E., and Meese, J. 1990. *The Self-Help Source Book: Finding and Forming Mutual Aid Self-Help Groups.* 3d ed. Denville, N.J.: American Self-Help Clearinghouse.

Mantell, J. 1983. Cancer patient visitor programs: A case for accountability. *Journal of Psychosocial Oncology* 1(1): 45–58.

Mantell, J.; Alexander, E.; and Kleiman, M. 1976. Social work and self-help groups. *Health and Social Work* 1(1): 86–100.

Marieskind, H. 1984. Women's self-help groups. In A. Gartner and F. Riesman, eds., *The Self-Help Revolution.* New York: Human Sciences Press.

Marris, P. 1974. *Loss and Change.* New York: Pantheon.

Martinson, I. 1976. The child with leukemia: Parents help each other. *American Journal of Nursing* 76(7): 1120–22.

Masiak, R.; Cain, M.; Yarbro, C.; and Josof, L. 1981. Evaluation of Touch: An oncology self-help group. *Oncology Nursing Forum* 8(3): 20–25.

Maslach, C. 1976. Burned Out. *Human Behavior* 5: 17–22.

Maton, K.; Leventhal, G.; Madara, E.; and Julien, M. 1990. The birth and death of self-help groups: A population ecology perspective. In A. Katz and E. Bender, eds., *Helping One Another: Self-Help Groups in a Changing World*. Oakland, Calif.: Third Party Publishing.

Maton, K., and Rappaport, J. 1984. Empowerment in a religious setting: A multivariate investigation. *Prevention in Human Services* 3: 37–72.

Mattlin, J.; Wethington, E.; and Kessler, R. 1990. Situational determinants of coping and coping effectiveness. *Journal of Health and Social Behavior* 31: 103–22.

McCarthy, J., and Wolfson, M. 1992. Consensus movements, conflict movements, and the cooptation of civic and state infrastructures. In A. Morris and C. Mueller, eds., *Frontiers of Social Movement Theory*. New Haven: Yale University Press.

McCarthy, J., and Zald, M. 1973. *The Trend of Social Movements in America: Professionalization and Resource Mobilization*. Morristown, N.J.: General Learning Press.

McCarthy, J., and Zald, M. 1977. Resource mobilization and social movements: A partial theory. *American Journal of Sociology* 82: 1212–41.

McCollum, A., and Schwartz, A. 1972. Social work and the mourning patient. *Social Work* 17(1): 25–36.

McGee, D. 1983. *What Murder Leaves Behind: The Victim's Family*. New York: Dodd-Mead.

McWhirter, B.; McWhirter, E.; and McWhirter, J. 1988. Groups in Latin America: *Comunidades Eclesial de Base* as mutual support groups. *Journal for Specialists in Group Work* 13: 70–76.

Meadow, R. 1968. Parental responses to the medical ambiguities of congenital deafness. *Journal of Health and Social Behavior* 9(4): 299–309.

Mechanic, D. 1964. The influence of mothers on their children's health attitudes and behaviors. *Pediatrics* 33: 444–53.

Mechanic, D. 1978. *Medical Sociology*. New York: Free Press.

Medvene, L. 1990. Family support organizations: The functions of similarity. In T. Powell, ed., *Working with Self-Help*. Washington, D.C.: NASW Press.

Medvene, L., and Krauss, D. 1989. Causal attributes and parent-child relationships in a self-help group for families of the mentally ill. *Journal of Applied Social Psychology* 19: 1413–30.

Meissen, G.; Mason, W.; and Gleason, B. 1991. Understanding the attitudes and intentions of future professional toward self-help. *American Journal of Community Psychology* 19(5): 699–714.

Mellor, M.; Rzetelny, H.; and Hudis, I. 1984. Self-help groups for caregivers of the aged. In A. Gartner and F. Riessman, eds., *The Self-Help Revolution*. New York: Human Sciences Press.

Melucci, A. 1985. The symbolic challenge of contemporary social movements. *Social Research* 54(Winter): 789–817.

Melucci, A. 1989. *Nomads of the Present: Social Movements and Individual Needs in Contemporary Society.* Philadelphia: Temple University Press.

Menaghan, E. 1983. Individual coping efforts: Moderators of the relationship between life stress and mental health outcomes. In H. Kaplan, ed., *Psychosocial Stress: Trends in Theory and Research.* New York: Academic Press.

Merton, R., and Kitt, A. 1950. Contributions to the theory of reference group behavior. In R. Merton and P. Lazarsfeld, eds., *Continuities in Social Research: Studies in the Scope and Method of the American Soldier.* Glencoe, Ill.: Free Press.

Merton, V.; Merton, R.; and Barber, E. 1983. Client ambivalence in professional relationships. In B. DePaulo, A. Nadler, and J. Fisher, eds., *New Directions in Helping.* Vol. 2. New York: Academic Press.

Miles, M. 1964. On temporary systems. In M. Miles, ed., *Innovation in Education.* New York: Teachers College Press.

Miles, M., and Huberman, M. 1984. *Qualitative Data Analysis: A Sourcebook of New Methods.* Beverly Hills: Sage, 1984.

Miller, P. 1985. Professional use of lay resources. *Social Work* 30(5): 61–67.

Monaco, G. 1988. Parent self-help groups for the families of children with cancer. *CA-A Cancer Journal for Clinicians* 38: 169–75.

Morrow, G.; Hoagland, A.; and Morse, I. 1982. Sources of support perceived by parents of children with cancer: implications for counseling. *Patient Counseling and Health Education* 4(1): 36–40.

Morrow, G.; Carpenter, P.; and Hoagland, A. 1984. The role of social support in parental adjustment to pediatric cancer. *Journal of Pediatric Psychology* 9: 317–29.

Mullan, F. 1992. Rewriting the social contract in health. In A. Katz, H. Hedrick, D. Isenberg, L. Thompson, T. Goodrich, and A. Kutscher, eds., *Self-Help: Concepts and Applications.* Philadelphia: The Charles Press.

Nadler, A. 1983. Personal characteristics and help-seeking. In B. DePaulo, A. Nadler, and J. Fisher, eds., *New Directions in Helping.* Vol. 2. New York: Academic Press.

Nash, K., and Kramer, K. 1993. Self-help for sickle-cell disease in African-American communities. *Journal of Applied Behavioral Science* 29(2): 257–71.

Nathanson, M. 1987. *Organizing and Maintaining Support Groups for Parents of Children with Chronic Illness and Handicapping Conditions.* Washington, D.C.: Association for the Care of Children's Health.

Neighbors, H., and Jackson, J. 1984. The use of informal and formal help: Four patterns of illness behavior in the black community. *American Journal of Community Psychology* 12(6): 629–44.

Neighbors, H.; Elliott, K.; and Gant, L. 1990. Self-help and Black Americans. In T. Powell, ed., *Working with Self-Help*. Washington, D.C.: NASW Press.

Newcomb, T. 1950. *Social Psychology.* New York: Dryden Press.

Newton, G. 1984. Self-help groups: Can they help? *Journal of Psychosocial Nursing* 22(7): 27–31.

Oncology Handbook for Parents. 1978. Cincinnati: COPE-Cincinnati Oncology Parents Endeavor.

Oncology Handbook for Parents. 1977. Milwaukee: LODAT-Living One Day At A Time.

Ortner, S. 1991. Narrativity in history, culture and lives. Working paper #66 (September). Ann Arbor: University of Michigan Center for the Study of Social Transformation.

Pancoast, D.; Parker, P.; and Froland, C., eds. *Rediscovering Self-Help*. Beverly Hills: Sage.

Parent/Child Handbook. 1980. Rochester, N.Y.: Strong Memorial Hospital & CURE.

Parker, P.; Pancoast, D.; and Froland, C. 1983. Wheels in motion. In D. Pancoast, P. Parker, and C. Froland, eds., *Rediscovering Self-Help*. Beverly Hills: Sage.

Parsons, T. 1951. *The Social System*, Glencoe, Ill.: The Free Press.

Pearlin, L. 1985. Social structure in processes of social support. In J. Sarason and B. Sarason, eds., *Social Support and Health*. The Hague: Martinus Nijoff.

Pearlin, L., and Schooler, C. 1978. The structure of coping. *Journal of Health and Social Behavior* 19(2): 2–21.

Pheifer, W. 1992. AIDS and bereavement: Support groups for survivors. In A. Katz, H. Hedrick, D. Isenberg, L. Thompson, T. Goodrich, and A. Kutscher, eds., *Self-Help: Concepts and Applications*. Philadelphia: The Charles Press.

Pilisuk, M., and Minkler, M. 1980. Supportive networks: Life ties for the elderly. *Journal of Social Issues* 36(2): 95–116.

Pilisuk, M., and Parks, S. 1980. Structural dimensions of social-support groups. *The Journal of Psychology* 106: 157–77.

Pitel, A.; Pitel, P.; Richards, H.; Benson, J.; Prince, J.; and Forman, E. 1985. Parent consultants in Pediatric Oncology. *Children's Health Care* 14(1): 46–51.

Polkinghorne, D. 1988. *Narrative Knowing and the Human Sciences*. Albany: State University of New York Press.

Potasznik, H., and Nelson, G. 1984. Stress and social support: The burden experienced by the family of a mentally ill person. *American Journal of Community Psychology* 12(5): 589–607.

Powell, T. 1975. The use of self-help groups as supportive reference communities. *American Journal of Orthopsychiatry* 45(5): 756–64.

Powell, T. 1985. Improving the effectiveness of self-help. *Social Policy* 16(2): 22–29.

Powell, T. 1987. *Self-help Organizations and Professional Practice.* Washington, D.C.: NASW Press.

Powell, T., ed. 1990. *Working with Self-Help.* Washington, D.C.: NASW Press.

Powell, T. 1993. Self-help research and policy issues. *Journal of Applied Behavioral Science* 29(2): 151–66.

Rait, D., and Lederberg, M. 1989. The family of the cancer patient. In J. Holland and J. Rowland, eds., *Handbook of PsychoOncology.* New York: Oxford University Press.

Rappaport, J. 1983–84. Studies in empowerment. *Prevention in Human Services* 3(2–3): 1–8.

Rappaport, J. 1985. The power of empowerment language. *Social Policy* 16(Fall): 15–22.

Rappaport, J. 1987. Terms of empowerment—exemplars of prevention: Toward a theory for community psychology. *American Journal of Community Psychology* 15: 121–44.

Rappaport, J. 1993. Narrative studies, personal stories, and identity transformation in the mutual help context. *Journal of Applied Behavioral Science* 29(2): 239–57.

Rappaport, J.; Seidman, E.; Toro, P.; McFadden, L.; Reischel, T.; Roberts, L.; Salem, D.; and Zimmerman, M. 1985. Collaborative research with a mutual help organization. *Social Policy* 15(3): 12–24.

Rappaport, J.; Swift, C.; and Hess, R., eds. 1984. *Studies in empowerment: Toward understanding and action.* New York: Haworth Press.

Reiff, R. 1974. The control of knowledge: The power of the helping professions. *Journal of Applied Behavioral Science* 10(3): 451–61.

Remine, D.; Rice, R.; and Ross, J. n.d. *Self-Help Groups and Human Service Agencies.* New York: Family Service of America.

Report of Consensus Conference on Principles of Family Research. 1989. Lawrence, Kans.: National Institute on Disability and Rehabilitative Programs and the Beach Center on Families and Disability.

Reynolds, J. 1982. Water for Karas: Harambee in West Pokot, Kenya. In G. Weber and L. Cohen, eds., *Beliefs and Self-Help: Cross-cultural Perspectives and Approaches.* New York: Human Services Press.

Richardson, A. 1983. English self-help: Varied patterns and practices. In D.

Pancoast, P. Parker, and C. Froland, eds., *Rediscovering Self-Help.* Beverly Hills: Sage.

Riessman, F. 1965. The "helper-therapy" principle. *Social Work* 10(2): 27–32.

Ringler, K.; Whitman, H.; Gustafson, J.; and Coleman, F. 1981. Technical advances in leading a cancer patient group. *International Journal of Group Psychotherapy* 31(3): 329–44.

Rodgers, A., and Tartaglia, L. 1990. Constricting resources: A Black self-help initiative. *Administration in Social Work* 14(2): 125–37.

Rodolfa, E., and Hungerford, L. 1982. Self-help groups: A referral resource for professional therapists. *Professional Psychology* 13(3): 345–53.

Romeder, J., ed. 1990. *The Self-Help Way: Mutual Aid and Health.* Ottawa: Canadian Council on Social Development.

Rosenberg, M. 1979. *Conceiving the Self.* New York: Basic Books.

Rosenberg, P. 1984. Support groups: A special therapeutic entity. *Small Group Behavior* 15(2): 173–86.

Ross, J. 1980. Childhood cancer: The parents, the patients, the professional. *Issues in Comprehensive Pediatric Nursing* 4(1): 7–16.

Rossi, P.; Wright, J.; and Wright, S. 1978. The theory and practice of applied social research. *Evaluation Quarterly* 2(2): 171–92.

Rothenberg, M. 1967. Reactions of those who treat children with cancer. *Pediatrics* 40: 507.

Rowan, J. 1981. A dialectical paradigm for research. In H. Reason and J. Rowan, eds., *Human Inquiry.* New York: Wiley.

Rowland, J. 1989. Interpersonal resources: Social support. In J. Holland and J. Rowland, eds., *Handbook of PsychoOncology.* New York: Oxford University Press.

Sanford, N. 1970. Whatever happened to action research? *Journal of Social Issues* 26: 3–23.

Schensul, S., and Schensul, J. 1982. Self-help groups and advocacy. In G. Weber and L. Cohen, eds., *Beliefs and Self-help.* New York: Human Sciences Press.

Schulz, A.; Israel, B.; Checkoway, B.; and Zimmerman, M. 1993. Empowerment as a multi-level construct: Perceived control at the individual, organizational and community levels. Program on Conflict Management Alternatives Working Paper #40 (March). Ann Arbor: University of Michigan.

Schweers, E.; Farnes, P.; and Foreman, E. 1977. *Parents' Handbook on Leukemia.* Providence, R.I.: American Cancer Society.

Scott, R. 1981. *Organizations: Rational, Natural and Open Systems.* Englewood Cliffs, N.J.: Prentice-Hall.

Scotch, R. 1988. Disability as the basis for a social movement: Advocacy and the politics of definition. *Journal of Social Issues* 14: 159–72.

Scott, S., and Doyle, P. 1984. Parent-to-parent support. *The Exceptional Parent* (Feb.): 15–22.

Sherif, M. 1953. The concept of reference groups in human relations. In M. Sherif and M. Wilson, eds., *Group Relations at the Crossroads.* New York: Harper & Row.

Sidel, R. 1976. Self-help and mutual aid in the People's Republic of China. In A. Katz and E. Bender, eds., *The Strength in Us.* New York: New Viewpoints/Vision Books.

Sidel, V., and Sidel, R. 1983. *A Healthy State.* New York: Pantheon Books.

Siegel, B. 1986. *Love, Medicine and Miracles.* New York: Harper & Row.

Silver, R., and Wortman, C. 1980. Coping with undesirable life events. In J. Garber and M. Seligman, eds., *Human Helplessness: Theory and Application.* New York: Academic Press.

Silverman, P. 1974. *Helping Each Other in Widowhood.* New York: Health Sciences.

Silverman, P. 1992. Critical aspects of the mutual help experience. In A. Katz, H. Hedrick, D. Isenberg, L. Thompson, T. Goodrich, and A. Kutscher, eds., *Self-Help: Concepts and Applications.* Philadelphia: The Charles Press.

Silverman, P., and Smith, D. 1984. Helping in mutual help groups for the physically disabled. In A. Gartner and F. Riessman, eds., *The Self-Help Revolution.* New York: Human Sciences Press.

Smith, D., and Pillemer, K. 1983. Self-help groups as social movement organizations: Social structure and social change. *Research in Social Movements, Conflict and Change.* 5: 203–33.

Snow, D., and Benford, R. 1988. Ideology, frame resonance, and participant mobilization. In B. Klandermans, H. Kriesi, and S. Tarrow, eds., *International Social Movement Research.* Vol. 1. Greenwich, Conn.: JAI Press.

Somers, P. 1992. Narrativity, narrative identity and social action: Rethinking English working-class formation. Working paper #484, Ann Arbor: University of Michigan Center for Research on Social Organization.

Spiegel, D. 1993. *Living Beyond Limits.* New York: Random House.

Spiegel, D.; Bloom, J.; Kraemer, H.; and Gottheil, E. 1989. Effect of psychosocial treatment on survival of patients with metastatic breast cancer. *Lancet* 2: 888–91.

Spinetta, J., and Deasy-Spinetta, P., eds. 1981. *Living with Childhood Cancer.* St. Louis: C. Mosby.

Starr, P. 1982. *The Social Transformation of American Medicine.* New York: Basic Books.

Stein, J. 1986. Support groups may benefit parents of children with cancer. *Oncology Times* 8 (11): 4, 20.

Steinman, R., and Traunstein, D. 1976. Redefining deviance: The self-help challenge to the human services. *Journal of Applied Behavioral Science* 12(3): 347–61.

Stewart, M. 1990. Expanding theoretical conceptualizations of self-help groups. *Social Science and Medicine* 31: 1057–66.

Stolberg, A., and Cunningham, J. 1980. Support groups for parents of leukemic children. In J. Schulman and M. Kupst, eds., *The Child With Cancer.* Springfield, Ill.: C.C. Thomas.

Stone, C. 1983. Whither the welfare state? Professionalization, bureaucracy, and the market alternative. *Ethics* 93: 588–95.

Stuetzer, C. 1980. Support Systems for Professionals. In J. Schulman and M. Kupst, eds., *The Child with Cancer.* Springfield, Ill.: Charles C. Thomas.

Suler, J. 1984. The role of ideology in self-help groups. *Social Policy* 14 (Winter): 29–36.

Sunderland, S. 1982. The strengths of compassionate friends: Enduring life following the death of a child. Mimeo. Cincinnati, Ohio: University of Cincinnati.

Sunderland, S. 1984. The parents of murdered children: Expanding the rights of the constitution to include the victims. Mimeo. Cincinnati, Ohio: University of Cincinnati.

Susman, G., and Evered, R. 1978. An assessment of the scientific merits of action research. *Administrative Science Quarterly* 23: 582–603.

Sutow, W. 1984. General aspects of childhood cancer. In W. Sutow, D. Fernbach, and T. Vietti, eds., *Clinical Pediatric Oncology.* St. Louis: C. V. Mosby.

Swift, C., and Levin, G. 1987. Empowerment: An emerging mental health technology. *Journal of Primary Prevention* 8: 71–94.

Szasz, T., and Hollender, M. 1956. A contribution to the philosophy of medicine: The basic models of doctor-patient relationships. *Archives of Internal Medicine* 97: 585–92.

Taylor, S. 1979. Hospital patient behavior: Reactance, helplessness, or control. *Journal of Social Issues* 35(1): 156–84.

Telch, C., and Telch, M. 1986. Group coping skills instruction and supportive group therapy for cancer patients: A comparison of strategies. *Journal of Consulting and Clinical Psychology* 54: 802–08.

Theirs, N. 1987. Self-help movement gains strength, offers hope. *Guidepost* 30(9): 1, 8, 16.

Thoits, P. 1986. Social support as coping assistance. *Journal of Consulting and Clinical Psychology* 54: 416–23.

Thoits, P. 1994. Stressors and problem-solving: The individual as psychological activist. *Journal of Health and Social Behavior* 35(2): 143–61.

Tichy, N., and Friedman, S. 1983. Institutional dynamics of action research. In R. Kilman and D. Thomas, eds., *Producing Useful Information for Organizations.* New York: Praeger.

Tiebes, J., and Kraemer, D. 1991. Quantitative and qualitative knowing in mutual support research. *American Journal of Community Psychology* 19(5): 739–56.

Toch, H. 1965. *The Social Psychology of Social Movements.* Indianapolis: Bobbs-Merrill.

Toseland, R., and Hacker, L. 1982. Self-help groups and professional involvement. *Social Work* 27: 341–47.

Touraine, A. 1985. An introduction to the study of social movements. *Social Research* 52: 749–87.

Touraine, A. 1988. *Return of the Actor: Social theory in Post-Industrial Society.* Minneapolis: University of Minnesota Press.

Trojan, A. 1983. Groupes De Santé: The users' movement in France. In S. Hatch and I. Kickbush, eds., *Self-help and Health in Europe: New Approaches in Health Care.* Copenhagen: WHO.

Trojan, A. 1989. Benefits of self-help groups: A survey of 232 members from 65 disease-related groups. *Social Science and Medicine* 29(2): 225–32.

Trojan, A.; Halves, E.; and Wetendorf, H. 1986. Self-help groups and consumer participation: A look at the German health care self-help movement. *Journal of Voluntary Action Research* 15(2): 14–23.

Tsouderos, J. 1955. Organizational change in terms of a series of selected variables. *American Sociological Review* 20: 206–10.

Tulsky, D., and Cella, D. 1992. Pilots in gliders: The professional's role in a cancer wellness group. In A. Katz, H. Hedrick, D. Isenberg, L. Thompson, T. Goodrich, and A. Kutscher, eds., *Self-Help: Concepts and Applications.* Philadelphia: The Charles Press.

Turner, R. 1956. Role-taking, role standpoint and reference group behavior. *American Journal of Sociology* 61 (January): 316–28.

Unell, J. 1987. *Help for Self-Help.* London: Bedford Square Press/NCVO.

U.S. Dept. of Commerce, Bureau of the Census. 1980. *1980 Census of the Population.* Washington, D.C.: U. S. Government Printing Office.

U.S. Dept. of Health and Human Services. 1992. *Health in the United States, 1992.* Washington, D.C.: U. S. Government Printing Office.

Vachon, M., Lyall, W., and Freeman, S. 1978. Measurement and management of stress in health professionals working with advanced cancer patients. *Death Education* 1: 365–75.

van Harberden, P. 1990. Self-help behind the dikes. In A. Katz and E. Bender, eds., *Helping One Another,* Oakland, Calif.: Third Party Publishing.

van Harberden, P., and Raymakers, T. 1986. Self-help and governmental policy in the Netherlands. *Journal of Voluntary Action Research* 15(2): 24–32.

Vaux, K. 1977. Life-threatening disease in children: The challenge to personal and institutional values. In J. Van Eys, ed., *The Truly Cured Child*. Baltimore: University Park Press.

Videka-Sherman, L. 1982. Effects of participation in a self-help group for bereaved parents: Compassionate Friends. *Prevention in Human Services* 1: 69–78.

Videka-Sherman, L. 1990. Bereavement self-help organizations. In T. Powell, ed., *Working with Self-Help*. Washington, D.C.: NASW Press.

Vine, P., and Beels, C. 1990. Support and advocacy groups for the mentally ill. In M. Herz, S. Keith, and J. Docherty, eds., *Handbook of Schizophrenia*. Vol. 4. *Psychosocial Treatment of Schizophrenia*. New York: Elsevier Science Publishers.

Voysey, M. 1972. Impression management by parents with disabled children. *Journal of Health and Social Behavior* 13(1): 80–89.

Vugia, H. 1991. Support groups in Oncology: Building hope through the human bond. *Journal of Psychosocial Oncology* 9(3): 89–105.

Waitzkin, H. 1983. *The Second Sickness: Contradictions of Capitalist Health Care*. New York: The Free Press.

Ware, J.; Davies-Avery, A.; and Stewart, A. 1978. The measurement and meaning of patient satisfaction. *Health and Medical Care Services Review* 1: 1–14.

Weber, G. 1982. Self-help and beliefs. In G. Weber and L. Cohen, eds., *Beliefs and Self-Help: Cross-cultural Perspectives and Approaches*. New York: Human Services Press.

Wechsler, H. 1976. The self-help organization in the mental health field: Recovery, Inc., a case study. In G. Caplan and M. Killilea, eds., *Support Systems and Mutual Help: Multidisciplinary Explorations*. New York: Grune & Stratton.

Wehr, P. 1979. *Conflict Regulation*. Boulder, Colo.: Westview Press.

Weigers, M. 1994. Meaning-making and childhood cancer. A study of structure and agency in the narratives of Mexican, Mexican-American and Anglo-American mothers of children with cancer. Unpublished doctoral dissertation. Ann Arbor: University of Michigan.

Weiss, R. 1976. The contributions of an organization of single parents to the well-being of its members. In G. Caplan and M. Killilea, eds., *Support Systems and Mutual Help: Multidisciplinary Explorations*. New York: Grune & Stratton.

Wempner, M. 1984. The role of social work in a model self-help organization. *Psychiatric Clinics of North America* 7(2): 395–403.

Wethington, E., and Kessler, R. 1986. Perceived support, received support, and adjustment to stressful life events. *Journal of Health and Social Behavior* 27: 78–89.

Wethington, E., and Kessler, R. 1991. Situations and processes of coping. In J. Eckenrode, ed., *The Social Context of Coping*. New York: Plenum.

Whyte, W. 1986. On the uses of social science research. *American Sociological Review* 51(4): 551–63.

Withorn, A. 1980. Helping ourselves: The limits and potentials of self help. *Social Policy* 11(3): 20–28.

Wollert, R., and Barron, N. 1983. Avenues of collaboration. In D. Pancoast, P. Parker, and C. Froland, eds., *Rediscovering Self-Help*. Beverly Hills: Sage.

Wollert, R.; Knight, B.; and Levy, L. 1984. Make Today Count: A collaborative model for professionals and self-help groups. In A. Gartner and F. Riessman, eds., *The Self-Help Revolution*. New York: Human Sciences Press.

Wortman, C., and Dunkel-Schetter, C. 1979. Interpersonal relationships and cancer: A theoretical analysis. *Journal of Social Issues* 35(1): 120–25.

Wuthnow, R. 1994. *Sharing the Journey*. New York: The Free Press.

Yoak, M., and Chesler, M. 1985. Alternative professional roles in health care delivery: Leadership patterns in self-help groups. *Journal of Applied Behavioral Science* 21(4): 427–44.

Yoak, M.; Chesney, B.; and Schwartz, N. 1985. Active roles in self-help groups for parents of children with cancer. *Children's Health Care* 14(1): 38–45.

Zimmerman, M. 1986. Citizen participation, perceived control, and psychological empowerment. Presented at the American Psychological Association. Washington, D.C.

Zimmerman, M. 1990. Taking aim on empowerment research: On the distinction between individual and psychological conceptions. *American Journal of Community Psychology* 18(1): 169–87.

Zimmerman, M. In press. Psychological, organizational and community empowerment: Directions for future research. In J. Rappaport and E. Seidman, eds., *The Handbook of Community Psychology*. New York: Plenum Press.

Index